# Discovering
# New Medicines

Careers in Pharmaceutical Research and Development

# Discovering New Medicines

• Careers in Pharmaceutical Research and Development •

Edited by

**Peter D. Stonier**

*Medical Director, Hoechst Roussel Limited, Denham, Middlesex, UK*

**JOHN WILEY & SONS**

Chichester · New York · Brisbane · Toronto · Singapore

*Other Wiley Editorial Offices*

John Wiley & Sons. Inc., 605 Third Avenue,
New York, NY 10158-0012, USA

Jacaranda Wiley Ltd, 33 Park Road, Milton,
Queensland 4064, Australia

John Wiley & Sons (Canada) Ltd, 22 Worcester Road,
Rexdale, Ontario M9W 1L1, Canada

John Wiley & Sons (SEA) Pte Ltd, 37 Jalan Pemimpin #05-04,
Block B, Union Industrial Building, Singapore 2057

*Library of Congress Cataloging-in-Publication Data*

Discovering new medicines : careers in pharmaceutical research and
  development / edited by P.D. Stonier.
    p.  cm.
  Includes bibliographical references and index.
  ISBN 0 471 94194 8
    1. Pharmacy—Vocational guidance.  2. Pharmacy—Research—
  Vocational guidance.  3. Pharmaceutical industry—Vocational
  guidance.  4. Pharmaceutical chemistry—Vocational guidance.
  I. Stonier, P.D.
  RS122.5.D57  1994
  615'.19'0023—dc20                                     94-16151
                                                             CIP

*British Library Cataloguing in Publication Data*

A catalogue record for this book is available from the British Library

ISBN 0 471 94194 8

Typeset in 10/12 pt Palatino by
Mathematical Composition Setters Ltd, Salisbury, Wiltshire.
Printed and bound in Great Britain by
Redwood Books, Trowbridge, Wiltshire

This book is dedicated to the memory of Dr Denis M. Burley, a physician whose career spanned the major landmarks in the evolution of pharmaceutical medicine. As an industry pharmaceutical physician, Denis Burley was deeply involved in the education and training of doctors and scientists who turned to a career in the development of medicines.

He was well known around the world for his efforts to communicate this growing speciality to students and to both lay and expert audiences. He recognised that pharmaceutical medicine bridged the discovery process, product development, licensing and eventual marketing—a sequence proven to be both logical and ethical in bringing new treatments to the patients who need them.

He recognised, too, the growing number of disciplines, both within and outside science, which make a contribution to the development of new medicines, and which this book endeavours to reflect. That the authors have given freely of their time and their chapters in the knowledge of this dedication is a further tribute to him.

Dr Denis Burley died on 19 August 1992, aged 65, whilst serving as President of the Faculty of Pharmaceutical Medicine of the Royal Colleges of Physicians of the UK.

# Contents

**V** GETTING STARTED

**VI** CHANGING COURSE

# List of Contributors

**Dr Nigel S. Baber**
Director of Clinical Pharmacology, Glaxo Research and Development, Stockley Park, West Uxbridge, Middlesex, UB11 1BT, UK

**Professor Nick Bosanquet**
Professor of Health Policy, Department of General Practice, Lisson Grove Health Centre, Gateforth Street, London NW8 8EG, UK

**Dr Tony Chandler**
Managing Director, Talentmark Recruitment Ltd, King House, 5–11 Westbourne Grove, London W2 4UA, UK

**Dr Ian Dews**
Medical Director, MCRC, Lewis House, 1 Mildmay Road, Romford, Essex RM7 7DA, UK

**Dr Geoffrey Diggle**
Head of Toxicology, Department of Health, Skipton House, 89 London Road, London SE1 6LW, UK

**Mr Ian Dodds-Smith**
Solicitor, McKenna & Co., Mitre House, 160 Aldersgate Street, London EC1A 4DD, UK

**Dr Jan I. Drayer**
Senior Vice President, Scientific Affairs, G.H. Besselaar Associates, 103 College Road East, Princeton, New Jersey 08543-5237, USA

**Dr David Ellis**
Consultant, Euromedica Ltd, 8 Enterprise House, Vision Park,
Histon, Cambridge CB4 4ZR, UK

**Dr John C. Emmett**
Consultant, Euromedica Ltd, 8 Enterprise House, Vision Park,
Histon, Cambridge CB4 4ZR, UK

**Dr Keith Fowler**
Medical Affairs Consultant, Roche Products Ltd, Broadwater Road,
Welwyn Garden City, Herts AL7 3AY, UK

**Dr Luciano M. Fuccella**
Director of Clinical Research, Tecnofarmaci, Via E. Noe 23, 20133
Milan, Italy

**Dr Felicity Gabbay**
Managing Director, Gabbay Group Ltd, Ambassador House, 8
Carlton Crescent, Southampton SO1 2EY, UK

**Dr Brian Gennery**
Consultant in Pharmaceutical Medicine, Gennery Associates,
6 Qualitas, Roman Hill, Bracknell, Berks RG12 4QG, UK

**Professor Charles F. George**
Professor of Clinical Pharmacology, University of Southampton,
Biomedical Sciences Building, Bassett Crescent East, Southampton
SO9 3TU, UK

**Dr John Hall**
Medical Director, Allen & Hanburys Ltd, Stockley Park, West
Uxbridge, Middlesex UB11 1BT, UK

**Dr John Hawkings**
Partner, Personnel Consultancy, Eames Jones Judge Hawkings, 29
High Street, Welwyn, Herts AL6 9EE, UK

**Dr David Jordan**
Head of Pharmaceutical Development, Hoechst Roussel Ltd,
Kingfisher Drive, Covingham, Swindon, Wilts SN3 5BZ, UK

**Ms Elizabeth Langley**
Independent Marketing Consultant, Langley Associates, 98 Shinfield
Road, Reading, Berks RG2 7DA, UK

**Dr Trevor Lewis**
Head of Biostatistics, Pfizer Ltd, Sandwich, Kent CT13 9NJ, UK

**Professor David K. Luscombe**
Director, Medicines Research Unit, Welsh School of Pharmacy, University of Wales, King Edward VII Avenue, Cardiff CF1 3XF, UK

**Dr Ronald D. Mann**
Director, Drug Safety Research Unit, Bursledon Hall, Southampton SO3 8BA, UK

**Ms Brenda M. Mullinger**
Editorial Consultant, 'Larches', Green Road, Shipbourne, Tonbridge, Kent TN11 9PL, UK

**Dr Richard K. Rondel**
Managing Director, Oxford Workshops, Dorna House, West End, Woking, Surrey GU24 9PW, UK

**Dr Marian Saunders**
Director & Vice President Resource Management Standards and Training, SmithKline Beecham Pharmaceuticals, Great Burgh, Yew Tree Bottom Road, Epsom, Surrey KT18 5XQ, UK

**Professor Paul S.J. Spencer**
Professor of Pharmacology and Head of School, Welsh School of Pharmacy, University of Wales, College of Cardiff, PO Box 13, Cardiff CF1 3XF, UK

**Dr Bert Spilker**
President, Orphan Medical, 13911 Ridgedale Drive, Minnetonka, Minnesota 55305, USA

**Mr Roger D. Stephens**
Director, Roger Stephens & Associates, Chequers House, 3 Park Street, Old Hatfield, Herts AL9 5AT, UK

**Dr Karen Summers**
Vice President and Director, Medical Research and Safety, Syntex Pharmaceuticals Ltd, St Ives Road, Maidenhead, Berks SL6 1RD, UK

**Ms Janet Taylor**
Information Manager, Shire Pharmaceutical Development Ltd, Fosse House, East Anton Court, Ickneild Way, Andover, Hants SP10 5RG, UK

**Dr Pat Turmer**
Registration Manager, Hoechst Roussel Ltd, Broadwater Park, North Orbital Road, Denham, Uxbridge, Middlesex UB9 5HP, UK

**Dr Malcolm J. VandenBurg**
MCRC, Lewis House, 1 Mildmay Road, Romford, Essex RM7 7DA, UK

**Ms Sheila Varley**
Head of Data Management, Clin Trials Ltd, Kings Chase, 107 King Street, Maidenhead SL6 1DP, UK

**Dr Colin Webb**
Director of Biometrics & IT, Amgen (UK) Ltd, 240 Cambridge Science Park, Milton Road, Cambridge CB4 4WD, UK

**Dr Frank Wells**
Director, Department of Medicine, Science and Technology, ABPI, 12 Whitehall, London SW1A 2DY, UK

**Professor Jenifer Wilson-Barnett**
Head of Division of Nursing & Midwifery and Head of Department of Nursing Studies, King's College London, Cornwall House Annex, Waterloo Road, London SE1 8TX, UK

**Dr Robyn Young**
Medical Editor, 8 McDermott Road, Borough Green, Kent TN15 8SA, UK

**Ms Anna Zajdler**
Research Fellow, Department of General Practice, Lisson Grove Health Centre, Gateforth Street, London NW8 8EG, UK

# Preface

The past 50 years has seen striking success and dramatic growth in the development of new medicines, both from naturally occurring substances in plants and animals, including human, and from purely chemical sources.

These new medicines have allowed doctors to manage a wide range of diseases for which, previously, there was no treatment.

At the same time, scientists have formed a deeper understanding of the normal functioning of the body and how normal processes are changed by illness and disease. Often these two areas of research have interacted so that the use of certain medicines has helped to unravel the workings of the body in health and disease.

Alongside the euphoria of such progress has come the recognition that no medicine is without hazard, at least in some patients. The benefits of successful treatment of an illness must always be balanced against the possible risk of an unwanted side-effect of the medicine. This was tragically illustrated by thalidomide in the early 1960s, when a sedative that appeared to be safer and better tolerated than those already available produced deformities in the babies of some women who had taken the drug for sleep disturbances during pregnancy.

These events more than any others marked a permanent change in the way the world saw medicines research. Government agencies acting in the public interest increased legislation regulating the development, licensing and marketing of medicines, and gradually the public itself was encouraged to take more interest in its health and the medicines used to preserve it. The age of innovation of the 1950s and 1960s gave way to the age of regulation in the 1970s and to the age of communication and accountability in the 1980s.

The coming era of biological innovation and biotechnology, of health care economics and of the application of modern management methods to the research and development process see the 1990s as continuing this evolution, and perhaps also being the start of a new age for medicines.

Whilst today scientific and medical achievements tend to be over-shadowed by political and economic considerations affecting medicine and health care services, more patient involvement in treatment and the international rationalisation of research may enable the true benefits of the last 50 years to be integrated with the selective demands of informed health care systems to enable progress in treating illness to be continued and to be brought to an even wider population around the world.

The field of pharmaceutical research and development remains one of the hallmarks of the technological age and continues to make innovative progress and to have a profound economic effect on those countries which embrace it. The institutions and companies involved in medicines research have themselves contributed greatly to the increasing standards of research through self-regulation and the imposition of good practices and standard procedures, including audit, to ensure high quality of work. Such actions have not dulled the intellect and skills of a highly trained work-force which forms the focus of so much hope for the future.

For medicines research to evolve and be responsive to the needs of patients and their doctors there must necessarily be an evolution in the breadth and sophistication of the scientific and medical disciplines involved and the teams of scientists, doctors and others contributing to this work. Thus to the research chemists and life scientists conducting basic research and the clinical pharmacologists, pharmacists, physicians and statisticians who traditionally were the conductors of clinical trials, have now been added many long-recognised and some newer specialists—clinical research scientists, data managers, medical writers, research nurses and, increasingly, management specialists, economists, accountants and lawyers.

In parallel with these developments in the scope of medicines research and its management has developed the speciality of pharmaceutical medicine, a discipline concerned with the discovery, development, evaluation and monitoring of medicines and the medical aspects of their marketing. This definition embraces a subject which is both scientific and clinical and includes the many professionals of varied backgrounds mentioned above.

This book contains views from many of the professional disciplines which contribute to pharmaceutical medicine about the jobs involved, and the careers open to those who wish to pursue medicines research in industry and in academia.

Even so, it cannot be all-embracing and, for instance, does not pretend to cover the many contributions made by practising physicians and others whose careful observations at the bedside and in the community have added so much to knowledge of the effects of medicines. Nor does it do justice to the many study volunteers and members of research ethics committees whose unpaid and often unsung work contributes so much to the effort.

Nevertheless it aims to open windows into the world of medicines research, a still widening and growing field, for those without ready information but with career options still unsatisfied and with their futures still to plan.

Peter D. Stonier

# Part I

# Background to Pharmaceutical Medicine

# 1
# Pharmaceutical Medicine— Development of a Global Medical Speciality

## Felicity Gabbay

Gabbay Group Ltd, Southampton, UK

It is difficult to define pharmaceutical medicine. It has much in common with clinical pharmacology, but includes the medical aspects of the work of the pharmaceutical industry which discovers and develops almost all new drugs. It also includes insight into the social and legal aspects of medicines and particularly the involvement of government through the regulatory authority and through various controls on labelling, prices and promotion.

Thus it could be said that pharmaceutical medicine occupies the area of common ground between the medical profession, the pharmaceutical industry and government.

Burley, Clarke and Lasagna (1993)

The above quotation is taken from the latest edition of *Pharmaceutical Medicine*, first published in 1985 and edited by Denis Burley and Terry Binns. These physicians joined the pharmaceutical industry in the 1950s and have seen dramatic changes in company and government structures to maintain the flow of valuable pharmaceutical products whilst ensuring maximum protection to the public. During this period specialist disciplines for physicians and scientists alike have emerged and it can be very confusing trying to understand the role of organisations and

*Discovering New Medicines: Careers in Pharmaceutical Research and Development.*
Edited by P.D. Stonier
© 1994 John Wiley & Sons Ltd

individuals within pharmaceutical medicine. The objective of this book is to give an overview of the different opportunities in pharmaceutical medicine, and of the scientific background and specialist training needed to accomplish them. The book is dedicated to Denis Burley, to whom pharmaceutical medicine owes a great deal. His many contributions to the development of the subject culminated in his election in 1991 to the Presidency of the Faculty of Pharmaceutical Medicine.

Pharmaceutical medicine was until recently considered to be outside the conventional medical and scientific professions. This was despite pharmaceutical physicians' ultimate responsibility for interpreting clinical data which determined whether or not drugs were, or continued to be, marketed. These considerable responsibilities extended nationally and for some pharmaceutical physicians internationally. The responsibility could be likened to signing prescriptions for whole countries, with some pharmaceutical physicians responsible for the actual signing, many for providing information to ensure the prescription was correct, and others for scrutinising the prescription (through government regulatory departments and committees) once it was written. As in most parts of the medical profession, pharmaceutical medicine is, and always has been, heavily dependent at all levels on non-medically qualified scientists. Even they were considered to have 'left' research when joining the pharmaceutical industry. This chapter attempts to summarise the key events which have led to their roles in the industry, and to pharmaceutical medicine becoming a respected and exciting discipline which, once they have joined it, few can bear to leave.

Pharmaceutical agents have always been at the foundation of medicine and therapeutics. As medicine became professionalised in Europe in the seventeenth, eighteenth and nineteenth centuries, lists of acceptable drugs appeared. The forerunner to the *British Pharmacopoeia* started life as the *London Pharmacopoeia* in 1618 (Adam and Passmore, 1980). It included nearly 2000 medicinal agents, few of which had a rationale for their action which we would recognise today.

The regulation of marketing of recognised medicinal agents was, until the nineteenth century, under the control of the physicians, surgeons and apothecaries. The General Medical Council (GMC), created by the Medical Reform Act (1858), subsequently approved compounds for listing in the *British Pharmacopoeia*. The amalgamation of physicians, surgeons and apothecaries as a single group of doctors created the need for specialist professionals to formulate and dispense drugs. This role became filled by pharmacists.

During the latter part of the nineteenth century when 'laboratory medicine' made substantial advances, scientists including chemists, pathologists, physiologists and microbiologists identified the causes of a number of diseases. The discoveries coincided with the emergence of large chemical industries utilising the scientific advances in chemistry. Other companies were already using scientific technology to make building materials, domestic items and improve transport. Scientists working in the new chemical companies began to turn their attention to applying medical research to develop pharmaceutical agents, and in 1890 general disinfectants, anaesthetics, antipyretics and hypnotics began to emerge.

The developments in the pharmaceutical industry around the turn of the century were not limited to national companies and the industry rapidly became an international one. For example, in 1901 Parke Davis, which had a British plant but was an American pharmaceutical company, introduced adrenalin into clinical practice and in 1914 it was agreed by the GMC to include the word 'adrenalin' in the *British Pharmacopoeia* (Parke Davis, 1939).

Pharmaceutical companies were chemical companies specialising in the production of medicinal agents and were largely run by pharmacists who had established themselves as formulators of medicines—the final stage before dispensing them. Other scientists were, however, also crucial to the work within the companies. These included chemists, toxicologists, pharmacologists and in some companies microbiologists.

Doctors played only a small part in the development of new drugs before the Second World War. Eminent physicians still questioned the value of statistics in the progress of medicine (Armitage and Berry, 1987). Doctors were, however, playing a role in pharmaceutical companies in medical information and clinical interpretation even though they conducted few clinical trials of new medicines. Sir Austin Bradford Hill's book on the *Principles of Medical Statistics*, published in 1937, was an important milestone (Bradford Hill, 1937).

The emergence of drugs which were clearly efficacious and the ability to demonstrate this in clinical medicine by combining clinical interpretation with medical statistics led to substantial investment, including some government subsidy in the pharmaceutical industry as it now was called (Cromie, 1993). By the 1940s and 1950s there were the first beginnings of clinical trial departments, many staffed by non-medical scientists (who had already been performing animal experiments), as well as physicians. Scientists originally trained in chemistry, biochemistry, pharmacology, pharmacy and many other medically allied sciences have remained to form the largest and one of the most valuable components of clinical research departments. They now fill roles at all staff and managerial levels and are known variously as clinical research associates, clinical scientists or by other titles describing the kind of work they perform.

Commercialisation of scientific discoveries led to patents becoming widely applied in many countries, and branding was introduced to protect companies' research and development (R&D) investments (Teeling Smith, 1992). This brought specialised lawyers into the pharmaceutical industry. Companies also now needed to know as soon as possible whether new therapeutic candidates showed clinical effects in patients. Doctors were increasingly recruited to the industry to conduct trials for evaluation of drugs in patients (Cromie, 1993). Branding also brought competition, and companies began to design studies to demonstrate the advantages of the newer therapies against their competitors. This brought physicians and other clinical research personnel into the area of sales and marketing.

An incident in the late 1930s in the USA had a major impact on the development of pharmaceutical medicine. In North America, where there had been relatively less professional control of marketing of pharmaceutical agents, an enterprising but misguided company dissolved sulphanilinamide in diethylene glycol, resulting in the deaths of 107 people (Lawrence, 1966a). The resulting furore led in 1938 to the setting up of the Food and Drug Administration (FDA), the first of the official full-time bureaucratic agencies dedicated to monitoring the development and marketing of pharmaceutical agents. Within this organisation was born a further specialist breed of physicians and scientists who were devoted to the assessment of new medicines and the control over the way in which they were marketed. At this stage Europe did not follow suit, thinking the existing controls to be adequate. In the UK these controls included pharmacopoeias, the Therapeutic Substances Act (1925), the Dangerous Drugs Act (1930) and the Cancer Act (1930), all of which were implemented to ensure quality of drugs, control dangerous drugs and protect the public from false claims (Cromie, 1993).

Regulation and patent control brought a national flavour to the companies, dividing up what had been a subject with few geographical boundaries to a subject where most companies now required local affiliates in order to fulfil the requirements for regulation and control in individual countries. Regulation also changed the nature of medical and research departments by demanding levels of evaluation in R&D hitherto not considered.

The impact of patents and branding changed the shape of the pharmaceutical industry (Teeling Smith, 1992). In the 1950s there was a dramatic increase in interest in the commercial behaviour of pharmaceutical companies. In that decade the first broad-spectrum antibiotics appeared in profusion, many patented by Lilly (a US pharmaceutical company), and were very expensive compared to the unpatented penicillin and spectinomycin. This generated concern in the USA as to whether patenting and branding were in the public interest or whether it might just lead to companies making huge profits from the sick. This was reported in 1961 by a Senate Committee and resulted in considerable antagonism to the pharmaceutical industry, not just in the USA but also in countries in Europe. Scientists and doctors working in the pharmaceutical industry already suffered a lower professional status than their counterparts in universities or other jobs outside the industry due to general antagonism of the professions to commerce and few would align themselves with the industry in the following decade.

In 1961 thalidomide, marketed in Germany and Great Britain, was shown to be responsible for phocomyelia. Not only was the pharmaceutical industry exploiting science by making profit out of the sick but it was also capable of marketing drugs which had major adverse effects. The physicians working at Distillers (the pharmaceutical company concerned), Denis Burley and Charles Brown, had to evaluate the tragic adverse events (Cromie, 1993). Denis Burley, to whom this book is dedicated, remained in the pharmaceutical industry until he retired in 1991. He devoted much of his life to professional organisations linked with pharmaceutical medicine to increase the standards of the subject. He subsequently became President of the Faculty of Pharmaceutical Medicine of the Royal Colleges of Physicians of the United Kingdom but sadly died during his term of office in 1992.

During Denis Burley's lifetime it was to become realised that even if drugs were put through greater toxicological screens than thalidomide, it was impossible to screen out all adverse effects. Furthermore the increased sophistication of data collection and tracking was able to detect effects occurring at very low frequencies (e.g. the effects of practolol in the elderly and the hepatic side-effects of benoxyprofen). A group of pharmaceutical physicians and scientists have devoted their discipline to investigating adverse event frequencies in the population after the drug has been given to tens of thousands of patients. They practise post-marketing surveillance.

During the 1960s, in response to the thalidomide-related events, regulatory agencies along the lines of the FDA were set up throughout Europe to ensure that rigorous pre-clinical and clinical study of new chemical entities was conducted before the drugs were marketed. In response, the European drug companies developed groups of clinical scientists who specialised in writing for the regulators (regulatory executives and medical writers), mirroring their American counterparts.

The thalidomide tragedy had damaged the image of the pharmaceutical industry still further and calls in the British parliament for nationalisation of all pharmaceutical companies in Great Britain were part of the Labour government manifesto when it was elected to power in 1964

(Teeling Smith, 1992). The committee set up to look into this in 1967, having examined in detail the economics of R&D and innovation, decided against nationalisation, stating that 'in the absence of the prospect of abnormal profits, private industry would have no special inducement to undertake research to which is attached an abnormal risk of failure'. The committee had discovered that the cost of R&D of a new medicine was extremely high, taking on average 8–10 years to recover from the market. Thousands of drugs may need to be screened to find one suitable candidate. With the introduction of ever more stringent regulations this cost was growing and it has now reached over £150 million for each new drug.

Concerns about the economics of the pharmaceutical industry and its commercial interests have remained and heightened. Ever since the formation of the National Health Service (NHS) in the UK in 1948, the government has been concerned by the cost of drugs, which was estimated to make up about 10% of the cost of health care (Lawrence, 1966b). In other countries, governments have introduced systems of reimbursement to help patients pay for drugs, and insurance schemes can also cover the cost of drugs as part of health care. Schemes were introduced to regulate prices of drugs and at the same time ensure continued investment in R&D and innovation by pharmaceutical companies. Tight regulatory systems now require companies in some countries to demonstrate economic benefit from new pharmacological advances before marketing. From this a whole discipline of pharmacoeconomics has developed.

The calls for nationalisation of the industry were accompanied by concerns from academic medicine about the standards of clinical research in industry, questioning the scientific impartiality of pharmaceutical physicians and scientists (Hampton and Julian, 1987). Clinical pharmacology had become a discipline in the 1950s and 1960s and some saw comprehensive drug development as its role. Whilst a symbiosis has developed between universities and industry, it has become clear that the size of the operation involved in the complete development of a new drug is outside the scope of a single university department. Clinical research departments in pharmaceutical companies include specialised clinical research associates, clinical scientists, nurses, data managers, data entry staff, archivists and statisticians, in addition to physicians. The size of one submission to the FDA had grown from about 30 pages in the early 1950s to the volume of paper which would fill a furniture removal van in the late 1970s; and the number of people working on one clinical research submission had increased to hundreds. The belief that the industry was likely to suffer from commercial bias did not, however, recede and the FDA increased their demand on the industry to open their databases for inspection. Now the USA requires Computer-

Assisted New Drug Applications (CANDAS). These applications involve the deposition with the regulatory agency of all data in electronic form for inspection and sometimes further evaluation. In addition, companies are also required to inspect all data and data collection procedures using independent auditors who comment on the quality of the data. Government inspectors also operate in some countries. The European Union, the USA and many individual countries require all research to be performed to minimum standards which are governed by working practices—rules dictated and written by the research group itself and called standard operating procedures (SOPs). This subdiscipline, audit in research, has become an important one. Ironically in addition to increasing standards in industry it has unearthed the fact that a small percentage of doctors working in clinical practice under grants are thought to submit fraudulent or severely substandard data (Wells, 1993a).

The necessity for the analysis of data by the pharmaceutical industry itself did not, however, usurp the role of the clinical pharmacologist but rather enhanced it. There are many interfaces between drug development and clinical medicine where they have a crucial role to play: the major one is the execution of specific individual research projects; another is training particularly within medicine; and a third is collaboration with pharmaceutical and regulatory physicians on the evaluation of drugs and methodology used in development.

The coordination of the large number of scientists and others involved in a single drug development programme required yet another group of people. Project managers are responsible for ensuring that the many different tasks during clinical development and marketing are achieved. Finance and administration people oversee resourcing of the projects, tracking finance and running the business side of the operation. Finally, and not least, there have to be specialist information technology staff running computer systems that track and integrate the vast amounts of data collected. Numerous other specialists are involved such as designers of case record forms and clinical trials supply pharmacists.

With all the scientific, political and economic evolutions in the pharmaceutical industry the structure of pharmaceutical medicine has become extremely complex and expensive. Small companies have been unable to withstand the expense and many of the compounds brought to the market worldwide are developed by the biggest pharmaceutical companies. Ninety-five per cent of drugs marketed in the world are developed by just six countries—USA, the UK, France, Germany, Switzerland and Sweden—nearly 50% being developed by American companies (Lis and Walker, 1989). Even such companies have found the cost and complexity hard to bear and mergers amongst the top companies have made them even bigger. An alternative solution has been the licensing or co-licensing of drugs between companies, from which a whole speciality of people working in licensing has developed.

Relations between those working in pharmaceutical medicine in the industry and in academia and government have improved beyond recognition in the last two decades. Regulators and academics have realised the immense burden on the industry for demonstrating efficacy and safety. This would clearly be eased if each country did not insist on its own stringent regulations for registering drugs. Pharmaceutical medicine has therefore returned to being a global speciality, most research being part of an overall plan to learn more about an individual drug, with little or no repetition of studies except for confirmatory purposes. The International Conferences on Harmonisation (ICH) are among the initiatives to bring all interested parties together to set standards for performing research on new developments. Other initiatives include working parties to produce guidelines for study designs, standard inclusion and exclusion criteria and analytical procedures for individual therapeutic research areas.

In the 1980s, led by a company from the USA, yet another solution to the monolithic pharmaceutical company came into being. This was the formation of smaller service and research companies performing individual activities in pharmaceutical medicine for the pharmaceutical industry as a whole. This has enabled many of the Japanese and smaller biotechnology companies, whose presence in Europe is less dominant than the big companies, to consider developing their own drugs. The service companies are loosely grouped together under the term contract research organisations (CROs), and their functions are as numerous and varied as those within the pharmaceutical industry itself. Some are run by people who have never been in the industry but can offer specialised services needed by the industry such as clinical pharmacology. Although there are estimated to be over a thousand worldwide only a handful offer complete clinical R&D, most specialising in a particular subdiscipline or therapeutic area in pharmaceutical medicine.

The development of pharmaceutical medicine has resulted in a number of subdisciplines described in the chapters of this book. R&D of drugs has changed dramatically in the last hundred years and, like other scientifically based commercial developments, the rate of change has increased faster as the twentieth century has progressed. In the last two decades there have been dramatic changes in companies, largely driven by developments in information technology, scientific methodology and economics. This has meant an international streamlining of larger companies and the career progression described, for example, in pamphlets in the late 1980s now bears little resemblance to that within the structure

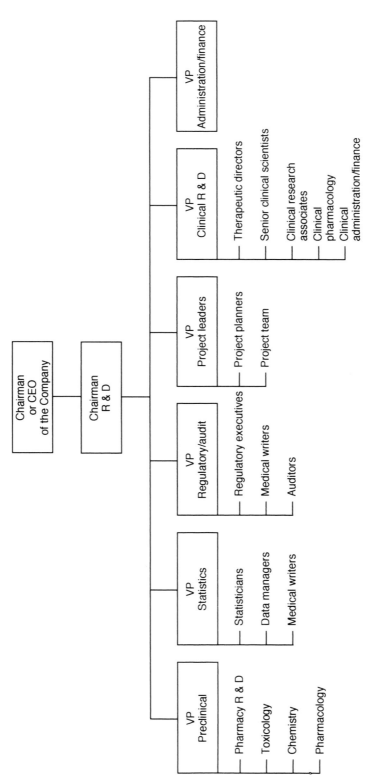

**Figure 1.** Research and development organisation. Management organisations are highly variable and frequently 'matrix' in nature, leading to complex organisations not easy to draw. The organisation chart here uses North American titles and a simplified structure for explanatory purposes only (VP, vice-president).

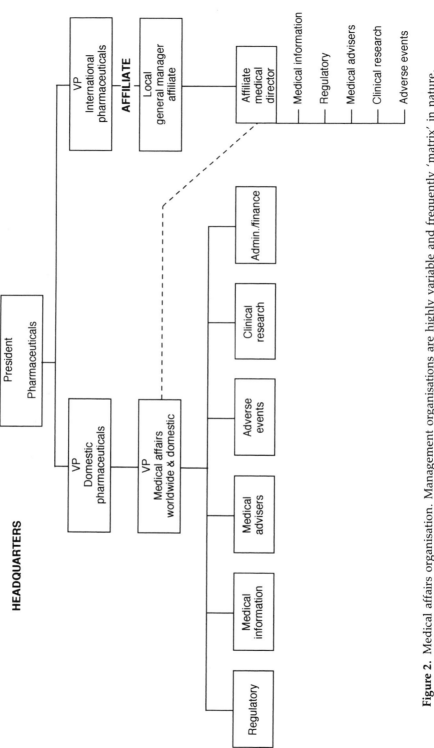

**Figure 2.** Medical affairs organisation. Management organisations are highly variable and frequently 'matrix' in nature, leading to complex organisations not easy to draw. The organisation chart here uses North American titles and a simplified structure for explanatory purposes only (VP, vice-president).

existing in the current pharmaceutical industry and its allied organisations. Figures 1 and 2 demonstrate, in summary, how pharmaceutical companies may be organised. They demonstrate how physicians and scientists working in different parts of the organisation have different highly specialised functions and cannot, as they could in times before, be interchanged. Similarly CROs will offer types of expertise orientated towards post-marketing R&D (often in particular therapeutic areas or specialist scientific disciplines, e.g. statistics and data analysis) but rarely all.

During the nineteenth and early twentieth centuries a number of professional and academic bodies sprang up to support standards in medicine. In addition, there was a burgeoning of the number of scientific bodies to encourage innovation in all scientific disciplines. Three types of professional organisation were formed to support the different medical and allied disciplines.

The first provides basic professional support for its members in the jobs that they do. It includes bodies such as the Association of Clinical Research in the Pharmaceutical Industry (ACRPI), originally founded to support clinical research associates and clinical scientists within clinical research groups in the pharmaceutical industry; the British Association of Pharmaceutical Physicians (BrAPP) and one of the first such organisations to support pharmaceutical physicians; Statisticians in the Pharmaceutical Industry (PSI), supporting statisticians; and many others supporting the different professional people within pharmaceutical medicine. All these organisations bring together professional scientists doing similar jobs, they offer symposia which keep their members up to date with necessary developments and they highlight professional issues which may need to be taken up by other bodies. The equivalent medical professional body which is the most obvious example of this is the British Medical Association. Table 1 lists the professional bodies which support the different career groups in pharmaceutical medicine.

The second type of organisation is a faculty, college or institute. Examples of these are the Royal Colleges and Faculties supporting the different disciplines in medicine, and the Institutes of Chartered Accountants and Surveyors. They are bodies who set competency standards usually through examinations. In pharmaceutical medicine the Faculty of Pharmaceutical Medicine exists to set standards for pharmaceutical physicians through its diploma, associateship and membership qualifications. The faculty came into being after its need was recognised by BrAPP. Other professional bodies have also recognised a need but in the absence of appropriate standard-setting bodies within the professional group they have delegated the control over the examinations to universities. Examples are ACRPI and the British Institute of

**Table 1.** Professional,  standard-setting  and  academic  bodies  in pharmaceutical medicine

| Professional | Standard setting | Academic |
|---|---|---|
| Association of Clinical Data Managers (ACDM) | Faculty of Pharmaceutical Medicine (RCP) | Society of Pharmaceutical Medicine |
| Association of Clinical Research in the Pharmaceutical Industry (ACRPI)[b] | Pharmaceutical Manufacturers Associations[c] | Drug Information Association |
| Association of Information Officers in the Pharmaceutical Industry (AIOPI) | | |
| British Association of Quality Assurers (BAQA) | | |
| British Association of Pharmaceutical Physicians (BrAPP)[a] | | |
| British Institute of Regulatory Affairs (BIRA)[b] | | |
| European Medical Writers Association (EMWA) | | |
| International Federation of Associations of Pharmaceutical Physicians (IFAPP) | | |
| Statisticians in the Pharmaceutical Industry (PSI) | | |

[a] There are similar organisations in most European countries, which are linked by IFAPP.
[b] Also perform standard-setting functions.
[c] Pharmaceutical manufacturers associations have a number of committees and produce standard-setting guidelines for the industry as a whole.

Regulatory Affairs (BIRA), whose diplomas are awarded by the University of Wales, Cardiff. The standard-setting bodies not only set examinations but also set a list of basic requirements for entry into the career grade. Pharmaceutical physicians need to have at least two years postregistration general clinical experience before entering pharmaceutical medicine and four years of experience in pharmaceutical medicine before achieving membership. A list of professional examinations is

**Table 2.** Diplomas and degrees in pharmaceutical medicine and related subjects

| Country | Issuing body |
| --- | --- |
| *Diplomas in pharmaceutical medicine* | |
| UK | Faculty of Pharmaceutical Medicine of the Royal College of Physicians (UK) |
| Belgium | Université Libre de Bruxelles |
| | Vrije Universiteit, Brussels |
| Spain | Complutense University, Madrid |
| | Autonomous University, Barcelona |
| *Master of Science degree in pharmaceutical medicine* | |
| UK | University of Surrey |
| *European course in pharmaceutical medicine* | |
| Switzerland | Upper Rhine Universities of Basle, Freiburg, Strasbourg |
| *Various courses in applied pharmacological sciences* | |
| France | Pharmacovigilance, Lyon |
| | Therapeutic Evaluation, University of Paris |
| | CESAM, Statistics, Paris |
| | IMS |
| Italy | School of Specialisation in Clinical Pharmacology, University of Milan |
| | Society for Applied Pharmacological Sciences, University of Milan |
| *Diploma in clinical science* | |
| UK | University of Wales, Cardiff |
| *Diploma in regulatory affairs* | |
| UK | University of Wales, Cardiff |

given in Table 2. Much of the subject matter is very similar and a summary of some of the common subjects in the syllabus is given in Table 3.

Finally, but perhaps most importantly, for it is the way in which any discipline moves forward, there is the academic society. Pharmaceutical medicine is a discipline which is largely concerned with research and development. What then is the role of an academic society doing research into R&D? It is not, as thought by some, to foster research into the therapeutic disciplines themselves as there are ample academic societies for this, but into the methods used to perform research and development. As has been explained in the early part of this chapter, the complex task of bringing together all the scientists and other

**Table 3.**   Syllabus subjects in pharmaceutical medicine.

| | |
|---|---|
| Pharmacology | Adverse reactions |
| Toxicology | Regulatory affairs |
| Clinical pharmacology | Medical information |
| Medical therapeutics | Ethical, legal aspects |
| Clinical trial methodology | Marketing and sales |
| Pharmacy | Management |
| Statistics | Economics |

professional staff involved in bringing a drug to the market-place requires sophisticated methodology and team-work. Many of the tasks must be performed by people who have a relatively underdeveloped approach to clinical trials. They have yet to understand the importance of minor changes in study design and the detail in Good Clinical Practice (GCP). For standards to be set, studies must be conducted to validate the methods we use. This is the 'R&D' of R&D. Academic societies provide a forum for the presentation of research into new and as yet unvalidated methods that challenge the way in which we currently work. It is quite difficult for each professional group to find the resource to support all the kinds of professional organisations described. Therefore, there is only one multidisciplinary academic society supporting pharmaceutical medicine for all career groups: the Society of Pharmaceutical Medicine.

In the last 50 years radical changes have occurred in pharmaceutical medicine. This is not unexpected when one considers that there have been dramatic changes in therapeutics over this period, the introduction of broad-spectrum antibiotics in the 1940s and 1950s, the introduction of drugs based on receptor theory in the 1970s, and in the 1980s the first biotechnology products. Pharmaceutical medicine is a discipline within which equal priority is given both to research and to development, whereas the latter often fails to be adequately executed in other medical scientific disciplines (House of Lords, 1988). The constant evaluation of the performance of medicines throughout their lifetime on the market has generated a group of highly skilled people whose sole task is to bring effective treatments to the market and to monitor their use.

# 2
# Development of Careers in Pharmaceutical Medicine

## Luciano M. Fuccella

Tecnofarmaci, Milan, Italy

The job descriptions of physicians and scientists joining the pharmaceutical industry in the mid-1990s are substantially different from those which applied in the mid-1960s, and this reflects the advances in pharmaceutical medicine over this time as well as great changes in the external environment in which research is conducted. This chapter discusses from a personal viewpoint some of these changes in the context of the evolving and broadening needs of medicines research programmes and the opportunities for career development.

## FIRST STEPS

The job description of a physician joining a pharmaceutical company 30 years ago was certainly different from that submitted to job candidates today. One major reason for this was the basic rationale for hiring physicians in the first place. Companies required a medically qualified person to represent them and visit clinicians whenever it was deemed important to discuss something considered to be outside the competence or remit of the sales representative or area marketing manager. Typical examples were requests for clinical studies coming either from the company itself or from the would-be investigator, or for discussions on

*Discovering New Medicines: Careers in Pharmaceutical Research and Development.*
Edited by P.D. Stonier
© 1994 John Wiley & Sons Ltd

actual adverse events or effects which might suggest unexpected pharmacological properties of the product.

This first and basic task of company physicians was often one requiring enormous diplomatic qualities, since marketing people were usually both sensitive and overly protective of their direct and special relationship with prescribing clinicians and tended to perceive the activity of the company physician as a fastidious intrusion. It was always clear that if a mutually satisfactory agreement was found for a study protocol then this was down to the special rapport with the salesman, whereas any problems encountered could only be attributable to the lack of 'savoir faire' and to the stubbornness of the company physician!

## EARLY CLINICAL TRIAL METHODOLOGY

The experimental approach to the clinical evaluation of new drugs was just beginning to be recognised and one of the main difficulties for a pharmaceutical physician was to struggle amiably to place proposals coming from often exceedingly creative clinicians into a basic, but essential, framework of principles of correct methodology.

Terms like *randomisation, placebo, control* and *double-blind* still sounded exotic to many. Suggestions to use placebo were often considered an overt challenge to the investigator's abilities to distinguish the real effects of a treatment from spontaneous fluctuations of the disease. The proposal 'Why don't we do it double-blind?' was immediately followed by the putative investigator's disappearing smile, to be replaced by the suggestive hostile stare implying 'Do you mean that I am unable to assess impartially the respective effects of the two treatments?'

At that time, international collaboration in clinical development of drugs was rather uncommon. The relatively short duration and limited costs of drug development compared to the present, combined with profound differences in local medical culture and with marked differences in procedures for marketing authorisation, made it preferable to follow a local, country by country approach to development and commercialisation. Multi-centre, multinational clinical trials were very rare and pharmaceutical physicians had very few opportunities for international exchange of experiences or for harmonised development of methods and measures for clinical trials.

## CHANGES IN DRUG DEVELOPMENT ENVIRONMENT

The scene for medicines development has changed quickly in recent years and is still evolving rapidly. In short, however, simultaneous and international clinical development is the approach most likely to be adopted by multinational companies today. This has brought pharmaceutical physicians from countries with different academic and medical traditions to collaborate closely and to elaborate common attitudes and strategies for timely and cost-effective drug development programmes.

## Harmonisation of Requirements

Faster communication in medicine and international development of drugs have contributed greatly to the merging of medical cultures and increasing disappearance of local traditions and therapeutic attitudes; new advances in therapy are now rapidly accepted worldwide.

At the same time, differences in regulatory requirements are also fast disappearing. Europe, once a typical mosaic in this respect, has made impressive progress towards harmonisation and is heading rapidly towards a central regulatory agency (European Medicines Evaluation Agency (EMEA) based in London). The International Conference on Harmonisation (ICH) process aims to address differences in approach to drug development and registration between Europe, USA and Japan and endeavours to harmonise them where possible.

## Professional Recognition and Standards

The introduction of Good Clinical (Research) Practice regulations in Europe and elsewhere is accelerating this process and, at the same time, is setting the stage for the recognition of pharmaceutical physicians and other professional and scientific groups involved in the drug development process.

On the one hand there will be a drive to reach a consensus on the conduct of scientific activities and the approach to problems amongst physicians working in Europe. Harmonisation in the European Union (EU) will accelerate this process also in countries not yet associated with the EU but strongly dependent on scientific, cultural and commercial interactions with it. This will help reduce differences between the USA and Europe, and ultimately between Japan and other world market sectors with whom it seeks to do business.

On the other hand, the relative lack of recognition which has so far characterised the role of the pharmaceutical physician within the medical world may turn gradually to acceptance of the professional part they play in the practice of pharmaceutical medicine, which becomes embodied in guidelines and regulations such as those relating to Good Clinical Practice in the EU.

This process is perhaps most advanced in the UK, which has inaugurated a Faculty of Pharmaceutical Medicine to establish and uphold standards within the speciality, to examine those standards in its membership examinations, and to present a public platform for the speciality in order to benefit the public with respect to medicines' development.

### The Clinical Trial Monitor

As the principal link between the sponsor and the investigator, the clinical monitor has the responsibility of taking all steps to ensure that clinical trials are conducted properly; that from a scientific and procedural point of view the methodology is appropriate and the data generated are of the required quality. This places the monitor in a pivotal role in the drug development process, both as a manager and a scientist.

The question remains, who is the monitor? There is no specification that he or she should be medically qualified. This is possibly due to the fact that a supranational body such as that which drafted the Good Clinical Practice guidelines did not wish to establish binding regulations for companies in different countries on how their infrastructures and personnel policies should be defined.

There is indeed much room for flexibility here, and from the definition of the monitor in the glossary of the EU Note for Guidance on Good Clinical Practice several types of medical and scientific or administrative training might be appropriate for clinical trial monitoring. Thus, 'Qualifications and experience to enable a knowledgeable supervision of a particular trial' (a physician? Perhaps a specialist in the clinical area) who may be helped by 'Trained technical assistants . . . in collection of documentation and subsequent processing' (the clinical research associate?).

Indeed it may be argued that such operational definitions of tasks and job functions coming to be written down in international documents, together with a genuine increase in scientific and organisational complexity of the clinical trial process itself, are responsible in part for the growth in professional specialities contributing to clinical research and for the evolution of the medical role away from conduct of clinical trials and back towards a more general professional facilitatory and consultative role characteristic of those physicians joining the industry in the 1960s.

## PHARMACEUTICAL PHYSICIANS

When considering how careers have developed in the international pharmaceutical industry, it is possible to ask: how many positions exist for pharmaceutical physicians, how are these distributed and how many new posts become available annually? Whilst exact figures do not exist, and not all doctors working in the industry are members of national associations of pharmaceutical physicians, useful information may be obtained from membership figures of these organisations.

Overall, total membership of the 26 associations affiliated to the International Federation of Associations of Pharmaceutical Physicians (IFAPP) is between 3500 and 4000. Adding the 2500 US physicians, who are not yet members of IFAPP, a total of 7000 is reached. Of the 3500 doctors affiliated to IFAPP, 75% are concentrated in the five largest European countries: UK, Germany, France, Italy and Spain. Holland, Belgium and Scandinavia account for a further 15%. Japan is a peculiar case since, in spite of the size of the population and of the importance of pharmaceutical research, the number of physicians in the industry is both totally and relatively small: around 70. Assuming that physician members of national associations represent on average 50% of those actually employed by pharmaceutical companies, overall there may be around 7000 physicians devoting their time to the discovery and development of new medicines in companies and in contract research organisations (CROs) in countries represented in IFAPP plus about 2500 physicians in the USA (total 9500). No information is available on the number of physicians working in the pharmaceutical industries of Eastern Europe and China, but it is unlikely that they would change substantially the above figures.

Assuming an attrition rate of 5% per year, around 500 positions should be available for new pharmaceutical physicians every year in the world (approximately 50 in the UK). This does not represent an impressive turnover; in addition, while in the last decade the number of physicians in the industry has grown, the trend might flatten or even decline in the next few years. The increasing cost of development of new drugs might force a reduction in fixed costs and overheads through the permanent employment of the smallest number of physicians compatible with the main development programmes, together with a shift towards use of CROs whenever the need arises. Of course, there might open more opportunities for physicians in these organisations.

In addition, the progressive shift towards biological approaches to treatment and disease prevention might change company structures substantially, as well as bring about the modification of research strategies and policies and development procedures in pharmaceutical companies in the foreseeable future.

## Career Change of Physicians

One important aspect of an industry career is that the job content for the pharmaceutical physician may undergo considerable change during the course of that career.

In the beginning, the scientific aspects predominate; clinical expertise in the assigned therapeutic area, combined with a good pharmacological background and a sound understanding of trials methodology and biometrics, represent the essential ingredients. Throughout the period with the company training and education continue through internal workshops and participation in courses held by a variety of academic and private organisations.

With time and a demonstration of satisfactory performance and potential for growth, the physician will perceive that the company expects him or her to move progressively from technical and scientific activities towards roles with a managerial content (project management or staff management), whether or not in the research domain.

There will be reduced time spent in organising and monitoring clinical trials and in assessing their results, and more time devoted to managing people, projects and resources; planning activities of individuals and groups; providing essential medical input to other company groups; participating in an increasing number of meetings, strategic and operational; and providing a contribution to decisions which go well beyond the pure clinical area.

Sometimes, this change in responsibilities and activities does not suit those physicians who are reluctant to abandon the scientific motivations which determined their original decision to embrace medical science as a career or, in more general terms, medicine as a profession. The extreme reaction may be a blunt refusal to change roles and responsibilities.

Of course, this attitude may be acceptable; the individual will grow in specific experience and competence, becoming an expert and 'guru' in a particular class of therapeutic products, but his or her vertical career development may be hindered. In large multinational companies, especially in the head office, it may be less difficult to find opportunities for development which are also satisfactory for those who wish to remain forever close to their initial field of scientific competence. In smaller companies and subsidiaries, however, pyramids are fewer and smaller in size so that often the movement upwards is prepared, as in chess, by a previous lateral movement to find an open career pathway.

The refusal to make this side-step may be detrimental to future career options. For instance, once someone else has taken a position, to find a new opportunity may take a long time. Meanwhile, the company may modify its views on such an individual, labelling him or her as intransigent, refractory or uncooperative.

Excessive technical specialisation is therefore a danger which a physician entering a pharmaceutical company should possibly avoid at all costs.

On the contrary, the need for flexibility and preparedness for change should be made clear to every aspiring pharmaceutical physician, whilst the company should plan appropriate training programmes contemplating not only biomedical subjects but also topics such as management, finance and marketing. These subjects should also receive appropriate coverage in every course on pharmaceutical medicine. In addition the harmonisation of such course programmes held in different countries seems to be desirable and useful also when a possible relocation within the company is being considered. This is becoming increasingly frequent at a time of progressive internationalisation and globalisation of the clinical development of medicines.

## CLINICAL SCIENTISTS

Clinical research scientists and other technical specialities nowadays find more opportunities within the company now that pharmaceutical medicine has become such a complex subject requiring a variety of professional contributions. Graduates in biology, pharmacy, biochemistry etc. usually take into consideration a pharmaceutical company as a suitable employer even during their university education. If they get a position in a medical department as a clinical research associate (CRA), or in the regulatory department as an assistant, they can expand their knowledge rapidly in areas such as clinical development of drugs, methodology, quality assurance and regulatory matters, whilst the frequent contacts with product managers open them up to new stimulating horizons in marketing, market analysis, project planning and coordination, sales, representative training and so on.

An intelligent and ambitious CRA can therefore find a number of stimulating opportunities for career development in the company, essentially because he or she may prove more adaptable than physicians, less dependent on traditions and more willing to take up new challenges in non-scientific areas.

There is of course the danger of 'emulation at all costs'. When a young and bright CRA moves to another department and is assigned a new, greater responsibility, and usually also a higher salary, other colleagues, sometimes more senior, feel frustrated and may decide they want to try the same experience—even, if necessary, in a different company. The results are sometimes good, but more often not because the person is an excellent, scrupulous, precise CRA but lacks some of the qualities required to be a good junior marketing manager.

In the last few years, the advent of Good Clinical Practice guidelines in several countries has opened, and is still broadening, new opportunities for development in a new area: clinical quality assurance. A clinical monitor or senior CRA with a sound experience in monitoring of clinical trials may become an excellent clinical quality assurance manager with a direct experience in the field certainly absent in other persons trained in quality assurance without prior experience in the field.

## CONCLUSION

Over many years careers have opened up for physicians and clinical scientists in the drug development process, notably in clinical research. Whilst physicians are filling a number of strategic, operational and managerial roles in drug development as a whole, clinical scientists and CRAs are managing an increasing proportion of the clinical trial procedures. Both are involved in information transfer within the company.

CRAs are now fulfilling broad scientific and clinical aims through a more defined and encapsulated job description at the heart of the research process, notably in the establishment, monitoring, analysis and reporting of clinical trials.

Industry physicians have grown as a profession, and may be reverting to the more general advisory and operational roles of the 1950s and 1960s, away from direct responsibility for the details of clinical trials.

Both groups, as well as many other ancillary groups, are responsible for a growing and valuable resource in any company's terms, namely the data from clinical experiments, the clinical trials!

# 3
# UK Trends in Employment in Pharmaceutical Medicine

## Tony Chandler

Talentmark Recruitment Consultants, London, UK

This chapter addresses employment trends within industry in relation to pharmaceutical medicine. It does not address pharmaceutical medicine in academia. As this chapter was prepared in August 1993 the figures given are best estimates as of that date unless otherwise stated.

### PHARMACEUTICAL MEDICINE

Let us first look at just what is meant by pharmaceutical medicine, as there are at least three accepted bases for defining it (Figure 1). In the narrow definition, as for instance that governing eligibility for membership of the Faculty for Pharmaceutical Medicine or the Postgraduate Course in Pharmaceutical Medicine, University of Wales, Cardiff, its practitioners are necessarily physicians. There is, however, a wider definition which embraces non-physicians of various other specialist disciplines, broadly understood to be part of the medical function within the pharmaceutical industry. And then there is a wider definition still, as for instance that adopted by the Society for Pharmaceutical Medicine, which extends to include toxicologists, discovery scientists and others involved in the pharmaceutical research and development (R&D) process.

*Discovering New Medicines: Careers in Pharmaceutical Research and Development.*
Edited by P.D. Stonier
© 1994 John Wiley & Sons Ltd

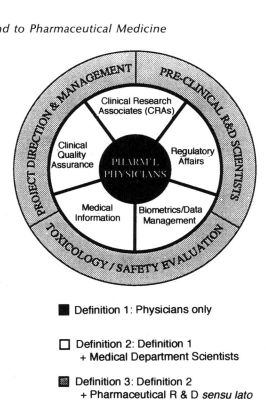

■ Definition 1: Physicians only

☐ Definition 2: Definition 1
+ Medical Department Scientists

▨ Definition 3: Definition 2
+ Pharmaceutical R & D *sensu lato*

**Figure 1.** Disciplines comprising pharmaceutical medicine.

## INCREASED PROFESSIONALISM AND SCOPE OF JOB FUNCTIONS

Over the last 20 years many factors have combined to change the inter-national operating environment of the pharmaceutical industry, and have thereby led to increasing professionalisation and specialisation within pharmaceutical medicine. Some of these are shown in Figure 2.

The thalidomide tragedy of 1961–1962 led to regulatory controls of growing stringency, with both increased costs and longer development time-scales in consequence. R&D in which the 'R' used to feature most prominently has increasingly given way to R&D in which the 'D' is ever larger. Tauter control of R&D programmes—with clearer decision points—became the name of the game. Clinical evaluation programmes were integrated on an international scale. Standard operating proce-dures and audits were introduced; data collection and information tech-nology mushroomed; all of which placed a greater premium on organisational and managerial skills, both to handle the burgeoning programmes and to try to contain the inexorable rise in costs.

- More stringent regulatory and political controls
- Emphasis of D over R
- Better evaluation procedures
- Sharper 'go/no go' focus and decision points
- Much longer development timescales
- Internationalisation of clinical R & D programmes
- Requirement for fuller documentation and audit trails: introduction of GCP, etc.
- Greater information-processing requirements
- Vastly increased costs
- Greater emphasis on organisational and people skills

**Figure 2.** Professional pressures on pharmaceutical medicine.

These influences have been matched by a vast increase in the range and sophistication of functions encompassed by pharmaceutical medicine (Figure 3) and also, of course, the demands made upon its practitioners.

- Medical services/medical affairs
- Clinical research
- Clinical pharmacology
- Drug surveillance
- Regulatory affairs
- Medicolegal

- Toxicology
- Professional relations
- Information/data management
- Project finance and management
- Quality assurance
- Pharmacoeconomics
- Contracts management

**Figure 3.** Extending the range of functions encompassed by pharmaceutical medicine.

## Tighter Selection Criteria

In view of this increase in sophistication, it is not surprising that the industry has become progressively more demanding and selective in the executives it recruits. For example, for physicians, 15 years ago, entrants were drawn more or less equally from general practice and hospital medicine and, in the main, not too much attention was paid to age or qualifications so long as presence, attitude and personality were acceptable. Today, new entrants are some five times more likely to come from hospital medicine or academia, are more likely to be in the approximate age range 28–35, and are also much more likely to have at least one higher qualification. Hand in hand with these changes, there is now a considerably more searching appraisal of personal qualities and potential for development.

## GROWTH IN NUMBERS EMPLOYED IN THE SPECIALITY

### Physicians

Another consequence of the increase in professionalism and range of activities undertaken within the speciality has been a substantial growth in the number of pharmaceutical physicians employed. My 'best estimate' is that this has increased over the last 20 years in the UK from around 265 in 1974 to 672 today.

It is interesting to try to put this growth into the context of the growth in other medical specialities over the same period. For the purposes of comparison, it seems reasonable to postulate, albeit somewhat arbitrarily, that a physician in the industry corresponds to a senior registrar or consultant in the National Health Service (NHS). Whilst that is quite a sweeping assumption in some cases, it is perhaps as good a basis for comparison as any, insofar as the typical level for entry into the industry now is as a well-experienced registrar with MRCP or equivalent.

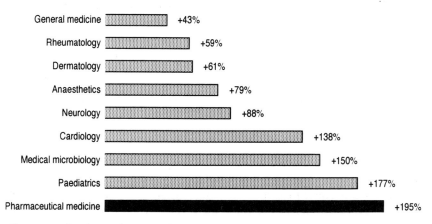

**Figure 4.** Growth in various UK medical specialities 1971–1991. (Data for NHS specialities from *Health Trends*, 1972, 1993; data for pharmaceutical medicine from own records.)

On this basis, pharmaceutical medicine has been one of the fastest-growing medical specialities over the last 10 years (Figure 4). It is now about the same size as rheumatology and cardiology put together (Figure 5).

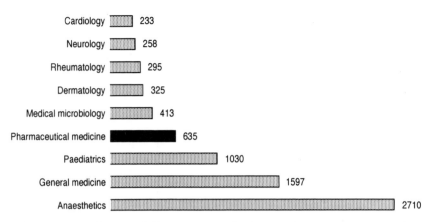

**Figure 5.** Numbers in different UK medical specialities in 1991. (Data for NHS specialities from *Health Trends*, 1993; data for pharmaceutical medicine from own records.)

Over recent years there has been an increasing tendency for physicians in the UK industry to develop their careers overseas. Since January 1989, I estimate that 98 physicians have left the UK industry for appointments overseas (44 in the USA alone), and this has been 'balanced' by an inflow of only 52 experienced pharmaceutical physicians entering the UK industry from overseas. The UK has therefore been acting as something of a training ground or provider for the industry internationally.

### Scientists and Other Professional Groups

If we take a broader look at pharmaceutical medicine (definition 2, Figure 1), which encompasses the new categories of professionals who have emerged alongside the physicians, it is clear that—substantial though the growth in employment of pharmaceutical physicians has been—it has been dwarfed by the growth in employment in pharmaceutical medicine within the medical function as a whole.

Thus, whilst the figure for the physicians' professional society membership has gone up by over 50% during the last 10 years, that for regulatory affairs executives has gone up by over 150%, that for clinical research associates (CRAs) has gone up by over 200%, that for

**Table 1.** Growth in pharmaceutical medicine specialities over the last 10 years

| Professional society[a] | Members served | Numbers | | Note | Growth over 10 years (%) | Estimate of 'true' UK numbers[b] |
|---|---|---|---|---|---|---|
| | | 1983/4 | 1992/3 | | | |
| BrAPP | Physicians | 442 | 676 | | +53 | 670 |
| ACRPI | CRAs | <353 | 1073 | | >200 | 2000+ |
| BIRA | Regulatory | 452 | 1290 | | +185 | 1400 |
| AIOPI | Information | 280E | 323E | 1 | +15 | 340 |
| ACDM | Data management | <274 | 760 | 2 | >175 | 1000 |
| PSI | Statisticians | 100E | 620 | | +520 | 500 |
| BARQA | Clinical QA | <10E | 240E | 3 | >1000 | 200 |
| Total | | <1911 | 4982 | | >160 | 6110 |

*Notes:*
1. E = estimate. Current membership figure = 404, of whom 80% are estimated to be research information scientists and are therefore excluded.
2. ACDM founded only at end of 1987; with a first-year (1988) membership of 274.
3. E = estimate. Current membership figure approx. 600, of whom 60% are estimated to be Good Laboratory Practice rather than Good Clinical Practice orientated, and are therefore excluded.
[a] See Acknowledgements section for full title of society.
[b] See text for explanation.

statisticians has gone up by over 500%, and that for clinical quality assurance specialists has gone up by over 1000% (Table 1). Moreover, such growth has happened at a time of relatively modest growth in overall numbers employed in the UK pharmaceutical industry. In the latest 10-year period for which figures are available (1980–1990), total numbers have gone up only from 73 000 to 76 000 (Office of Health Economics, 1993, personal communication).

Membership of the appropriate professional society is not, of course, synonymous with the number of executives practising full-time in that speciality in the industry in the UK. For example, membership lists usually include overseas members and associates, including those who may once have been working in the speciality but now no longer do so, part-timers, retired members and so on. There is also the question as to what 'the industry' comprises. There seems general agreement that it includes biotechnology companies, but there is much less accord over whether it includes the contract research industry which services the pharmaceutical industry (of which more later), and whether it includes such fields as medical devices, medical computing, and medical advertising and communications. There is also the question as to how many executives there are who are practising in the speciality and/or who are eligible for membership, but have not taken up membership of the appropriate professional body.

Any attempt to quantify the number of pharmaceutical medicine specialists working in, or directly serving, the UK pharmaceutical industry on a full-time basis must therefore be highly tentative. However, in consultation with leading members of the various professional associations, I have endeavoured to reach a best estimate of the number of people currently actively engaged in the major constituent specialities in the UK. This is given in the final column of Table 1. To the total of some 6100 must be added perhaps another 400 to take account of smaller specialities, such as medical writers and contract managers, and others not conveniently fitting into any particular speciality, to give a grand total of some 6500.

## Outsourcing and Contract Hire

A trend which has been emerging strongly over recent years, and stands to grow even more strongly over the coming years, is outsourcing. Companies are tending to keep their head-counts and establishment down by employing on a permanent and full-time basis only those essential skills needed all the time, and contracting out non-core activities. One consequence of this is more flexible staffing arrangements, with the ability to call on extra resource and expertise only when needed.

This has resulted in a massive growth in the service sector, and particularly dramatic within this has been the development of the contract research industry. Twenty years ago there were only 31 contract research organisations (CROs) in the UK, 10 years ago there were 81, and there are now over 170, employing between them over 7000 full-time staff, with at least another 1000 part-time (Technomark, 1993, personal communication). Such growth has drawn heavily on the industry itself for experienced staff.

In relation to this, there has also been a strong trend for executives within the industry, and notably physicians, to break away and establish their own independent consultancy or join with others, to provide drug development or clinical research-related services to the industry.

There has been a 10-fold greater increase in the numbers engaged in independent consultancy and in clinically related contract research over the last 10 years than in the numbers of full-time pharmaceutical physicians in the mainline pharmaceutical (and biotechnology) industry over the same period (Table 2). Of these, I calculate that the majority (88 out of the 129) came from the industry—41 of the 45 consultants and 37 of the 84 working in CROs. Indeed, over a quarter of pharmaceutical physicians are now employed outside the medical functions in the mainline pharmaceutical industry. This proportion is likely to grow.

A further trend has been the growth in contract hire and non-permanent employment. Contract hire typically entails the hiring of executives on a fixed-term contract basis from a service provider company, for a fixed period of time. Such executives remain employees of the provider but may otherwise be almost fully integrated into the hiring company for the duration of the contract.

By non-permanent employment I refer to freelancer and locum appointments, and to full- or part-time short- and fixed-term contracts arranged individually between the employer and the executive concerned. All these are strongly on the increase. Indeed, the medical department of the UK subsidiary of one major pharmaceutical company

**Table 2.**  Growth of pharmaceutical physicians in independent consultancy and contract research

|  | 1983 | 1989 | 1993 | 10-year growth |
|---|---|---|---|---|
| Mainline Pharmaceutical/ Biotech Industry | 390 | 454 | 516 | +32% |
| Consultancy/Contract Research | 25 | 94 | 129 | +416% |

now has an establishment of some 70 people, of whom only about 30 are permanent employees. The remainder are consultants, contract hire executives, freelancers (including ex-staff), short-term contract staff and so on, on a variety of different contractual arrangements.

Such 'arm's length' employment need not be in any way less satisfactory to the staff concerned, or detrimental to their career interests. They may enjoy the same benefits of service as the permanent staff, but be in a better position to manage their own careers. In the computer industry, where such arrangements have generally been in existence longer, some of the best software developers, for instance, will *only* work on a short-term contract basis.

Such arrangements also benefit staff who have gained the relevant experience and have left the company to start a family. They provide such people with career continuation possibilities which would earlier have been much more difficult to realise.

Continuing pressures on the industry to achieve flexibility, economy and efficiency on the one hand, and new evolving patterns of personal lifestyle preference and possibility on the other, make such company executive arrangements win–win situations for particular types of people, and further growth in such flexible employment alliances is certain.

## EMERGENCE OF BIOTECHNOLOGY COMPANIES

As biotechnology companies mature and research products enter the clinic for evaluation, so they have started to employ pharmaceutical physicians. Ten years ago no such physicians were employed within the UK biotech industry; five years ago there were five; and today I am aware of 15. This trend is set to continue, but the growth is not likely to be dramatic—partly because biotech companies will overwhelmingly choose to make extensive use of CROs rather than building up their own clinical research departments beyond core levels, and partly because biotechnology companies will work hard to transform themselves into fully fledged pharmaceutical companies.

## CONCLUSION

This chapter has touched on some of the major trends in employment in pharmaceutical medicine, and attempted to give some factual overview of the size of the industry. There are other trends, some of which are quite important, and these will be picked up and elaborated, in context, in later chapters.

## ACKNOWLEDGEMENTS

I acknowledge with thanks the information and advice provided by the following, notably in relation to the compilation of Table 1, for which the data were compiled in late July/early August 1993: A. Leslie of the British Association of Pharmaceutical Physicians (BrAPP); T. Scane of the Association of Clinical Research Associates in the Pharmaceutical Industry (ACRPI); C. Griffett of the British Institute of Regulatory Affairs (BIRA); M. Collins of Statisticians in the Pharmaceutical Industry (PSI); S. Lacey of the Association of Information Officers in the Pharmaceutical Industry (AIOPI); S. Cummings and J. Collard of the Association of Clinical Data Management (ACDM); N. Dent of the British Association of Research Quality Assurance (BARQA); and S. Ankier of the Society for Pharmaceutical Medicine. I record my regret that shortage of space precluded my developing many of the interesting themes arising in my discussions with them.

# 4

# Contributions of Schools of Pharmacy to the Pharmaceutical Industry

Paul S.J. Spencer

Welsh School of Pharmacy, University of Wales, Cardiff, UK

In summary, this chapter reviews the breadth of potential contributions the UK schools of pharmacy make to the international pharmaceutical industry. The schools produce some 1250 pharmacy graduates each year, a small but significant number taking up posts in industry (the vast majority choosing to enter professional pharmacy in hospital or primary (community) sectors where early salaries are better).

The very strong emphasis in their undergraduate courses on the pharmaceutical sciences, together with their knowledge of health care delivery systems and patient needs, fits these graduates for virtually any type of career in industry. Because of pharmacy graduates' disinterest generally in industrial careers, the industry has recently made wider use of graduates in chemistry, biochemistry and pharmacology who have been easier to recruit.

The schools of pharmacy also produce significant numbers of higher graduands (PhDs and MPhils) by research, most of whom find careers in the pharmaceutical industry, notably in pharmacology and toxicology, drug formulation and development, product information and other product support functions. The schools of pharmacy provide other 'services'. Many schools offer one or more specialist postgraduate

*Discovering New Medicines: Careers in Pharmaceutical Research and Development.*
Edited by P.D. Stonier
© 1994 John Wiley & Sons Ltd

courses for the industry, for example to support 'qualified person' training, training in regulatory affairs, clinical trials support and in analytical work.

Finally, there are the many services provided within the schools themselves. These include conduct of industry-financed research and development, analytical services and human volunteer studies on new or modified products.

The purpose of this review is to examine the variety of scholarly and other academic activities being pursued within the schools of pharmacy, and to show how these activities are, or could be, of service to the pharmaceutical industry. Looking at the graduates in pharmacy as perhaps the single most significant product of these schools, it must be emphasised that no other first degree in the chemical, biological or medical sciences (notwithstanding medical and veterinary degrees) can provide such a firm foundation in the very sciences that underpin the discovery, development and manufacture of today's medicines. Indeed, it was the pharmacists of the nineteenth century from whom today's international pharmaceutical industry sprang.

Before looking in some detail at the schools of pharmacy and the products and services they provide, two general comments should be made. Firstly, cooperation and interaction between university and industry are not something eccentric or unique about the schools of pharmacy and the drug industry. A former minister of state for higher education once remarked, 'education cannot prosper in isolation from the community that encircles it', adding 'active measures are needed to promote more fruitful interaction between education and society, including its industrial and commercial aspects'. Some progress has been made in the 16 years that have elapsed: today, both industry and higher education recognise the importance of one to the health and progress of the other, and increasingly the flow of help and services is a two-way phenomenon.

The second general comment relates to the meaning of the word 'pharmacy'. To the majority of people working in industry (and including perhaps the pharmaceutical physicians), the word 'pharmacy' describes a particular stage in a new drug or product's development, when substantial experimental work is carried out to define the exact nature and properties of the dosage form the new product will take, for example tablet or capsule or injection. Considerable control can be exerted over a drug's rate and extent of absorption, distribution and persistence in the body; to many, the application of these skills during drug development is 'pharmacy'. Outside of the pharmaceutical industry, the word means something very much broader: one of the four major health care professions, whose primary role is to bring about the safe and effective distribution and use of medicines. Schools of pharmacy were established to provide qualifying courses leading to pharmaceutical registration, and consequently the breadth or range of scientific and professional resources in the schools is very substantially wider than that required in the formulation and development of new drug candidates.

## ABOUT THE SCHOOLS OF PHARMACY

Organised pharmaceutical education in the UK followed upon the establishment of the Pharmaceutical Society and the granting of its Royal Charter in 1842, and the schools of pharmacy were subsequently created at the end of the nineteenth or in the first two decades of the twentieth centuries. Today, there are 16 schools of pharmacy in the UK, and one in the Irish Republic (see Table 1). Each school was originally established to provide local facilities for teaching courses leading to the recognised professional qualifications of the professional bodies in Britain, Northern and Southern Ireland. Subsequently, professional diploma courses were progressively replaced by university degrees (e.g. Bachelor

**Table 1.** Distribution of schools of pharmacy in Britain, Northern Ireland and the Irish Republic

| Country | University |
|---|---|
| England (12) | Aston |
| | Bath |
| | Bradford |
| | Brighton |
| | Leicester (de Montfort) |
| | Liverpool (John Moores) |
| | London (School of Pharmacy) |
| | London (King's College) |
| | Manchester |
| | Nottingham |
| | Portsmouth |
| | Sunderland |
| Wales (1) | Cardiff (Wales) |
| Scotland (2) | Aberdeen (Robert Gordon) |
| | Strathclyde |
| Northern Ireland (1) | Belfast (Queen's University) |
| Irish Republic (1) | Dublin (Trinity College) |

of Pharmacy (BPharm)), and by 1966 pharmacy had become a degree-entry profession. Furthermore, the schools of pharmacy had ceased to serve their local or regional functions, but increasingly admitted students from all over the UK (and from overseas) and were also engaged in increasingly wider postgraduate activities with a full international role.

The schools of pharmacy based in the established red-brick universities established research schools during the 1930s, often in close association with adjacent schools of chemistry. Later, and particularly since the Second World War, research broadened to include the new pharmaceutical sciences such as applied microbiology, pharmacology, pharmaceutics (studies on formulation and delivery systems), and more recently pharmacoepidemiology and pharmacoeconomics. Today, eight or nine schools of pharmacy have research schools numbering about 100 personnel—testimony to the nature and extent of their postgraduate development during the last 40 years.

It is possible to create an image of a 'typical' school of pharmacy. At the undergraduate level, there will be perhaps 1000–2000 applications every year for 80 places on the BPharm programme, so that high entry level qualifications are demanded. These are often comparable with those in medicine and veterinary medicine. Data from the Royal Pharmaceutical Society of Great Britain (RPSGB) reveal that 97% of the annual output of graduates will seek to register as pharmacists (in addition to a pharmacy degree, the potential pharmacists must complete a year's pre-registration programme under approved supervision and reach an acceptable standard in the Society's newly introduced (1993) professional qualifying examination (PQE). The most recently published manpower data (see Table 2) show that about 70% of pharmacists make careers in community (retail) pharmacy, 17% in the hospital sector and only 5% in some area of the pharmaceutical industry.

At the postgraduate level, schools of pharmacy are involved in a very wide portfolio of activities, including basic research in pharmacology,

**Table 2.** Distribution of British pharmacists in employment by different sectors

| | |
|---|---|
| Community (retail) practice | 71.6% |
| Hospital sector | 17.4% |
| University | 1.2% |
| Pharmaceutical industry | 5.3% |
| Other | 4.3% |

Source: Royal Pharmaceutical Society of Great Britain, 1992 Manpower Survey data

medicinal, physical and analytical chemistry, in pharmaceutics (drug formulation and delivery systems) and microbiology. In the typical school, research projects will largely be interdisciplinary, and research objectives may be described in general terms, such as 'drug design', 'drug discovery', 'drug targeting' and 'drug usage'. Perhaps in excess of 200 PhDs and MPhils by research emerge from these research schools each year, and the vast majority (in contrast to first-degree careers) will find careers in the pharmaceutical industry, increasingly in the international sphere. The spectrum of postgraduate activities is completed with the offer of various specialist postgraduate courses, the provision of continuing education programmes, and consultancy and other commercial services. In the typical school, fully 60% of external support of research and other postgraduate activities will come from the industry.

It is interesting to speculate on the relative unattractiveness of a career in the pharmaceutical industry for basic graduates in pharmacy. Despite the interest of doctoral graduates in the industry (not all of these will have a pharmacy first degree anyway), fewer than 5% of graduates from schools of pharmacy are joining the industry, and the number of industrial pharmacists today is smaller than in the 1960s. Initial salaries for the new pharmacist are better in professional sectors such as hospital and community; on the other hand, industry has been able to appoint substantially greater numbers of graduates in chemistry, biochemistry and pharmacology at more modest salaries. (It would be interesting nevertheless to imagine the consequences of trying to recruit medical graduates at similar salary levels!). In describing the schools of pharmacy contributions to the industry, one must be careful to differentiate between service/products 'on offer' and those with no possibility of realisation.

## THE SCHOOLS' CONTRIBUTIONS TO INDUSTRY

The schools of pharmacy produce first-degree and other graduands; they engage in research and development work, in the course of which they provide research training for PhDs; academic staff provide consultancy services; they offer specialist courses—and involvement in all of these activities properly constitutes the 'compleat school of pharmacy'. Table 3 gives a fuller analysis of these potential contributions to the industry.

### Graduates in Pharmacy

In the UK, some 1250 pharmacy graduates are produced each year. These go on to a pre-registration year before contemplating a career in

**Table 3.**  Outline of services and products from the schools of pharmacy, with the pharmaceutical industry as prospective clients

---

*Undergraduate teaching*
(a) First degree in pharmacy (BPharm, BSc(Pharm) etc.)
(b) Other first degrees (pharmacology, toxicology, neuroscience, medical sciences etc.)

*Postgraduate teaching*
(a) Provision of specialist award-bearing courses, of one or two years duration, full- or part-time, leading to postgraduate diploma or MSc, in subject areas meeting specialist needs of the pharmaceutical industry (e.g. to meet needs of 'qualified persons'; those working as clinical research associates; or in the drug registration/regulatory fields)
(b) Provision of specialist non-award-bearing short courses, to meet the negotiated requirements of an individual company (e.g. on laboratory safety, Good Laboratory Practice requirements or new analytical techniques)
(c) Provision of continuing education (updating) programmes, following an outline syllabus from a professional body (e.g. RPSGB or College of Pharmacy Practice) to meet the needs of pharmacists

*Research and development*
(a) Engage in 'blue skies' research or applied research, with support from a research council, charity or individual drug company
(b) In association with (a) above, provide research training programme for graduates, leading to PhD or MPhil degrees (part- or full-time)
(c) Engage in overtly commercial activities (e.g. through the provision of experimental data on new products or formulations, using unique or specialist skills and/or facilities such as gamma scintigraphy or bioanalytical data)

*Miscellaneous*
(a) Provision of general advice or consultancy to individual companies
(b) Provision of focus, venue and/or facilities for conferences and workshops
(c) Provision of specialist library or other bibliographic facilities
(d) Make general contributions to the scientific literature

---

industry (it remains possible for them to spend half of their pre-registration year in an industrial placement, and 50–60 do so each year). With the exception of Bradford (four-year sandwich course) and the two Scottish schools (Aberdeen and Strathclyde), British pharmacy degrees are typical science-based three-year honours degrees, although there are also significant additional professional and clinical subjects taught in this programme. The pharmacy programme is thus extraordinarily broad: the sciences range from physical, organic and analytical chemistry, to applied microbiology, the materials science of drugs, their excipients and packaging; to pathology, biochemistry, physiology, pharmacology and therapeutics. The professional subjects include forensic studies, behavioural science, pharmacoeconomics and pharmacoepidemiology. These lists of subjects do not constitute the syllabus but serve merely to illustrate the range of disciplines included in the pharmacy programme. The opportunities for students to integrate subjects such as organic chemistry with molecular and pharmacological modelling, and the potentially useful and harmful clinical effects that a single chemical species might induce, are very considerable; much recent development of the pharmacy degree curriculum has sought to enhance the amount of interdisciplinary teaching and subject integration throughout the syllabus.

Every facet of the drug industry is appropriate for these graduates when considering employment. Many pharmacists are found in pharmacological and formulation research, but novel synthetic chemistry, chemical development and toxicology are also targeted by these graduates. Significant numbers of pharmacy graduates also work in manufacturing plants (where they may be 'qualified persons') and a whole range of product support and information services attached to the pharmaceutical industry.

The RPSGB publishes and regularly updates its accreditation document, 'Criteria for Accreditation of Degrees in Pharmacy' (1992), which specifies the core content of pharmacy degrees in the UK. For their part, schools of pharmacy must submit to a re-accreditation process on a 5-year cycle. Most schools offer their students an optional element or specialist material during the final undergraduate year, although the extent and nature of such optional syllabuses vary between schools. Much of this optional material relates closely to industry; in particular it is in the final-year projects that the 'research school' and 'undergraduate school' find their greatest common ground. Consequently, many of these graduates gain a considerable, albeit narrow, insight into chemical, pharmacological or pharmaceutics research, using and developing skills of direct relevance to industry's research and development (R&D).

## Other Science Graduates

For professional reasons, schools of pharmacy have exercised considerable restraint in the growth of their 'pharmacy undergraduate populations', and one by-product has been the diversification of schools of pharmacy into new or parallel degree schemes with a 'pharmaceutical flavour', often in collaboration with another university department. Examples of other types of first degrees are pharmacology, toxicology, medical sciences and neuroscience, with the industry having actively encouraged several of these developments.

Two further developments are clearly of importance to the pharmaceutical industry. First, it is likely that the whole of the UK range of degree schemes will be organised on a modular basis by the end of the 1990s. Briefly, this means that current undergraduate programmes of about 1800 hours of student/staff contact will be subdivided into 'modules' of about 50 hours each, so that 36 completed modules will form the basis of a degree qualification. The concept of modularisation will facilitate assessment of student progress in a far more thorough manner (down to individual modules); it will also promote the movement of students between departments, and even between institutions—it is well within possibilities that by the year 2000 pharmaceutical companies will be receiving applications for employment from graduates who have studied at three separate institutions, mixing say biochemistry, physiology, pharmacology and toxicology; or graduates in chemistry with say three modules in pharmacology— students who may well have developed interdisciplinary skills, such as the molecular modelling of biologically active molecules. If industry was now to specify the types of skills it will need in the twenty-first-century drug developers, they could bring considerable favourable influence to bear on universities in the way in which final-year modules might be parcelled together, to the advantage of both potential graduate and industry (Watson, 1989).

Second, is the whole question of quality assurance in higher education, and the process of 'academic audit'. The 'audit' or assessment of research in universities has occurred twice with consideration being given to the range and quality of research, and the proportion of staff engaged in research in any given institution. Table 4 lists the results of the recent research assessment exercise applied to the UK schools of pharmacy (grade 5 is the highest, whilst the letter 'A' signifies that not less than 85% of academic staff are engaged in research).

Government-derived support of research in universities will be governed increasingly by the 'grading' and the proportion of academic staff actively engaged in research, and it is expected that the major share of government support for research in schools of pharmacy will be focused on just five or six schools (see Table 4) (Research Assessment Exercise, 1992).

In parallel, academic audit of undergraduate courses and procedures is now well advanced (The Measurement of Value Added in Higher Education, 1989; Teaching Standards and Excellence in Higher Education, 1991; Spencer, 1992). Whilst attempts to model quality assurance procedures on BS 5750 have been abandoned (at least, temporarily), there remains an ongoing careful examination of the quality assurance procedures operating in the delivery of undergraduate schemes. Quality

**Table 4.** Summary of assessments of schools of pharmacy research at the most recent assessment exercise (1992). The 'grading' number refers to quality, quantity and standing of the research, a '5' indicating research quality that equates to international excellence in some areas of the school, national excellence in all others. The letter 'A' indicates that more than 85% of academic staff have been included in the assessment. Government funding of research in universities is quantitatively determined from both the grading number and letter. (Data from Research Assessment Exercise, 1992: The Outcome, UFC Circular 26/92, December 1992)

| School of pharmacy, at the University of: | Research assessment | |
|---|---|---|
| | Grading | Proportion of staff |
| Aston | 4 | B |
| Bath | 5 | B |
| Bradford | 3 | B |
| Brighton | 2 | D |
| Leicester (de Montfort) | 2 | C |
| Liverpool (John Moores) | 1 | D |
| London (School of Pharmacy) | 5 | B |
| London (King's College) | 4 | B |
| Manchester | 4 | B |
| Nottingham | 5 | A |
| Portsmouth | 2 | C |
| Sunderland | 2 | D |
| Aberdeen (Robert Gordon) | 1 | C |
| Strathclyde | 3 | B |
| Cardiff (University of Wales) | 4 | A |
| Belfast (Queen's University) | 2 | B |

assurance, and the associated audit procedures, are linked to modularisation, because the latter facilitates the provision of very detailed assessment documents on a range of subjects studied by graduates, including how studied, where and at what level the 'credits' were obtained. Indications from industry generally suggest that employers will welcome detailed analyses of a prospective employee's academic performance across the breadth of disciplines, but universities need further guidance of preferred combinations of subjects which graduates should offer prospective employers.

Modularisation of degree schemes will also foster part-time study. Whilst many research degrees (PhD and MPhil) are already obtained over a five-year period, it seems increasingly likely that first degrees will also be attained through part-time study (financial and other personal circumstances may demand that the study of a 36-module programme is best studied over a six- or seven-year period, with modules or 'credits' accumulated slowly over this period). Although it seems unlikely that the main thrust of pharmacists' education will take this course, it is clear in subjects such as pharmacology or toxicology that qualifications could be gained by a mixture of directly taught material (attendance at planned modules) and on-the-job experience gained whilst working in the laboratories of a pharmaceutical company—new opportunities perhaps which show great similarity with study through the Open University or, more closely, with the earlier part-time University of London general degrees in science which many technicians pursued during the 1950s and 1960s.

## Postgraduate Courses

Some but not all of the schools of pharmacy have offered conventional part taught, part research, one-year full-time courses leading to MSc, but with no great enthusiasm, mainly because it has proved so difficult to obtain student grants and stipends for such postgraduate courses; support by the research councils has been welcome but too little, and usually directed at just one or two university departments. Pursuance of a similar MSc through part-time study taking, say, three years requires that the postgraduate student has reasonable geographical access to the university mounting the course.

More recently, schools of pharmacy have developed specialist part-time postgraduate courses on a slightly different basis. First, the driving force for the introduction of such courses, and in particular for defining the syllabus, has come from the pharmaceutical industry as 'customers' of such schemes. Moreover, part-time study has taken a new form, when course material is provided in one-week bursts, for example four or five one-week courses or modules in each year, with industry providing a day-to-day overseeing of private study and project work. Eight to ten such modules provide a total programme of about 300 hours plus the directed private study. Examples of such courses currently available to industry include: 'qualified persons' programme at Brighton; the programme for clinical research associates at Cardiff; and also the scheme for graduates working in regulatory affairs. Professional bodies contribute to the development of syllabuses and overseeing of student assessments and standards, whilst the 'cooperating' employers provide time off for the modules, participants' other costs and usually some on-site supervision of private study within the company. One of these programmes currently registers 65 students over a two-year programme, every student being supported by his or her employer.

Taking these examples as a baseline, it means that schools of pharmacy can respond to individual company initiatives, providing a minimum of, say, 12 participants a year could be guaranteed. Recently, a company with multiple community (retail) pharmacy stores has done just this, to provide specific postgraduate training for their junior pharmacists, with the 'contract' going to just one school of pharmacy. Such company-specific courses should be award-bearing (since this encourages completion of the programme), but could take many forms—from just a few hours leading to a certificate; or several hundred hours, leading to a postgraduate diploma or master's degree.

## THE SCHOOLS' RESEARCH AND INDUSTRY

The universities' funding councils continue to provide a foundation for research, although the level of support (as a proportion of a school's government-derived income) will vary from about 5% to 60%, depending on the school's research grading. Put another way, a school of pharmacy may have almost half of its tenured academic staff funded on the basis of their contribution to research—or the school may have no such 'research-funded' staff.

Increasingly, research is carried out within the framework of a major research programme whose workers share similar resources; a large research school, notwithstanding academic, academic-related, research students and technicians numbering about 100 workers, may have just three or four main areas or programmes of research. Within each programme there may be eight to ten individual but closely related projects—individual because each project may reflect the special interests of one or two individual staff, or the way the project is funded. For example, specific resources may have been provided through a research grant from a research council, national charity or individual pharmaceutical company. A major service to the industry is the training of PhD students, and the major research school with 100 personnel may actually 'graduate' 15 or 20 successful PhDs each year. The vast majority of these go into the pharmaceutical industry in the UK and, increasingly, in Europe or the USA. The CASE scheme (Cooperative Awards in Science and Engineering) operated by the Science and Engineering Research Council (SERC) is particularly suited to PhD students intending to pursue their careers in industry—it is a pity therefore that support for this scheme by SERC and the industry is not given more priority. The major research skills these PhDs possess will be focused on the pharmaceutical sciences: synthetic and analytical chemistry, drug targeting and formulation, and experimental pharmacology—but schools of pharmacy have also developed research in clinical pharmaceutical practice, with studies on drug utilisation focusing upon pharmacoeconomic or phamacoepidemiological aspects. Most major drug companies now have sections in R&D studying the potential benefits/costs of new products, and pharmacy-based PhDs with drug utilisation and pharmacoeconomic skills would surely provide a major extension of the current research-training roles of the schools of pharmacy.

## COMMERCIAL ACTIVITIES OF SCHOOLS OF PHARMACY

The schools have traditionally provided consultancy advice and related services, particularly in the fields of drug formulation and targeting, and in experimental pharmacology; these consultancies sometimes are in association with industry-supported research on a specific project carried out within the school. Increasingly, schools recognise that there may be purely 'service' roles they can play, when the intellectual challenge of the work may be limited but 'in-house' skills may be well suited to providing data in a specific field, vital to a new product's continuing development. Examples of such 'commercial roles' are in the provision of analytical services, whether developing new analytical methods or carrying out routine analyses, the provision of gamma scintigraphy studies in laboratory animals or human volunteers, or studies on drug-induced cognitive effects, again in human volunteers. In fact, the examples of such commercial services are growing, since the schools have recognised that 'profits' from such activities may in part be ploughed back into the school to underpin provision for its basic research.

## FUTURE DEVELOPMENTS

Considerable changes have occurred in universities during the last two decades, most particularly in the level of funding of both undergraduate and postgraduate activities from government sources. The consequences will be that major research programmes will be focused in fewer but larger research schools; the costing of either research or purely commercial services will become increasingly 'realistic'. At the undergraduate level, there will be downward pressure on the breadth and extent of laboratory skills that are developed in first degrees, whilst there will be increasing 'opportunity' for undergraduate students to offer 'pick and mix' degrees based on the developing modular concept. Whilst individual university departments will place some restraint on the possible combination of modules, industry could seriously influence such degrees by indicating special skills they seek in new graduates.

The output of schools of pharmacy, currently about 1250 pharmacy graduates each year, is unlikely to increase significantly because of restraint requested by the professional body, RPSGB. Indeed, current discussions with the Department of Health and the universities' funding councils in the hope of extending the BPharm degree from three to four years, if successful, may have to be implemented through a spreading of existing resources over four instead of three years, effectively reducing the number of graduates each year by 25%. Under these circumstances, recruitment of pharmacy graduates by the pharmaceutical industry would be depressed further. There will need to be discussions between the industry, the RPSGB and schools of pharmacy about the industry's future needs of pharmacists (or pharmacy graduates), both in numerical and qualitative terms. Failing this, we could arrive at a UK industry almost devoid of pharmacists—which would be in marked contrast to current trends in Europe and the USA.

# 5

# The Contribution of Academic Clinical Pharmacology to Medicines Research

## Charles F. George

### University of Southampton, UK

Clinical pharmacologists have a major role to play in the pre-marketing phase of drug development. Specifically, their knowledge and skills equip them for:

1. studies on dose–response relationships;
2. studies in special groups, e.g. the elderly, those with liver or renal disease; and of pharmacogenetics;
3. studies of drug interactions;
4. the estimation of compliance;
5. other activities.

## DOSE–RESPONSE RELATIONSHIPS

Although policies within individual companies differ one from another, there can be no doubt that the industry and the recipients of their products have suffered when new chemical entities have been used in too high a dose. There are many examples which could be cited but I shall confine myself to two. The first example is the treatment of

*Discovering New Medicines: Careers in Pharmaceutical Research and Development.*
Edited by P.D. Stonier
© 1994 John Wiley & Sons Ltd

hypertension with benzothiadiazine (thiazide) diuretics. Despite careful studies by Cranston *et al.* (1963) showing that low, intermediate and high doses of bendrofluazide, cyclopenthiazide and chlorthalidone were equi-effective in lowering blood pressure, most doctors prescribed intermediate or high doses for their patients. Diuretics of this type produce hypokalaemia but the significance of the latter and the risks of long-term glucose intolerance were not appreciated until much later (Murphy *et al.*, 1982; Lant, 1987). Nevertheless, when used in low dose diuretics remain an effective, economic and simple treatment for hypertension, while their risks are minimised.

Similarly, the first angiotensin-converting enzyme inhibitor to be marketed, captopril, was initially given in large doses (Lant, 1987), often to people in whom we would now prefer to avoid its use, e.g. those with renal artery stenosis and collagen vascular disease. Problems such as rashes and agranulocytosis arose as a consequence of the high doses used compared with those now recommended (Romankiewicj *et al.*, 1983). Modern methodology (Wellstein *et al.*, 1987) should allow a more detailed study of the extent of inhibition of the angiotensin-converting enzyme *in vivo*. Such information is of use in exploring the dose–effect relationship and deciding upon an appropriate one (as well as the dosing interval for a new compound).

By contrast, in the sphere of angina pectoris (and hypertension) Prichard and Gillam (1971) carried out pioneering studies to show the importance of dosage titration. Thus, in angina pectoris studies comparing the efficacy of full dose (average 417 mg/day; range 80–1280 mg) a half, one-quarter and one-eighth of that amount showed a clear-cut dose–response relationship. Originally, it was thought that this might be a reflection of poor absorption in some patients. However, studies by Paterson *et al.* (1970) using radiolabelled propranolol showed that the absorption was almost complete.

Subsequently, Shand *et al.* (1970) demonstrated identical plasma concentration–time curves after intravenous administration to five healthy volunteers but sevenfold differences in the plasma concentrations obtained after oral dosing. This provided evidence for extensive pre-systemic drug metabolism and marked interindividual differences in its extent. This knowledge was used subsequently to demonstrate the importance of dosage titration in the control of cardiac arrhythmias (Woosley *et al.*, 1979).

The identification of pre-systemic drug metabolism and the likelihood of a short duration of action (as well as individual variability) led to subsequent more rational investigation of other cardiovascular acting drugs. Thus, in my laboratories we have worked extensively on the dihydropyridine calcium channel-blocking drug, nifedipine. We demonstrated

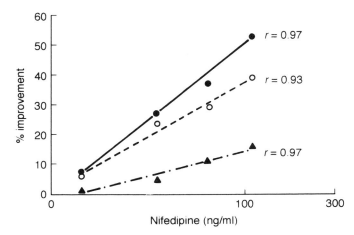

**Figure 1.** Relationship between plasma nifedipine concentration and antianginal effects in patients already receiving atenolol. •–•, time to pain; o– – –o, time to 1 mm ST depression; ▲–··–▲, maximal exercise tolerance. Reproduced from the *British Journal of Clinical Pharmacology*, with kind permission of the editor (Challenor *et al.*, 1989).

a close relationship between the response in angina pectoris (time to onset of pain, time to 1 mm ST segment depression and the maximum duration of exercise) and the logarithm of the plasma nifedipine concentration (Challenor *et al.*, 1989) (Figure 1). However, even with modified release preparations, twice-daily dosing was insufficient to produce an adequate response throughout a 24-hour day, the benefits wearing off by 12 hours after dosing.

## STUDIES IN SPECIAL GROUPS

### The Elderly

The elderly consume a disproportionate number of medicines (Ridout *et al.*, 1986; Cartwright and Smith, 1988). This is particularly true of drugs intended for use in cardiovascular medicine, others with an action on the central nervous system (e.g. anti-Parkinsonian remedies) and for agents with an action on the musculoskeletal system.

Historically, the elderly have run into problems with agents with an action on each of these three systems. Examples include various anti-hypertensives (Jackson *et al.*, 1976), anti-Parkinsonian therapy (Williamson and Chopin, 1980), benzodiazepines (Castleden *et al.*, 1977; Greenblatt *et al.*, 1991) and benoxaprofen (Hamdy *et al.*, 1982). If it is likely that a new medicine will be used by old people then it is essential to perform adequate studies of its pharmacology in that population.

Within my own group we (Robertson *et al.*, 1988) have performed studies of nifedipine's pharmacology in this age group. After an intravenous dose the initial concentrations achieved were similar to those in healthy young individuals but the clearance was diminished from 519 ml/min to 348 ml/min ($P < 0.05$). After oral administration, plasma concentrations were higher in the elderly than in young people due, in part, to an increased bioavailability from 46% to 61% consequent upon diminished pre-systemic metabolism. But the area under the concentration–time curve was increased also by delayed systemic clearance.

In addition to these age-related variations in pharmacokinetics, the drug had different effects after intravenous administration. In young people it produced a brisk tachycardia with no drop in blood pressure (Figure 2). By contrast, in the elderly there was no increase in heart rate but a pronounced reduction in blood pressure. Such differences reflect not only a decline in baroreceptor function with age (Reid *et al.*, 1971) but also altered adrenoceptor sensitivity (Buckley *et al.*, 1986; Scarpace, 1986; Montamat and Davies, 1989).

Given the increased prevalence of Parkinson's disease in the elderly (Robertson and George, 1990), it is perhaps surprising how little was done to examine the pharmacology of L-dopa in this age group until recently. There are, however, major differences in the pharmacokinetics of L-dopa (Robertson *et al.*, 1989) which, in part, explain the increased incidence of adverse effects encountered.

The elderly tend to complain more about problems with sleeping than do younger people. This is partly because their pattern of sleep is different and because they take 'cat naps' during the day, use less energy than their younger counterparts and require less sleep. Many studies have shown that the elderly are at greater risk from hypnotic drugs than are younger persons, and Greenblatt *et al.* (1991) have made elegant studies of the effects of benzodiazepines in this age group. They have demonstrated that the plasma concentration of triazolam needed to produce a particular effect is roughly one-half of that which would produce the same action in younger persons. In addition, hangover effects of benzodiazepines are more common in this age group (Castleden *et al.*, 1977).

The prevalence of arthritis, particularly osteoarthritis of the knee, increases markedly with age (Blackburn *et al.*, in press). As a consequence elderly people suffer considerable pain and limitation of their mobility. They therefore seek refuge in analgesic compounds. Although there is relatively little evidence that the non-steroidal anti-inflammatory

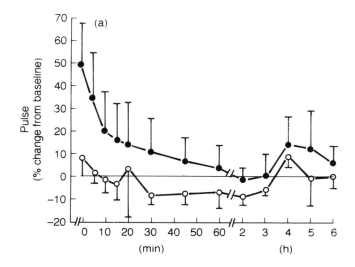

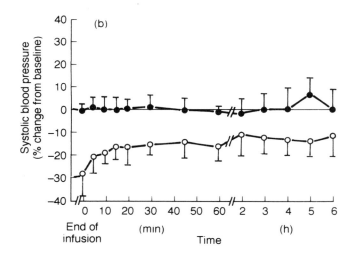

**Figure 2.** Effects of nifedipine on (a) heart rate and (b) systolic blood pressure in young (•) and elderly (○) subjects. Reproduced from the *British Journal of Clinical Pharmacology*, with kind permission of the editor (Robertson *et al.*, 1989).

drugs are required they are nonetheless frequently prescribed for patients in this age group. It is therefore vitally important that such agents are properly studied in healthy old people, those who have disease and others who are taking additional drug therapy. In collaboration with three other centres we (George *et al.*, 1986) studied the new compound isoxicam in 108 people, of whom half were elderly. Half of the old people were healthy volunteers, while the remainder were patients taking other treatments. Despite differences in age and concurrent disease, there were no significant differences in the pharmacokinetics of this compound between young and old people. By contrast, benoxaprofen was particularly hazardous for old people, especially those with renal dysfunction (Hamdy *et al.*, 1982).

## Renal Failure

Studies could be undertaken either by nephrologists or clinical pharmacologists. The important point is to define the proportion of drug (or active metabolite) excreted in the urine, and to document any changes in systemic clearance with renal dysfunction so as to make appropriate dosage modification in patients with renal failure. Amiloride is a good example of an initial failure to act upon these principles. The drug is cleared unchanged via the kidneys (George, 1980) and will accumulate in patients with renal disease. Such patients are at risk of hyperkalaemia, and death occurred in a few during the early stages of drug development. Similarly, the acetyl metabolite of acebutolol is active and its clearance is diminished in patients with significant renal disease (Smith *et al.*, 1983), thereby contributing to its overall effects and long duration of action. Other water-soluble $\beta$-adrenoceptor antagonists have produced problems in patients with renal dysfunction. Although attempts were made to identify the most appropriate dose and dose frequency for atenolol in hypertension, when it was first marketed it was available only in 100 mg doses. The prescription of these to old patients sometimes produced profound bradycardia and syncope. Only subsequently have 50 mg and 25 mg tablets become available.

## Liver Disease

The majority of drugs which are subject to metabolism within the human organism meet their fate in the liver. Disease of the latter organ can lead to:

1. diminished albumin synthesis and hence protein binding;

2. reduced metabolising capabilities due, in part, to shunting of blood through portosystemic anastomoses;
3. increased end-organ effects.

It is necessary to address most, if not all, of these parameters if a new chemical entity is likely to be used in people with hepatic disease. Clinical pharmacologists may have access to such patients and can certainly help with the design and interpretation of such studies. However, in general it is patients who show diminished synthetic ability for albumin, who are jaundiced or show evidence of liver failure with ascites and encephalopathy who are particularly at risk (George *et al.*, 1992).

### Genetic Polymorphism

Until comparatively recently there were few examples of how genetic mutations could result in subpopulations with quite widely differing abilities to carry out certain metabolic reactions. Among these, variations in the activity of N-acetyltransferase were the best documented. Genetic polymorphism in this case affects the metabolism of substrates, which include hydralazine, isoniazid, procainamide and sulphonamides (George and Waller, 1993).

More recently, it has become clear that genetic polymorphism occurs also with drug oxidation reactions. Thus, in 1977 'abnormalities' of 4-hydroxylation of debrisoquine were described (Mahgoub *et al.*, 1977; Tucker *et al.*, 1977). Since then, studies have identified numerous drugs which are subject to metabolism by the cytochrome P450 isoenzyme known as CYP2D6. Phenotypically poor metabolisers are subject to a variety of adverse effects, such as orthostatic hypotension from debrisoquine, nausea and vomiting from bufuralol, excessive duration of action of metoprolol and propranolol and possible central nervous system toxicity from a variety of tricyclic antidepressants (George *et al.*, 1992). Most of these discoveries have stemmed from work in academic departments of clinical/biochemical pharmacology. Several departments have established banks of human liver tissue, cell lines, purified enzymes and specific antibodies which allow the detection of potential metabolic pathways. Moreover, selective inhibitors of CYP2D6, including quinidine and propafenone, have been identified which allow the significance of this enzyme to be studied *in vivo*.

Twenty human isozymes have been cloned and characterised/sequenced in full. Among the most important ones to exhibit genetic polymorphisms are CYP1A2, CYP2B6, CYP2C, CYP2D6 (see above), CYP2E1 and CYP3A4, all of which have been shown to metabolise clinically important drugs (Cholerton *et al.*, 1992). Substrates for these enzymes include caffeine, theophylline; testosterone, tolbutamide and phenytoin; debrisoquine, metoprolol; chlorzoxazone; and nifedipine, erythromycin and cyclosporin.

An alternative technique for defining genetic polymorphism is based upon statistical/modelling approaches for data obtained *in vivo* on large populations (Jackson *et al.*, 1989). Clinical pharmacologists (mostly based in academia) have contributed much to our understanding of the appropriate use of these techniques (Grevel *et al.*, 1989).

The significance of genetic polymorphism is further developed in the next section.

## DRUG INTERACTIONS

Traditionally, interactions have been studied in 'blunderbuss' fashion. As a consequence, pharmaceutical companies have undertaken expensive, sometimes meaningless, studies of around 50 compounds with which their product might, in theory, interact. It is my belief, and that of colleagues both in academic clinical pharmacology and in the pharmaceutical industry, that we need to target our studies more meaningfully. In so doing, we should not only satisfy regulatory authorities but also undertake a more informed, ethical and appropriate series of studies. Hopefully, these should be cheaper and take less time than the more traditional approach.

When studying the fate of a new chemical entity in man it should be possible (by a combination of studies performed *in vivo* and in *vitro*) to establish the major pathways of metabolism/elimination. Thus, the demonstration that a new benzodiazepine is, like triazolam, metabolised by CYP3A (Kronbach *et al.*, 1989; Gascon and Dayer, 1991) should lead to the initiation of specific interaction studies. Firstly, enzyme inducers such as carbamazepine will need to be studied—perhaps in epileptics, since we know that this same enzyme is responsible for the metabolic degradation of felodipine (Capewell *et al.*, 1988). Interactions with citrus juices may need to be undertaken (Bailey *et al.*, 1991) and a variety of other inhibitors studied, e.g. cimetidine, calcium channel-blocking drugs, ketoconazole and the macrolides, e.g. erythromycin. Interactions may need to be undertaken also with non-sedative antihistamines, with the selective serotonin reuptake inhibitors and cyclosporin. Had it been recognised that astemizole and terfenadine were metabolised by this same cytochrome P450 system, studies might have been undertaken with specific inhibitors, e.g. erythomycin, and the torsade de pointes form of ventricular tachycardia recognised earlier than 1992 (Honig *et al.*, 1992).


## COMPLIANCE


There are four main variables which influence the effects of medicines:

- pharmaceutical, e.g. the formulation;
- pharmacokinetic factors,
- pharmacodynamic factors;
- patient's medicine-taking behaviour (compliance).

Non-compliance can take several forms, including not taking enough medicine, not observing the correct intervals between doses, not observing the correct duration of treatment, and taking additional medication (either prescribed or non-prescribed). Each of these forms of non-compliance can affect the outcome of drug treatment and is particularly important when assessing the effects of new treatments. Traditionally, physicians have relied on their patients giving honest answers to questions such as 'Do you ever forget to take your medicine?' Answers to these and other questions have been supplemented by pill counts which estimate the amount removed from the container. However, this technique assumes that whatever has left the bottle goes through the patient and this may not always be the case.

In recent years blood and urine tests have been used to identify the likely causes of failure to respond to drug treatment. Low blood concentrations mean either a failure to comply with treatment or poor absorption due to pharmaceutical factors and/or extensive pre-systemic drug metabolism. Repetition of the measurement under a period of supervised medication intake can lead to a more accurate assessment of the contribution of non-compliance to the low blood concentrations found. More recently, Feely *et al.* (1987) have pioneered the incorporation of a tracer dose of phenobarbitone. The presence or absence of the latter in blood indicates the extent of patient compliance. Compliance with other drug therapy has been assessed by the incorporation of a substance such as riboflavin which is excreted in urine. Subsequent screening of urine for the presence of riboflavin (by fluorescence under ultraviolet light) has been used extensively in the USA to select patients for inclusion in trials of antihypertensive medication (Veterans Administration Cooperative Study Group on Antihypertensive Agents, 1967). Finally, in recent times attempts have been made to identify non-compliant patients by examining the ratio of metabolite to parent drug as an indicator of whether or not patients have been indulging in 'drug holidays' (Ilett *et al.*, 1993).

## OTHER ACTIVITIES

In this chapter I have attempted to show some of the ways in which clinical pharmacologists can contribute to the development of new chemical entities. There are, however, other ways in which they contribute to the development of new medicines. First, many act as consultants to the pharmaceutical industry. Second, they contribute also to drug development through their activities as members of ethics committees and drug-regulatory bodies such as the Committee on Safety of Medicines and the Medicines Commission. Third, they have devised new techniques for the study of medicines in man. In general, however, the latter area is less specific to clinical pharmacologists than it is to electronic experts, psychologists and consultants in the various subspecialities of medicine. For that reason I will not attempt to enumerate them here. Readers interested in the subject are referred to the methods series run by the *British Journal of Clinical Pharmacology*.

# 6
# The Contribution of Nursing to Pharmaceutical Medicine

Jenifer Wilson-Barnett

King's College, London, UK

Although many nurses have worked in the pharmaceutical medicine field, there has been little awareness or professional recognition of their potential contribution and relevant educational background. This is a great oversight, as many employers have now realised. Their skills and understanding are particularly useful to the discipline and industry in many ways, and from their standpoint this career pathway offers advantages and opportunities not available within a conventional clinical career

## NURSING EDUCATION

The discipline of nursing is gradually developing from research using a mix of applied subjects relevant to medicine, and from a complementary perspective. Recently a more defined curriculum and preparation prepares nurses for a wide variety of roles and settings. Underpinning practice, a reformed educational process is providing nurses with a new confidence and a greater gamut of skills, many of which are general and necessary to survive in a competitive world but many more are particularly relevant to dealing with patients or clients.

*Discovering New Medicines: Careers in Pharmaceutical Research and Development.*
Edited by P.D. Stonier
© 1994 John Wiley & Sons Ltd

Above all, nursing is based on the premise that it is necessary to understand the 'whole person', to appreciate the factors that affect their life, health status and responses to illness if this occurs. From this holistic perspective it is possible to assess how factors affecting health interact and how external agents impinge on individuals and their families. Unlike medicine, nurses have resisted the temptation to specialise according to parts or systems of the body or diseases. They have sometimes followed medical specialisms but always aimed to concentrate on the individual's unique and total environment. With the intention of building on strengths within this 'personal environment', nurses have tried to augment the patient's available support systems and reduce the stresses and risk factors. Complex assessments are necessary in order to have an accurate picture of such relevant factors. They are also necessary as a baseline from which to monitor changes.

Such assessments require a sophisticated level of knowledge in many subjects and subtle and well-honed skills of communication and observation. Nurses therefore need a good understanding of many basic medical sciences combined with social sciences, psychology and ethics applied to health and illness. Increasingly nursing courses at pre- and post-registration level are including both pure and applied coverage of these contributory subjects. This breadth of coverage is quite demanding and many students seem to gain quite an aptitude for understanding different research approaches to increasing knowledge in these areas.

Two recent trends in nursing education are pertinent to a new confidence in the discipline and the skills which a whole new generation of graduates will possess. An increasing emphasis on health promotion is now expected by the statutory bodies and reinforced by Department of Health policy. This philosophy is fundamental to both the role and styles of communication adopted with individual patients and client groups, enhancing independence, self-care and confidence to improve health or manage problems. Providing support and information when needed becomes a prime responsibility for practitioners. Yet in reality the extent to which nurses have adopted this ideal practice is extremely limited (Macleod Clark *et al.*, 1992). Hopefully more recently qualified practitioners will have greater understanding and application and certainly this research indicated that more highly educated nurses had a more advanced propensity to give patients and their relations more opportunities to ask questions and express preferences for care and treatments.

Secondly, research understanding and an expectation that practice is based on research evidence underpins all curricula. Most courses include specific research methodology elements and encourage a critical appraisal of studies reported in the press. Many senior nurses are now

expected to appreciate the different contributions of major epistem-
ologies and select the most appropriate methods to address specific
research questions. Different levels of understanding and application
are expected for grades of staff and areas of practice as many senior
nursing posts now encompass quality assurance and evaluation of new
interventions.

## NURSING ROLES

These many strands of education prepare nurses for complex roles
which should exploit an egalitarian philosophy of health and research.
All this is contained in the work of assessing needs and providing care
and treatments. The technical skills are equally important, and dexterity
and the ability to manipulate equipment and understand its functioning
become second nature to nurses in high-technology areas. A sound
knowledge of treatment goals and drug actions is also essential in all
practice. In order to explain to patients and observe for side-effects and
therapeutic results a working application of pharmaceuticals is very
necessary to all in the profession. Data entry on to computers and in-
stant analysis also means that nurses learn to dispel any anxiety they
may feel about working with VDUs.

Developing roles in nursing requires excellent knowledge and skills
over a wide range, and the education which prepares nurses is often
praised by medical educationalists. In particular, graduates are highly
successful in health service and other careers. The expected roles they
will perform require clinical acumen, judgement and decision-making
but they also rest on a foundation of open and interactive communication skills. This last aspect is usually taught through video feedback
and role-play but also assessed in clinical settings through observation
and evaluation of practice by tutors.

## NURSING SKILLS

Through extensive and intensive contact with patients, clients and the
general public, nurses should gain confidence and ease in most settings.
Many challenges are faced throughout training and after qualifying,
such as dealing with very distressed people or those who are angry or
disorientated. This range of practical and emotionally demanding
difficulties prepares nurses for most challenges in life. It is probably this
ability to cope with the unpredictable and stressful which epitomises the
perception of the nurse's role for many people.

Even more relevant to a wider career choice is the emphasis on communication skills in all nursing work. Although much research indicates that practitioners could do better and patient complaints tend to focus on poor communications (Macleod Clark *et al.*, 1993), this may often be due to pressure of speed and workload in the acute sector. Given time and motivation it is unusual for nurses now not to be able to analyse patterns of communication and identify which elements promote interaction and encourage and satisfy patients and relatives.

Inter-professional communication is also part and parcel of practice. The nurse's role in representing patients and reporting pertinent changes in their condition is vital. Although this is sometimes apparently done in a rather non-assertive manner (Porter, 1992), doctors consistently rely on this information. Once more nurses are used to dealing with conflict and differences in professional opinions. Not all cope well with this but ward sisters generally function as an important arbiter and facilitator for most staff. Their confidence and understanding are generally respected by other staff.

In an increasingly complex and changing health service, nurses working in each sector need to have a sound understanding of the overall structure and a network of colleagues. Without the ability to contact those in the community, hospital nurses cannot achieve continuity of care for their patients. A knowledge of the respective roles of community agents, the statutory financial benefits and of the most efficient services needed to help patients is essential for practising nurses. This type of background is also invaluable to many research or development projects.

In general the ability to coordinate staff, initiate contacts and administer much that is complicated and sensitive is often undervalued. This hidden aspect of nurses' roles makes them capable and organised colleagues. Their capacity to deal with many issues simultaneously, stay calm and coordinate people tactfully is notorious (Pembrey, 1980). The energy required, mentally and physically, is immense and staying in a clinical career for many years is very demanding, especially when poorly remunerated.

It is possible that this portrait is slightly idealised: there are levels of practice which may be routine and unskilful. However, one can have confidence in the qualified nurse as their preparation has been rigorous and plans for compulsory continuing professional education will ensure that updating and performance are monitored. In whatever role they practice nurses are seen as responsible, the public continue to respect them (Clay, 1990) and their broad-based knowledge and background make them accessible to the lay person and professional alike.

## NURSING CAREERS IN PHARMACEUTICAL MEDICINE

When considering how nursing may contribute to pharmaceutical medicine it is probably necessary to analyse the many different levels and areas in which nurses work in order to have a realistic impression of how they may fit into the whole enterprise. The varying preparation and roles would necessitate a careful matching. From data collector to manager in the industry requires a different level of nurse from first clinical post to executive position. It is also obvious that those recently graduated from an honours course in nursing studies would be more able to cope with some research tasks than an experienced community nurse who would be ideal for home-to-home data collection but unprepared for data analysis or marketing.

In the last decade graduates in nursing have doubled in number (Hayward, 1992). The success of these bachelor degrees is clear, indicated by the retention of graduates within the health service, by their interesting career posts and by the satisfaction of employers. They have confidence and a knowledge level and intellectual performance equal to other professions, but it is their capacity to relate to others and understand their feelings which is so often distinguishable (Crow, 1980). All four-year, pre-registration degrees include a research dissertation. These have been praised by many an external examiner and instil a decision to do more research later. This research understanding is at quite an advanced level and many of the pilot studies they undertake involve designing questionnaires or interview schedules. However, it is still quite exceptional for students to undertake an experiment within this final year, as the time period is not sufficient.

Graduates who have not continued in nursing and have moved to another career have been followed up by most university departments. Although the numbers are relatively small they have achieved substantial success in personnel, business management and journalism. Graduates are also much more likely than other nurses to return to a career after rearing their children.

The diploma courses introduced three years ago have the goal of producing well-educated nurses, able to work in hospital or community posts. Their health promotion orientation and full student status are heralded as an advance. They should be independent, reflective and eager to research the literature to support their practice. If the employment situation in the health service permits they could be an invaluable resource, namely to endorse a more consumer-orientated focus to practice and to provide a continuity of care for patients either during hospital care or in the community. However, they should also be potentially good candidates for the early stages of a career in the industry.

Community nursing practice, as previously mentioned, is a popular choice amongst the higher-educated nurses. Many say they value the independence of district nursing or health visiting and find the team-work satisfying in many locations. They can also become known within a community and have the skills to win acceptance and access to patients who need, but do not readily ask, for assistance. Their know-ledge of social services and health resources becomes very extensive over time, as does their knowledge of the limited list for prescribers. In future their right to prescribe should be expanded and they will hope-fully be able to influence more direct and sensitive treatments. Top-up courses to ensure they are prepared for this prescribing role are already designed, many with input from lecturers in medical pharmaceutics. This extremely relevant background would make them ideal coordi-nators for projects in primary care.

Of note also is the fully trained intensive care nurse. His or her (90% of nurses are female) knowledge of drug actions and sensitive aware-ness of physiological reactions are finer than in many more senior physi-cians. The capacity to collate data to build up a complete picture of the health status of the patients is often masterful. Ongoing work at King's College Nursing Studies Department by King (1993) attests to this. Nurses are able to analyse and recount their assessment procedures and split-second actions very fully. They are conversant with the rapidly developing range of drugs and procedures related to intensive care and manage to sustain very full professional relationships with clinical col-leagues. Such staff would certainly instil confidence among medical staff in many spheres of practice.

From this account of what nurses do and how they are prepared one must conclude that within pharmaceutical medicine there are many challenging roles for which nurses are admirably suited. Within research, marketing or management, nurses have contributed in the past but are now even better prepared. Their personal and intellectual skills are valuable and the sadness is that so many of them feel under-valued in their health service posts. Importantly, moving into this area should not be seen as leaving nursing, just as teaching or research in nursing should not be seen as a total redirection. As long as their pro-fessional background is exploited and appreciated by employers it should be seen as influencing an important area of health care. Nurses' humanitarian approach to issues and their understanding of ethical principles of pressurising individual rights and autonomy should be invaluable to an industry devoted to beneficence.

## THE NURSE'S ROLE IN RESEARCH

In addressing the research role it is important to realise that the current emphasis on research methods in nursing really makes nurses akin to some psychologists in terms of their expertise on graduation. The eclectic approach to research taken by teachers in this field lends an adaptability and flexibility to graduates' thinking. To balance this, however, they may hold a slight bias against randomised controlled trials which do not allow for the process and response to treatments to be recorded. Consumer choice is also seen as essential, and the more progressive research designs enabling subjects to become more involved in the process of research group selection are preferred by most knowledgeable nurses. Their familiarity with qualitative approaches and the complex analysis pathways required may also serve to complement any research team. New research assessing the quality of life, making great efforts to include the consumer's perspective on drug therapy, would surely require this type of researcher on the team.

Classically nurses have served as efficient and sensitive data collectors; as well as this they now rightly request more involvement in the whole design and research process, including publication. With their enhanced skills this should present no difficulties to a multidisciplinary team. Indeed the very emphasis on inter-professional collaboration in research would endorse this. Many more nurses are also now much more confident in using computerisation for data analysis, and having produced a score of essays on word processors during their courses also find this becomes an inevitable part of their work!

Of interest to research teams is the more recent tendency for graduate and diploma courses to include a substantial component of professional and research ethics. Ensuring that the subject is well understood and that proposals represent a full consideration of such concerns is vital to success. The creativity and level of sophistication achieved by some nurses in this field are impressive and would make a real contribution to applications for study approval.

Perhaps one of the difficulties which should be mentioned to prevent all managers in the industry wondering why they have not got a complete team of nurses is their attitude to animal experimentation. Classes of undergraduates have been known to be substantially diminished where tetratogenic effects of drugs are demonstrated, and given the scale of such research testing it would be wise to assess their attitudes to this. Debates in the press are also fairly emotional, which may indicate that the profession at large has a problem with this activity.

This may well be balanced by the competence demonstrated by nurses employed as research assistants. In medical research in clinical settings there are several proven examples of nurses acting as superb interviewers, coordinators and data processors. Not only are they skilled but many academics have been impressed at their salaries—that is, how extremely economical it is to have nurses rather than doctors as researchers! Above all, the comfortable, easy way that nurses are able to locate patients within hospitals or at home, to provide clear information about a study in a way which is totally acceptable to respondents and therefore gain fully informed consent is impressive.

Communication skills are certainly needed when conducting research interviews or when requesting that respondents complete self-report instruments. Good nurses seem able to do this admirably, their warmth and confidence are appreciated and rapport is established early on in the process. Many patients find interviews in which they themselves provide most of the information actually very helpful. An opportunity to discuss issues and their feelings seems to be therapeutic in itself. Many nurse researchers feel the need to support patients during the research process (Webb, 1993) and after formal data collection many spend time 'chatting'. Not only does this help individuals in need, but it may also serve to enhance the reputation of the research team and the supporting organisation.

## MARKETING POTENTIAL

In marketing nurses are well tried and tested, their background knowledge and confidence to approach staff are clearly demonstrated. Sales representatives tend to be received better if they have an awareness of clinical schedules and appreciate how clinicians work and what information they require. The advanced educational support provided by the industry is now much more recognised amongst the professions. Contacts with sales staff are important but the back-up and resources available are also vital to keep pace with all the new drugs available.

Nurses' skills in personal communication, both written and through interviews, are also frequently matched by teaching skills in formal presentation. Newly qualified nurses have now all been through the challenging trial of presenting papers and their own research studies to both their peers and larger audiences. As this gives a good grounding (and the first time is always the worst) this should be recognised. Quite often their charm and confidence are quite inspiring, and combined with a special and often quite deep knowledge of their subject they do extremely well in such meetings.

As patient and colleague teaching is also expected nurses tend to have acquired the skill to prepare and present information in a clear and

orderly manner. Their understanding that learning only occurs if participation is encouraged provides a much more mature understanding of
possible ways to offer information. This type of skill may be exploited
to help train others and to present findings at various conferences.

## MANAGEMENT ROLES

Given the ambitions, experiences and skills of many senior nurses,
careers in management are an attractive proposition although so far few
nurses seem to be selected for the so-called 'top jobs' in the National
Health Service (NHS). This may be due to the inadequacies of the established health services management training schemes available or to
certain prejudices on the part of many ambitious male-orientated
management selection panels. However, there are many contributions
that mature well-educated nurses could make to the whole field of
pharmaceutical medicine.

Throughout their clinical education nurses have come into contact
with many different management styles. Their experience at the
receiving end and the organisation end of the spectrum increases their
awareness of the effects of management and of the importance of staff
support, direction and facilitation. Even at the staff nurse, newly qualified, level of practice staff fulfil a management function. Not only do
they organise the ward team and attempt to provide mentorship for students, but they also have the responsibility for coordinating the work of
others. Once appointed to a sister level increased responsibility is
encouraged. Many are now budget-holders and control both staff and
non-pay budgets. This prepares them ideally for senior managerial
positions.

One also has to realise that the added stresses of clinical practice
require a wider range of coping skills to preserve personal and team harmony. Such capabilities are certainly not achieved by all, but the most
able senior nurses could well function in many arenas equally well. With
the added dimension of deeply ingrained altruism many staff can take
instruction from such a person and feel strongly motivated to achieve
higher standards. More systematic staff appraisal systems throughout
the NHS afford good training in such practices; senior nurses becoming
well versed in the principles and applications.

## CONCLUSION

It would seem that nurses who function well at any level of the health
service should be able to make a substantial contribution to phar-

maceutical medicine. Their prospects may seem much more positive at this time than those presently offered in a troubled NHS, but perhaps it is not only the individuals who would do well but also the general perspective or philosophy of nursing which could be advantageous to this field. The values inherent in nursing would confirm the goals of therapeutic and investigative medical science. The influence of nursing through encouraging more consumer-orientated approaches to research, to science in general and to therapeutic approaches in particular may help to humanise this whole field. The popular esteem with which nurses are held and the trust they engender may reflect favourably on the drug industry, the image of which needs to be more positive. In turn this field offers respect for their professional background and skills and they themselves will probably learn to appreciate their own wide range of expertise. They need to be valued and rewarded more and this field may offer a superb avenue for this much needed fillip.

# Part II

# Careers in Pre-clinical Research and Development

# 7
# A Career in Drug Discovery

## David Ellis and John C. Emmett

Euromedica Ltd, Cambridge, UK

It is generally acknowledged that the modern life-saving pill, which is the product of the therapeutic revolution of the last 50 years, is a symbol of the innovative success of research conducted mainly in the pharmaceutical industry. Despite this inventive track record, however, the challenge for drug researchers to find new and improved therapies has never been greater, due to the combination of rapidly changing economic and social pressures and an ever-increasing complexity of science and technology.

Thus, on the one hand, the cost constraints imposed by finite national health care budgets will tend to favour the prescribing of cheaper, generic or over-the-counter (OTC) products rather than the usually higher priced new drugs, unless the latter have a demonstrated therapeutic advantage. On the other hand, to achieve the scientific breakthroughs required for the discovery of genuinely more effective new drugs, pharmaceutical companies will feel the need to increase their research and development budgets dramatically, in order to meet the challenges presented by more complex biological and chemical problems. *A priori*, it follows that in the future only those pharmaceutical companies which are able to address major medical needs, through harnessing the results of innovative, cost-effective research and development, will survive.

Innovativeness, in the context of addressing major medical needs, is

*Discovering New Medicines: Careers in Pharmaceutical Research and Development.*
Edited by P.D. Stonier
© 1994 John Wiley & Sons Ltd

essentially linked to the discovery of:

- safer and more effective variants of known therapies;
- alternative drugs acting by novel biochemical or pharmacological mechanisms;
- novel therapies for major untreatable diseases such as cancer, AIDS, neurodegenerative diseases, osteoporosis and immune-inflammatory diseases.

Consequently, the survival and growth of pharmaceutical companies will depend on their ability to discover, develop and market products which fall into one or more of these three categories.

This presents an exhilarating challenge for scientists interested in embarking on a career in drug discovery. Thus, although the major costs of research and development (R&D) are biased towards development rather than research, and these are increasing dramatically due to a more demanding regulatory environment, the fact remains that the improved effectiveness of research in discovering new chemical entities (NCEs) with different and/or more selective biological properties will favour the focus of development resources on new agents likely to lead to quantifiable therapeutic benefits. In addition to this clear justification and need for their innovative contributions, drug researchers in the pharmaceutical industry are also able to contribute to and taste the excitement of current international biological research, which is surely undergoing the most explosive growth in its history.

## KEY ELEMENTS IN PHARMACEUTICAL R&D STRATEGY

Presently, there is intense debate in the pharmaceutical industry concerning the possible strategies to be adopted to favour or ensure R&D success. Although it is inappropriate in this chapter to dwell at length on this continuing debate it is worth noting some of the key elements which are generally accepted to contribute to the creation of a successful R&D capability.

First of all, it is instructive to provide some definitions for the broad activities encompassed by drug discovery and drug development. The discovery phase of R&D is normally considered to involve all of the research activities which culminate in the identification of a lead compound with a sufficient combination of potency and selectivity, as defined by specific biological tests in animals, for it to have the potential to become a new medicine. The development phase of R&D (both non-clinical and clinical) includes the complex interwoven sequence of activities required to convert a chemical lead into a marketable medicine, which is both safe and effective in man.

The precise demarcation between discovery and development activities will vary in different companies. Thus, in some companies development encompasses all activities (including safety studies and clinical pharmacology) after the primary biological activity has been established in *in vitro* and *in vivo* tests in animals. In other R&D groups it will commence after clinical pharmacology has established safety and pharmacokinetics in man. Perhaps the most important consideration, however, is not the definition of the precise demarcation but the need to ensure that scientists in discovery research collaborate very closely with clinical pharmacologists, toxicologists and process research chemists in defining the critical path for the rapid evaluation of new compounds in exploratory development. The most important hurdle for a new compound to overcome before it is a serious development candidate is its assessment up to the end of phase I studies and, therefore, it is vital to obtain this assessment as quickly as possible. The close involvement of discovery scientists is likely to aid this fast-track development phase, since the chemical and biological knowledge gained in discovery will be critical in establishing the parameters and check-points in the early development plan.

## Drug Discovery

The most important ingredient for successful drug discovery is probably the most difficult and intangible to define, namely the presence of an innovative working climate within the research group. In our opinion, some or all of the following elements are necessary to produce this environment and it will be the recognised responsibility of senior management to encourage its creation and survival. These include:

- freedom for senior scientists to choose projects or areas of research;
- effective collaboration between scientists in different disciplines, particularly between chemists and biologists;
- concentration and focus of research resources to acquire knowledge and critical mass;
- creation of small, highly interactive teams within the overall resource, i.e. to reproduce the biotechnology company culture;
- informal communication and decision-making to minimise organisational and bureaucratic impact;
- encouragement of professional recognition;
- collaboration with external groups to broaden the scientific base of experimental activities;
- encouragement of peer group evaluation and criticism;
- condoning of 'risky research' and receptivity to new ideas;
- toleration of non-conformity;

- company recognition for project success;
- interactive, challenging and interested research management;
- motivation driven by both individual and team goals.

Many of these are recognisable ingredients in successful academic research groups. However, the fact that the pharmaceutical industry research group has a primary objective, namely the discovery of a new drug, differentiates it from the normally less goal orientated endeavour of academic research.

## Development

The development process is inherently different in its aims and modus operandi from that of discovery research. The main objective of drug development is to assess the therapeutic potential and obtain marketing approval for new chemical entities with maximum speed, optimum cost and high quality of the package submitted to regulatory authorities. Key ingredients include:

- detailed planning with fast track to phase I studies in man;
- product profiles clearly defined and agreed with marketing;
- strong input from regulatory affairs and medical marketing;
- project managers with good organisational, communication and analytical skills;
- project team members with good technical, problem-solving and communication skills, coupled with follow-through ability;
- check-points, milestones and management systems to assess project progress;
- effective use of information technology;
- flexible use of resources to create and disband teams when required;
- effective links between process research and production to aid the early involvement of production.

In addition to the need to plan and organise the development process there is also a clear need for innovation and creativity in the solving of defined, but often technically difficult, problems associated with developing a new drug. Thus, although the need for an innovative climate is not as critical as in discovery, it is recognised that development scientists must be given the opportunity to stay at the forefront of their disciplines through the practice of state-of-the-art science and publication of research findings as well as via collaborative interaction with other scientists in R&D.

## Management of Discovery and Development

The view has been expressed by many senior scientists and pharmaceutical industry analysts that small, flexible, highly interactive research groups are the most successful, at least in the discovery phase of R&D. Although it is difficult to find comparative data to aid an objective assessment, it is true that many of the major top-selling drugs (such as penicillins, cephalosporins, $\beta$-blockers, antiasthma drugs and $H_2$-receptor antagonists), discovered and developed by UK-based pharmaceutical R&D groups, were invented by relatively small, informally managed research teams.

In addition, the inventive success of the US biotechnology sector, as evidenced by the large number of clinical candidates currently awaiting Food and Drug Administration (FDA) regulatory approval, is probably linked to the fact that research in these companies is conducted by small, entrepreneurial and highly interactive teams, which have close links with academic centres of excellence.

This recognition that an innovative climate is often produced in smaller, less tightly managed research groups has led some of the larger pharmaceutical companies to separate discovery activities from the rest of the company organisation (including development) and, at the same time, give some autonomy to relatively small research programme teams, therapeutic area teams or satellite research groups, with encouragement to establish close working interactions with academic groups.

However, there could be inherent dangers in separating discovery from other company activities and in particular the development process. Thus: (1) the critical collaborative interaction between scientists in discovery and development could be diminished or lost; (2) there is a potential to create an 'ivory tower' mentality in discovery, if links with the 'real world' are made more tenuous; and (3) development will be less accessible as a future career opportunity to scientists from discovery. In fact, the success of biotechnology companies in exploiting basic science is almost certainly partly dependent on the close link between the research and business objectives of these companies. The challenge, therefore, for the large R&D groups is to create the required interactive, innovative teams within all parts of R&D, while retaining the ability to organise critical mass resources (particularly in development) to bring products to the market-place. Increasingly, it is recognised that this may be achieved more easily and with greater in-house flexibility by contracting out large parts of the more routine development work under the tight control of experienced company project managers, while solving critical development problems in-house through the creation of specific 'ad hoc' project teams comprised of scientists selected from both discovery and development on the basis of their relevant skills. As with the biotechnology sector, this might then lead to much more overlap between scientists from all areas of

R&D with a possible benefit to overall R&D effectiveness. One corollary, and possible additional benefit, of this approach is the resulting reduction in the total numbers of permanently employed staff in R&D and the increased flexibility in the spending choices for sizeable development budgets.

## Core Technologies

The complexity of modern-day science demands that discovery and development programmes will only be successful if 'state-of-the-art' scientific knowledge is brought to bear effectively on the problems to be addressed. This requires a realisation that all R&D groups require to build, develop and exploit a range of core technologies relevant to their scientific focus. These technologies may form an integral part of each department or project team involved in R&D or, alternatively, may exist separately as a broad-ranging support function which provides a collaborative resource to project teams as and when required. Examples of such core technologies might include biotechnology, computational chemistry or macromolecular science. Whatever the method of involvement of technologies of this type any successful R&D strategy must address the need to utilise them and ensure that the scientists involved are sufficiently well resourced to remain at the forefront of the development of their respective technology.

## Research Alliances and Product Licensing

Most R&D groups in the pharmaceutical industry recognise that, however large their resources, there is a need to network efficiently with other research groups in order to increase the options for the selection of development candidates. This interaction with outside groups may take the form of a collaborative strategic research alliance with another company, close involvement with an academic research group or simply the in-licensing of intellectual property or candidate compounds for development. These activities are now accepted as an essential part of R&D strategy for most pharmaceutical companies and represent the method by which the R&D resource can be broadened without necessarily increasing in-house R&D facilities.

For scientists in discovery research these activities present exciting opportunities to establish links with other research groups and expand their expertise and knowledge into new areas of research.

# THE DISCOVERY PROCESS

## Organisation and Management of Research

In practice there are two main ways of organising and managing drug discovery research within a pharmaceutical R&D group. These are: (1) via project or programme teams consisting of scientists drawn from different discipline departments such as medicinal chemistry, pharmacology and biochemistry; and (2) via project or programme teams created from larger multidisciplinary therapeutic area teams which assume most of the additional functions normally associated with separate departments.

In the first approach a matrix project management system runs across a primary department structure within research. Recruitment, training, staff development, technical performance and resource allocation are the prime remit of departments, while the remit of the research project teams is to conduct the collaborative research aimed at discovering a specific type of new drug. Project teams are managed by project leaders who are accountable, in turn, to the research director, usually via a research committee. In some organisations department heads also act as project leaders for specific research projects.

Both systems of managing discovery research have potential advantages and disadvantages. Thus, powerful departments can subvert and frustrate the work of project teams through the emphasis of overriding and often conflicting loyalties. On the other hand, the absence of a department structure can lead to a drop in scientific standards since peer group interaction and criticism are diminished. In addition, departments provide a natural focus for creative interaction between members of different project teams.

The non-departmental approach to managing research is, to some extent, a contrived one since most project teams will include certain key members who will also work in discipline-based departments. For instance, in particular, support scientists such as physical organic chemists, molecular modellers and molecular biologists may provide critical input, as a more central resource, to more than one project in discovery research. Consequently, provided that the matrix project system is given strong support from the research directorate, there appears to be no reason to dispense with a primary department system since this provides an important additional input in the organisation and management of research, the maintenance of professional standards and productive interaction between scientists working in different project areas.

## The Birth of Research Projects

Most research in the pharmaceutical industry starts from an idea based on published or patented results or in-house or academic research findings. The idea could come from any member of a research group or team and in most progressive organisations encouragement is given to younger scientists to suggest new ideas or approaches which may lead to new research proposals. For instance, based on the selective effects of known or newly synthesised molecules acting on pharmacological receptors or cellular enzymes, the relevance of a particular biological mechanism to an important physiological process in man may be suggested. Often the idea will relate to a way of improving the properties of a known drug or a compound being developed by a competitor company. Alternatively, a company may decide that some commitment to basic research in a particular biological field or therapeutic area is required to generate the essential new research results which will lead, in turn, to the specific goal to find a new drug.

Invariably, the first phase of any research project will involve a feasibility study (which may include further basic research) conducted by biologists to establish sufficiently sensitive and effective assays for measuring biological activity. The basic hypothesis, which may require receptor subtypes or specific isozymes to be identified, will need to be verified first of all. At this early stage one or two biologists (usually pharmacologists, biochemists or cell biologists) will be involved and contributions from a collaborative academic research group may be important. Medicinal chemistry will synthesise key compounds such as active prototypes, natural transmitters, hormones or substrates. Once the biological basis for the proposal has been proved (by establishing the importance of a particular mechanism) and a possible method of testing the hypothesis in man identified, medicinal chemists will be in a position to propose a chemical strategy aimed at designing novel compounds which will act selectively on a specific biological target (e.g. as a receptor antagonist or enzyme inhibitor). At this point a new research project is born and the project team formed with a nominated project leader.

## The Work of the Project Team

The engine which drives research forward in the search for a new drug is the collaborative interaction between medicinal chemists, who propose and synthesise new molecules, and biologists (pharmacologists, biochemists and cell biologists), who evaluate the biological properties of these molecules using a range of molecular, cellular, tissue and whole-animal assay procedures. Biological activities of compounds in these assays are measured quantitatively and structure–activity relationships (SARs) are defined by the medicinal chemists using molecular parameters measured or calculated by physical organic chemists who will also participate actively in the project team.

Other key members of the project team are likely to include:

- molecular biologists who will clone specific genes for the expression of new target proteins which will be utilised for *in vitro* assay measurements;
- molecular modellers (usually trained as organic or theoretical chemists) who will assist in understanding three-dimensional interactions of molecules;
- protein chemists who will characterise, isolate and purify target proteins;
- biochemists or chemists with expertise in drug metabolism who will provide early assessment of the biotransformation and fate of selected compounds, both *in vitro* and *in vivo*.

In addition, depending on the nature of the research, the team may require crucial input from specialist biologists such as electrophysiologists, immunologists and microbiologists. Then, as research progresses, with compounds nearing exploratory development, the team will be expanded to involve representatives from process research, clinical research, analytical chemistry, pharmacy and toxicology.

There are two main objectives which drive the creative dialogue between chemists and biologists. The first involves the attempt to relate affinity for the target receptor or enzyme (derived from primary ligand binding, enzyme, isolated cell or organ bath assays) to chemical structure, with the aim of designing new compounds with increased affinity and activity. Molecular modelling techniques and the measurement or calculation of physicochemical properties (e.g. lipophilicity, $pK_a$, electrostatic potential) are routinely used to develop and exploit this link between structure and ligand affinity. The second involves optimising *in vivo* activity (usually after oral administration) by utilising an understanding of those chemical properties which influence drug absorption, distribution, metabolism and elimination. Again, this is likely to utilise selected physicochemical parameters, together with some additional biological *in vivo* measurements such as blood levels.

In essence, drug research is an interactive team game, but with a large amount of freedom for each discipline group (and scientist within each group) to develop new ideas and approaches. Once reliable assays are established, the emphasis moves to the search for active leads, and the screening of new compounds may require automation and computer control to assist this process. In fact, a separate capability may be established to screen large numbers of compounds, with the purpose of identifying novel leads, using a high-throughput variation of one of the *in vitro* assays. Once the leads are identified, the excitement in the research team is derived from the discovery of more selective and more active compounds. As these emerge, the biologists are presented then with the new challenge of characterising their biological properties more exactly and deciding whether the central biological hypothesis needs to be modified. Assuming that these later compounds possess the required activity profile, further structural modification will then be undertaken to provide a drug candidate with the right profile for exploratory development.

## ENTRY REQUIREMENTS FOR A CAREER IN DISCOVERY

With a few exceptions a career in discovery research requires a graduate qualification. A small number of researchers join the industry after A-levels but, to progress, they should aspire to gaining a degree by part-time study, usually involving day release. A useful way to obtain research experience is via a sandwich degree course, which allows students to spend a year in industry as part of their training.

At graduate level, scientists will join research programmes as biologists or chemists and, through assignment to a particular discipline, will become medicinal chemists, physical organic chemists, pharmacologists, enzymologists, biochemists etc.

To progress to positions of scientific leadership a postgraduate research qualification (ideally to PhD level) is almost always required. Occasionally, companies will provide opportunities for outstanding graduates to undertake PhD training utilising results obtained from an in-house research project and collaborative help from an external supervisor and academic establishment.

## CAREER DEVELOPMENT

### Within Research

The pharmaceutical industry is generally considered to provide scientists in research with excellent opportunities for further training and personal development. For the bench scientist, budgets will usually allow for the purchase of state-of-the-art instrumentation and equipment and off-site training on specialised courses organised by academic centres. In addition, experienced scientists are encouraged to attend scientific conferences and present posters and papers, and the publication of original research results is usually encouraged, although important inventions relating to the biological activities of new compounds will need to be patented before disclosure. These activities establish links with the outside research community and assist in building an independent scientific reputation.

In most progressive organisations researchers at all levels will be encouraged to develop as experimental scientists and research leaders, with emphasis on individual decision-making and creative input to the team effort. Once supervisory and strategic skills are evident the responsibility for managing a small team will usually follow.

Biologists are often employed initially, particularly at the postdoctoral level, because of their specific expertise. This specialisation may continue and, although it will encourage the development of in-depth expertise, it may lead to over-specialisation, such that difficulty can be experienced in switching from one therapeutic area/research programme to another. Chemists, on the other hand, usually move more readily between research programmes since their skills and experience as synthetic and/or medicinal chemists are more easily transferred.

Career development is usually linked either to leadership of a discipline team or a multidisciplinary project team. In some organisations a separate scientific ladder will exist to allow for the recognition of gifted creative scientists who may not necessarily wish to manage large resources. Undoubtedly, though, promotion to senior positions (department head, project leader, therapeutic area head) will require an established track record as a creative scientist and the ability to lead others and manage resources. Such positions might be attainable within a period of 10 years after joining the industry for outstanding individuals.

Discovery scientists often find attractive opportunities for career advancement within research by moving from one company to another. For example, a move from a large multinational to a smaller company (start-up, biotechnology or single-country institute) will offer the chance to utilise much valued expertise in a wider and more varied role. Increasingly, also, the flow is no longer one way, since the specialised expertise gained in a biotechnology company is often in demand in the major ethical pharmaceutical companies.

## Careers Leading on from Discovery

For many scientists the opportunity to lead a small team and manage a laboratory, while staying closely in touch with science as a hands-on experimentalist, provides a supremely satisfying career. However, the increasing specialisation and inevitable focus of a research role of this type is often perceived as too narrow for other scientists, particularly in the longer term. It is appropriate, therefore, to consider the various alternative career options outside research for the discovery scientist.

Discovery usually provides excellent training and experience for a career move into other divisions within a pharmaceutical company, especially where the discipline overlap is significant. Thus, various options are available in development, particularly for those who are interested in seeing more tangible results of their work. Some examples include medicinal chemists moving to process research, physical organic chemists to analytical chemistry, biochemists and pharmacologists to clinical research and chemists or biochemists to drug metabolism and pharmacokinetics. Regulatory affairs also offers a good career move for scientists from all disciplines. Major developments in Europe and moves towards international harmonisation between Europe, the USA and Japan make regulatory affairs a particularly interesting and important area of activity within the development sphere.

Project management is a growing and vital activity at the heart of the development process. Increasingly, companies are appointing professional full-time project managers who have broad experience and knowledge of project management in discovery or development, coupled with good organisational and communication skills.

Alternative opportunities exist outside R&D for the discovery scientist and should be considered seriously as career options. Thus, chemists who are interested in moving away from the bench are often able to move into the legal department as a patent agent. This will require obtaining further qualifications as a chartered patent agent (CPA) and European patent agent (EPA) in order to rise to senior positions. Trademarks are often handled by the same department and give an added dimension to the work.

Increasingly, scientists are finding that successful alternative careers can be pursued in the commercial arena. The usual route has been via an early move into a medical representative position and then promotion up the sales and marketing ladder. However, scientists are finding that business development or licensing can also offer both an alternative career option and pave the way to promotion to other senior positions in marketing and general management.

## THE FUTURE

Scientific, regulatory and commercial pressures will lead to a greater diversity and flexibility in the way research is conducted in the future. Large R&D groups will reduce their in-house staff and budgets but will increase alliances with smaller companies, research institutes and universities. This, in turn, will expand research opportunities but will also require an increasingly risk-averse approach to career planning including the consideration of options outside research.

# 8
# The Toxicologist in Pharmaceutical Medicine[*]

## Geoffrey Diggle

Department of Health, London, UK

Interest in toxicology often starts at school. Those who study chemistry soon appreciate, during laboratory sessions, that chemical substances can have unpleasant effects. A drop of sodium hydroxide solution on the skin is enough to draw attention to *cutaneous irritancy*. The rule that some reactions must only be conducted in the fume cupboard is readily accepted when the noxious nature of some evolved gases is appreciated. In practical biology classes it is realised that the acute lethality of some chemicals enables them to be used to immobilise protozoa prior to microscopic study, and to kill metazoan animals humanely and efficiently before dissection.

While chemistry and biology are the foundation sciences underlying modern toxicology, the field has no fixed definition. Toxicology is developing and expanding, and is perhaps best described in terms of what those who call themselves toxicologists actually do. Even this pragmatic approach has its difficulties, however. First, the problem of inconsistency: some of those who do not regard themselves as toxicologists carry out work and follow approaches indistinguishable from those who

---

[*] The views expressed in this chapter are those of the author, and do not commit the Department of Health in any way.

*Discovering New Medicines: Careers in Pharmaceutical Research and Development.*
Edited by P.D. Stonier
© 1994 John Wiley & Sons Ltd

do. Second, there have been profound changes in the activities of toxicologists over time. However, there is general agreement about the role of modern toxicologists who work with pharmaceutical products, who are in fact the inheritors of an ancient tradition. It was appreciated in classical times that medicines and toxins had much in common, and that many substances had the qualities of both, although it was left to the great Paracelsus (1493–1541) to remind Western science of this. For the Greeks, both drugs and poisons were denoted by *pharmakon* (φαρμακον), which also translates as dye, spell and a concealed thing used to bring about certain effects. The archer's bow was toxon (τοξον) and these two words were combined to give the term for arrow poison, toxicon pharmakon (τοξικον φαρμακον). The English *toxicology* is in turn derived from this.

The earliest men knew of and used the toxic effects of animal venoms and poisonous plants, such as *Aconitum* spp. The knowledge of these early toxicologists was of value in hunting, in warfare and for getting rid of enemies. Some therapeutic properties of plant substances, such as the analgesic and euphoriant effects of opium from *Papaver somniferum*, were appreciated in the ancient world. In classical times, the poisoner was well established and there is much literature on the subject from the period. By 399 BC (the date of Socrates' death, allegedly following the administration of *Conium maculatum*) poisoning had become an official method of execution. By the Roman period, poisoners such as Locusta had become specialists in preparing and advising on the use of lethal substances, and their skills were much used by the imperial families, among others. Toxicology, in this sense, continued to develop through the Middle Ages, when specialists such as Catherine de Medici and Lucretia Borgia earned their reputations. The most infamous case on record is that of a professional poisoner known as *La Voisine* (The Neighbour), who was found guilty of poisoning many people, including 2000 children.

Today, however, most recognised toxicologists are concerned with the safety aspects of the subject, although a small minority deal with chemical weapons, riot control agents etc. The main focus of toxicological safety is on the individual and on human populations, although this includes environmental effects mediated through the actions of toxic chemicals on plants and animals. All medicines are capable of producing adverse effects. For a pharmaceutical product, the key question is whether its toxicological effects are outweighed by its therapeutic benefits. The role of the toxicologist working in this area is, ultimately, to make the best possible prediction of what those effects will be.

## THE WORK OF THE TOXICOLOGIST

The role of the toxicologist is of particular importance in research-based pharmaceutical companies in a number of areas, and especially in the testing of new active substances, in animals and *in vitro* to ensure eventual safety in use. The standard and thoroughness of pharmaceutical toxicology have been developed greatly since 1961, when the thalidomide tragedy came to light. In addition to the toxicological testing of candidate new drugs, the toxicologist may also be concerned with the correlation of animal and human pharmacology, the selection of compounds for exploratory human investigation and the planning of the developmental work required before initial human exposure can occur. The toxicologist also requires an adequate understanding of the issues involved in the identification of promising candidate compounds; these include factors related to therapeutic indications and efficacy endpoints, as well as safety aspects.

In toxicity testing, the fundamental differences (and similarities) between the toxicology of compounds in animals and in man must be explored and assessed, by qualitative and quantitative methods. The comparative toxicity of metabolites, as well as parent compounds, must also be studied. The pharmacological differences, as between test species and humans, must be examined.

New candidate drugs are subjected to a wide range of toxicological studies, many of which are carried out in laboratory animals, such as rats, mice and dogs. The studies are designed to investigate the drug's potential to cause harm to any organ or physiological process. Short-term tests (e.g. 14-day tests) aim to identify the target organ(s) in which damage occurs, and assist in selecting dose levels for longer-term studies. A range of special studies is used to investigate the potential for damage to any part of the reproductive cycle. Lifetime studies in rodents are used to assess carcinogenic potential. Expertise in the choice of testing methods and a full understanding of their predictive value are needed. Information about the absorption, distribution, metabolism and excretion of the test compound in the species studied is very relevant to the toxicological assessment, and must be considered alongside similar data from human subjects before early dose-ranging in man is undertaken, prior to the first clinical trials.

In many toxicological studies in animals, the expertise of the pathologist is essential. A pathologist must carry out (or at least supervise closely) the histological examinations required at the conclusion of such studies, although much of the routine work of general post-mortem examination may be carried out by expert toxicology technicians, with the guidance of the pathologist as necessary. If the study director (i.e. the toxicologist responsible for the study) is not a qualified pathologist, then suitable arrangements will have to be made to obtain the services of a pathologist, perhaps someone on the company's staff or an independent expert on a consultancy basis. (The pathologists who undertake this work include veterinary surgeons, doctors and graduates in other sciences who have obtained appropriate specialist qualifications in pathology.) The toxicologist must possess the qualities needed to establish and maintain effective collaboration with pathologists and specialists in other fields.

Toxicological programmes must be managed strategically in order to ensure that they fit smoothly with clinical and other lines of development, that unnecessary delays are avoided and that timely planning allows for the unexpected. This requires a clear grasp of the regulatory requirements laid down by government agencies for clinical trials and eventual marketing approval, including the preparation and submission of marketing applications, and the approval and appeal processes in the relevant countries.

The development of a new medicine requires an integrated approach at corporate and, often, at international level. The toxicologist must be fully aware of the operational issues involved, including those concerned with the medical aspects of product development, and especially the production of the toxicological and toxicokinetic supporting information needed before the first studies in man can take place. In this context, it is advantageous if the toxicologist has some general appreciation of such matters as the arrangements for compensation of healthy volunteers and patients in pre-marketing studies, the consent procedures employed in volunteer work and clinical trials and issues of confidentiality. Some awareness of the arrangements for indemnifying companies and investigators, the ethical review process, as well as problems of patenting and the contractual arrangements with external consultants, clinical investigators and contract research organisations can also be useful, although these matters are generally outside the domain of the toxicologist.

The development of new pharmaceutical products is not the only area in which the company may put the knowledge of the toxicologist to work. Employers must assess the risks, including the toxicological risks, to which their own employees are exposed and the availability of in-house toxicological expertise may be particularly advantageous in risk assessment in relation, for example, to production workers in the pharmaceutical industry. Similarly, the advice of company toxicologists may be sought occasionally on questions about the environmental impact of chemical effluents from production plants etc., although these are properly questions for ecotoxicologists.

Even the most well-established medicines are monitored for their safety in use. Toxicological expertise may be crucial in interpreting reports of adverse reactions, overdosage and interactions with other drugs. The advice of the toxicologist may be sought on mechanisms, the feasibility of re-challenge, predisposing factors and methods for assessing adverse reactions.

Senior toxicologists frequently undertake staff management responsibilities, and may act as line managers of other toxicologists and toxicology technicians. Staff may require further training and their needs may be met, for example, by means of day-release courses, as well as by on-the-job training. Animal technicians, however, generally work under veterinary supervision. Animal technicians carry out important, labour-intensive tasks such as ensuring the welfare and accurate dosing of animals, and this work is not of course restricted to normal working hours. Veterinary supervision must ensure that the standard of animal care is high and that the animal technicians are properly trained in matters of animal welfare and husbandry.

The toxicologist who acts as the study director for a particular test is responsible for its planning, preparation of the protocol, overall conduct and preparation of the report which will be submitted eventually to the regulatory agency as part of the application for clinical trial or marketing approval. Many of the study director's functions are coordinating ones, involving liaison with specialist sections of the company such as the laboratories responsible for carrying out the haematological and biochemical analyses of blood samples taken from the animals under test, and the pharmacy charged with providing adequate and timely amounts of the test substance. Supervision of the toxicology technicians who obtain blood and urine samples from the test animals and monitor their clinical condition, all in compliance with Good Laboratory Practice (GLP), is a particular responsibility of the study director.

The study director must be a competent and resourceful scientist who is able, for example, to respond quickly and appropriately when untoward or unexpected findings emerge which call for additional investigations. It may be necessary to devise special experiments to follow up adverse findings in animal studies and assess whether they are predictive for a risk to humans. (While a protocol may be amended *formally* to take account of significant changes in the course of a study, undocumented, informal alterations following the emergence of adverse effects are subject to possible misinterpretations in the future, and must not be permitted.) Good documentation ensures that the unpredictable events which may always occur in the course of studies do not lead to subsequent difficulties and queries. Suppose, for example, that a protocol specifies that blood sampling is to be carried out at the seventh week, from a group of animals in a long-term study, with the work scheduled for a Monday and Tuesday: because of unforeseen staffing problems, the samples are all taken on Tuesday. The competent study director will ensure that a file note of this departure from the protocol, *and the reason for it*, is made. Adequate records of this kind can be of great importance when the results of reports of studies are eventually considered by regulatory assessors and GLP inspectors. When, for instance, a technical mishap (such as equipment breakdown) makes it necessary to abandon part of a study and start again, a clear note in the record is all that is needed to avert any future misunderstanding of what happened.

All experienced toxicologists are aware of the need to minimise the distress suffered by animals, and the conscientious professional will be at pains to ensure that unnecessary suffering is avoided, consistent with the need to establish the safety of medicines for human use. Occasionally there is a need to take difficult decisions in this area, although this is often best done in consultation with the appropriate regulatory agency. Suppose, for example, that a new substance is being developed for use as a general anaesthetic or as a muscle relaxant for use during surgical operations. If it is to be effective, it must be capable of inducing deep anaesthesia, or of paralysing the muscles, including those which are used to breathe. Safety must of course be assessed before use in man can be contemplated, and this would normally be achieved by means of studies in animals (including repeated-dose studies and evaluations in pregnant animals) at various dose levels well above the intended human dose. Examples of this kind illustrate the difficulty of the problems which may on occasion confront the toxicologist.

In addition to the need, for humane reasons, to minimise the numbers of living animals used in toxicity testing there are also economically important reasons. Some methods, such as those used to assess carcinogenic potential, are extremely expensive because of the numbers of animals which must be used if reliable information is to be obtained. In most areas of toxicology the development of alternative methods using fewer animals has been slow, although a notable advance is a new test for acute (single-dose) toxicity known as the *fixed dose procedure*, as an alternative to the traditional $LD_{50}$ method. Another approach is the attempt to develop *in vitro* techniques employing cultured cells or tissues, or very small metazoan animals such as *Hydra*. Impressive development of *in vitro* approaches has taken place in genetic toxicology, in contrast to other specialised areas. Testing for genetic toxicity has been revolutionised by the development of standardised *in vitro* mutagenicity tests for detecting gene mutations caused by test substances in bacteria and in the cultured cells of higher organisms; reliable methods for revealing chromosome damage in cultured cells have also been achieved. The *in vitro* approach has made little headway in general toxicology because so many possible mechanisms of damage exist (unlike genetic toxicology, where there is a single underlying mechanism: damage to DNA). *In vitro* methods sometimes have a place in the further exploration of specific effects revealed by the general toxicity studies carried out in whole animals. Localised effects, such as cutaneous and ocular irritancy, also lend themselves to *in vitro* assays.

## THE QUALITIES AND ABILITIES NEEDED

It is possible to identify a number of personal qualities which are desirable, and some of them indispensable, in the toxicologist working in today's pharmaceutical industry. The ability to work well with other specialists, both within and outside line management relationships, is essential. A thorough grasp of the biology, of experimental methods and of regulatory guidelines is of course a *sine qua non*. Although this seems obvious, testing is sometimes carried out with an apparent disregard for biological common sense. (One still sees bacterial tests for point mutation carried out on compounds having inhibitory properties which prevent the use of adequate dose levels, for example.) It is essential that a 'check-list' implementation of guidelines be avoided.

The toxicologist must be comfortable with the meticulous approach needed when carrying out studies which meet the standards demanded by modern GLP. There can be no return to the working methods which necessitated the creation of the international GLP system. Nevertheless, the ability to carry out work meticulously is not the same as obsessionalism and rigidity; a flexible approach is needed when interpreting guidelines and deciding the programme of studies to be carried out. The toxicologist must be able to respond to guidelines as *guidelines*, when deciding which studies will be appropriate and when designing experimental protocols.

Allied to this is the ability to write clearly. For example, commentaries on the tests undertaken must be clear and unambiguous. If there are, for good scientific reasons, departures from regulatory guidelines, then the underlying thinking should be explained clearly and the assessors in the regulatory agencies who must eventually evaluate the data should be left in no doubt about the scientific reasons and reasoning involved. Pre-clinical reports are sometimes put together in final submissions by staff who are not fully conversant with the science, and the toxicologist's ability to write in such a way that the likelihood of misunderstanding is minimised is invaluable.

Investigative ability is an important quality, and of course this often requires intuition based on experience, as well as deduction. When a study suggests that there is an adverse effect which calls for an explanation, both time and money are saved when the toxicologist is able to distinguish promptly between experimental error (e.g. errors of measurement, of allocation of animals to test groups, of dosing etc.) and genuine findings. Such a situation might arise when, for example, a test for fertility and general reproductive performance seems to show reduced fertility in terms of numbers of offspring. The ability to confirm that a real effect is occurring, perhaps by recognising and focusing on the relevant part of the reproductive cycle, is clearly important. The same investigative ability is required in the elucidation of genuine but unexplained findings. When, for example, a compound has shown no DNA-damaging potential in the standard mutagenicity tests, but has produced tumours at a single site in a lifespan rodent bioassay, much skill may be needed to establish without undue delay that the substance is really non-genotoxic and that the mechanism of tumorigenesis poses no hazard for patients.

Planning ability is of particular importance. Toxicological studies must be so planned that bottlenecks in the drug development process are avoided. Planning must also ensure that the requirements of different regulatory agencies are satisfied, if appropriate, without undue duplication of work. Of course, this in turn calls for the ability to work harmoniously with other departments concerned with the product, such as the medical and regulatory affairs departments. An understanding of methods such as critical path analysis may be important in setting the timing of toxicological work, to ensure that it does not hold up other essential streams of interrelated activity. Carcinogenicity studies, for example, are lengthy and the results which they produce are not always conclusive; they are also extremely expensive. Once it has become clear that they will be needed, ample time for them must be allowed, in order to ensure that they do not delay eventual marketing authorisation.

Of all personal qualities, sound judgement is perhaps the most important to the toxicologist, and above all in the area of risk assessment. There is an extraordinary amount of public confusion about the safety of drugs and other chemical products, such as food additives and pesticides. Chemophobia is encouraged by irresponsible, alarmist media coverage (especially in the UK) and by the activities of certain interest groups, some politicians and members of the legal profession (especially in the USA). At the same time, there is relatively much less concern about agents (e.g. tobacco smoke) which are associated with real, substantial health risks. The balanced judgements of the professional toxicologist are indispensable in this atmosphere of mis-information and flawed perceptions. Toxicological risk assessment calls for the application of objective judgement and common sense to the question: how likely is it that the toxicological effect concerned could occur in patients receiving the medicine at the intended maximum dosage? In approaching this question, the toxicologist is at pains to establish the target organ toxicity for the compound under test in animals, as well as the maximum dose levels at which these effects cannot be observed. These levels are then compared with the proposed maximum therapeutic dose for patients, in order to judge whether the margins of safety are adequate. (The corresponding *blood* levels are often compared as well.) This judgement is essentially *qualitative*, although it is informed by much quantitative information. It must take into account many factors, including the toxicokinetics of the compound in the test species and in man. It must give due weight, for example, to inter-species differences in absorption, metabolism etc.

To illustrate this by means of a somewhat simplified example, consider a new active substance intended for eventual marketing as a non-steroidal anti-inflammatory product. Among its toxicological effects it is found to cause gastric mucosal erosions and renal papillary necrosis in laboratory animals, in routine medium-term studies. The most sensitive species for the effect on the kidney is found to be the dog, in which this effect is still seen at doses which are too low to produce other toxicological effects. Further work establishes that the maximum level to which the dose can be raised without affecting the dog kidney is one-hundredth of the intended maximum dose for the treatment of patients with arthritis: the question at issue, then, is whether there is any significant risk of renal damage in patients. Clearly, much experience is needed in making reliable assessments of this kind; the ability to arrive at sound judgements and give reliable, informed advice in areas such as these is the hallmark of the professional toxicologist.

## TRAINING AND CAREERS IN TOXICOLOGY

The educational routes leading to toxicology as a profession are varied, and each has merits and disadvantages. In many cases, a first degree in a biological science is followed by some form of specialised training. For the graduate seeking introductory or part-time training in toxicology, suitable courses now exist in many countries. First degrees in toxicology are being introduced slowly. Postgraduate courses are also available for science graduates wishing to obtain higher and more specialised degrees, such as the Master of Science (MSc) in toxicology, or in combinations of subjects which embody a toxicological component.

Suitably qualified scientists having at least five years relevant experience may enter for the UK Diploma of the Institute of Biology (DIBT) and, in certain circumstances, membership of the Royal College of Pathologists (MRCPath) can sometimes be obtained by non-medical graduates. Similar qualifications conferred by professional bodies are available in some other countries.

Various career outlets are available to trained toxicologists interested in pharmaceutical work. In addition to the companies which develop and market medicinal products, contract research laboratories and government regulatory agencies also employ such specialists. For those whose interests extend to other, non-pharmaceutical products, similar posts both in industry and regulatory work are available in relation to agrochemicals including pesticides, consumer products including cosmetics, industrial chemicals and other groups. Career moves between these areas are not unusual, sometimes within the same large company.

A company toxicologist sometimes undertakes a complete career change within the same organisation, moving for example to the department responsible for dealing with regulatory agencies. There is also some movement between 'product-based' and other forms of toxicology, including forensic toxicology, ecotoxicology, clinical toxicology, occupational toxicology and, of course, academic work.

# 9
# The Role of the Pharmacist in Health Care

## David Jordan

Hoechst Roussel Ltd, Swindon, UK

One of the many factors which contribute towards the special role of the pharmacist in health care generally, is its multifaceted and multidirectional image. There is no single description of the role of the pharmacist. By the very nature of the education process (see later sections), the subject matter in the pharmacy degree course covers many areas normally regarded as being pure subjects in themselves, e.g. chemistry, biochemistry, radiochemistry, metabolism and analysis. This allows the graduate pharmacist then to take on a plethora of roles in health care which could be deemed to be the domain of the specialist but which the pharmacist can add to by bringing in other impinging, yet relevant, sciences to achieve overall added value to the service provided.

## JOB DESCRIPTION

Perhaps the best-known role of the pharmacist is that of the community pharmacist, maybe better known still by the lay-person as the 'high street chemist'. In such a job, the pharmacist acts as the supplier of a prescribed medicine and as adviser on its best use and storage. He or she should be aware of the reason for that particular medication having

*Discovering New Medicines: Careers in Pharmaceutical Research and Development.*
Edited by P.D. Stonier
© 1994 John Wiley & Sons Ltd

been prescribed and be able to counsel the patient on matters such as side-effects, other drug or food interactions and correct disposal route of any unused medicine.

Internationally, these pharmacist roles are more or less equivalent and the experienced traveller will have noticed a certain similarity in professional approach, advice-giving and even displayed pharmacy symbol throughout the world, whether described by the word 'Pharmacy' or 'Apotheke', for example!

To expand on the job description of community pharmacists, responsibility is also accepted for behind-the-scenes activities such as stock control, purchasing from wholesalers, communication with GPs, dentists and often hospital doctors, and for the training of postgraduate pharmacists undertaking their one-year pre-registration experience prior to becoming members of the Royal Pharmaceutical Society.

Nowadays, links between the prescriber and the pharmacist are improved with the availability of computer-generated prescriptions which are associated with patient record software. This innovation has largely obviated the need for the pharmacist to double-check the often indecipherable handwriting of the prescriber to avoid mistakes of confusion such as supplying Losec instead of Lasix, or Danol for Daonil. Likewise, the pharmacist increasingly has patient record software at his disposal in order to help check for consistency and regularity of medication supply, drug interactions and even to computer generate the label for the medicine, again overcoming possible problems of illegible handwriting.

Computers also aid in speeding up the process of dispensing, especially in a busy pharmacy. After possibly waiting in the GP's surgery for some time, the last thing a sick person wants is to be kept waiting again at the pharmacy. For this reason, the advent and growth of health centres, incorporating a GP surgery with possibly a dental practitioner, chiropodist and pharmacy, must be beneficial to the patient, although they can always reserve the right to have their prescriptions dealt with at any pharmacy of their choice; this factor alone prevents the logical linking of prescriber and pharmacist computer systems.

Since community pharmacy accounts for about 70% of all pharmacists in the UK, it is justifiable to have spent a little longer than average to describe their roles in pharmaceutical medicine. Also, some of the basic principles involved in the supply of medicines to the community continue to apply in other areas of pharmacy too, namely in hospital pharmacy environments. Here, pharmacy services are organised into regions to provide a total drug supply function to nursing homes as well as hospitals and clinics in a given region.

Due to the greater complexity of this organisation compared with community pharmacy, career structures are involved, allowing pharmacists to progress from basic grade to staff and principal pharmacists, and up to district or regional pharmaceutical managers. One added characteristic of hospital pharmacists (which differentiates them from other branches of pharmacy) is their proximity to hospital medics which, therefore, enables them to provide *in situ* advisory services in terms of drug information directly to the doctor. Over the years this has led to the concept of ward pharmacy, where pharmacists not only control the supply, storage and use of medicines, but can also advise doctors on specific drug matters, often on the spot during routine ward rounds or emergency situations. A significant proportion (about 20%) of graduate pharmacists enter the hospital pharmacy service and the more senior or specialist (e.g. radiopharmaceuticals) roles are often held by those holding a doctorate (PhD).

Last, but not least, approximately 5% of the graduate pharmacy population take up posts in the pharmaceutical industry, usually to work on the formulation or analytical development aspects of new drug compounds. Except when formulations are being prepared for clinical investigations (phases I–III), the main activities of the industrial pharmacist do not involve any direct contact with members of the public, which differentiates this role from the greater majority of pharmacists working in health care.

During the drug development process, the pharmacist would be expected to become involved in the formulation of a wide variety of dosage forms and to carry out research into novel ways of delivering drugs, new or existing, to the body. They could also be expected to work on the development of stability-indicating analytical methods, leading ultimately to quality control tests, perform stability tests under simulated conditions of extreme climate, carry out quality reviews of existing products on the market, prepare clinical trial formulations and those suited to animal or human metabolism studies, scale up manufacturing procedures on to production plant, and so on. The list and variety seem endless. Within most large pharmaceutical companies, e.g. Merck, Glaxo, Hoechst, Bristol-Myers-Squibb, there are many opportunities for pharmacists to expand their broad knowledge base outside these areas also and these possibilities will be explored later in this chapter.

The remaining 5% of pharmacists find themselves working in academic life mainly or other associated pharmaceutical activities, e.g. wholesaling or consulting. Academics generally, apart from their teaching commitments, would normally pioneer research into relevant areas of pharmaceutical science, including subjects such as drug targeting to receptors, improvement in bioavailability, timed release and the extension of the duration of effects of drugs (so reducing dose frequency). Others, maybe more process orientated, choose to investigate such issues as tablet compression and coating, powder technology or capsule filling.

Whatever the chosen subject, there is no doubt that the newly graduated pharmacist has a wide choice of career directions and resultant job descriptions available, ranging from community/business management orientation to a more scientific or academic one. The ways in which these various options may be exploited by the individual will be discussed in detail in the remaining sections of this chapter.

## BACKGROUND TO THE PROFESSION OF PHARMACY

Presently (1993), there are 20 000 pharmacists practising in the UK, distributed among the various branches of the profession as indicated earlier. A more international figure is difficult to obtain but it may well be fair to assume that the same picture is reflected in other developed countries around the world.

Historically, the pharmacist, identified better as the apothecary in former times, received his training from an experienced father figure or mentor according to an apprenticeship style of learning. Such training would have included bizarre practices not associated with modern-day pharmacists, namely the production of concoctions according to folklore remedies, tooth extractions or even minor surgery. Latterly, the more appropriately trained apprentice would be granted the status of Pharmaceutical Chemist (PhC), the forerunner to membership of the Pharmaceutical Society of Great Britain, now the Royal Pharmaceutical Society since 1991 (MRPhS).

Bringing us up to date, pharmacists nowadays are trained in schools of pharmacy throughout England, Wales and Scotland to degree level (honours in many of these). Entry requirements are normally three 'A'-level passes in relevant subjects including chemistry, plus other science subjects such as physics, mathematics or biology, although this may vary from establishment to establishment. Good standard pass grades would be expected. The subject matter contained in these courses covers pharmaceutical chemistry (organic, inorganic and analytical), the science of the physicochemical properties of drugs along with processing methods for the preparation of medicines (pharmaceutics), the study of the action of drugs on the body (pharmacology), awareness of the potential of drugs from plants (pharmacognosy) and the law and practice relating to pharmacy. A modern approach in degree courses these days, in the more progressive universities, is to combine these course elements in order to teach the overall concept of, for example, stability studies of drugs extracted from plants (e.g. digoxin), which would bring in some pure chemistry, pharmaceutics, drug design/formulation and analytical chemistry, under a single heading.

Pharmacists would, almost exclusively, undertake an immediate post-graduate, practical training year in order to gain membership of the Royal Pharmaceutical Society. This is only achieved after a taxing 12 months of working under the supervision of a qualified and experienced pharmacist tutor, gaining knowledge about a range of core and specialist (depending on the area of pharmacy in which the training is taking place) subjects and successfully undertaking a relevant examination paper at the end of this pre-registration year.

Membership of the society is a legal requirement for pharmacists working in contact with the public, which chiefly covers the community and hospital roles, although it is taken to be a very significant expression of professional commitment in other roles too, where patient contact is not so great, e.g. in the pharmaceutical industry. For this reason, the pre-registration year may be undertaken exclusively in a community pharmacy or hospital pharmacy department but is limited to a maximum of six months if undertaken in the pharmaceutical industry, regulatory body (e.g. Medicines Control Agency) or university.

Furthermore, within the European Union, reciprocation exists to enable the pharmacist to receive bona fide training in Germany or France, for example. It is felt that there is a need in the future for pharmacy qualifications to be more tailored to the chosen direction although, due to the fact that it would seem unfairly limiting to confine future pharmacists to only a narrow area of the profession from early on in their degree course, it is difficult to envisage how this could be implemented practically and satisfactorily.

## ROLE AND RESPONSIBILITIES IN MEDICINES RESEARCH AND DEVELOPMENT

In any publication dealing primarily with careers in pharmaceutical medicine, great emphasis must be placed on the important minority of pharmacists working in research and development, in order to complete the chain of pharmacist involvement from 'creation' to supply. For this purpose, comment will be restricted to research and development (R&D) in the pharmaceutical industry since the commercial slant of such a role is often seen as the trigger for the process of new product development and ultimate availability to the medical practitioner to prescribe to his or her patients. The academic research scenario will not be discussed here.

In contrast to this statement, the overriding, or at least joint, responsibility of medical scientists to identify new therapeutic areas of benefit to mankind generally is perhaps a more realistic view of how drug discovery and development activities are initiated within the industry, followed then by the complex and often frustrating period (in the range of 5–15 years) of evaluating safety and clinical efficacy until sufficient evidence exists to justify a registration submission to the licensing body. Both in the pre-clinical and clinical phases of this process, the pharmacist can be involved for reasons highlighted earlier in this chapter. It is perhaps not too surprising that pharmacists are sometimes labelled with the descriptor 'Jack of all trades . . . ', although professional pride prevents me from completing this well-known phrase!

More often than not, however, the pharmacist will enter the pharmaceutical industry, and pursue a career in R&D in order to achieve scientific ambitions rather than community health care ones. This ought not to create the impression of an unprofessional, uncaring boffin, but rather someone who believes that their talents are best directed towards scientific challenges in order to benefit their profession and their 'customers', in this case the patient. Within this role, activities can be categorised under the following headings of formulation design, pharmaceutical analysis and clinical supplies, each of which will be discussed separately.

## Formulation Design

Pharmacists working in the first of these categories must be highly innovative individuals, self-motivated and capable of high levels of problem-solving skills and creativity. Such people will utilise these skills to generate new product ideas, contribute to the development of new drug delivery systems and liaise closely with contract university departments to achieve these goals as appropriate. Although this may appear to have at least one foot in the area of blue-sky research, it is often from such starting points, and very much by joint or later collaboration with other pharmaceutical scientists, clinical pharmacologists, kineticists and marketing executives, that valuable and beneficial new products are born.

From such beginnings, radical innovations such as transdermal patches, contraceptive implants, insulin pens and breath-activated aerosols for asthma have arisen. More routinely, however, such individuals will be involved in the task of formulating the dosage forms (e.g. tablets, capsules, injections, creams and suppositories) suitable for the dose and route of administration of new chemical entities. By optimising these activities with patient benefit in mind, it is normally possible to provide a convenient product for the market, to be used at a kinetically relevant dose frequency; daily would be regarded as convenient, whereas dosing every alternate day or seven times a day, for example, would be highly inconvenient to the patient.

A range of knowledge is required by the formulating pharmacist, from the microphysics of materials used in the product to ensure that manufacturability on a large scale and using rapidly working machinery is a possibility, to the effects of the formulation on the availability, bio-availability and pharmacokinetics/dynamics of the drug in question. More examples of disasters in these areas spring to mind than those where no problems were encountered at all, not due to their alarming frequency but more because of their impact on personal pride and damaged ego!

Cases where tranquillisers have been miraculously transformed into incredibly fast-acting hypnotics (hardly enough time to climb the stairs to bed before falling asleep!), improved hypoglycaemic products which produced impressive pharmacokinetics but no pharmacodynamic changes (due to the now-known limiting effect of the diabetic pancreas regardless of formulation), and nasal products containing drug absorption enhancers capable of effectively encouraging the reverse transport of cerebrospinal fluid into the nasal cavity, are all experiences which the formulator would prefer to be forgotten but which highlight the importance and influence of this activity in pharmaceutical development. Fortunately, there are many more examples of successful work in this field resulting in effective and convenient medication.

### Pharmaceutical Analysis

It is the role of a pharmacist, working in the area of pharmaceutical analysis, to ensure that developed formulations are stable, both physically and chemically, under a series of extreme temperature, light and humidity conditions. Resulting data, along with corresponding formulation details, form the core of the chemistry and pharmacy section of the regulatory submission, once combined with synthesis details of the drug substance itself. Far from being the domain of the pharmacist this time, the responsibilities of this role are very much shared with the analytical chemists, having much more fundamental chemistry training perhaps, although again the all-round experience of the pharmacist plays an important part of the overall product development objective. Together, analysts generate official data for regulatory approval based on individual country requirements. There are still large differences in these requirements, the temperature/humidity conditions, number of batches to be tested, the duration of the test and so on, and this whole issue is now an important part of the negotiations at the International Conferences on Harmonization (ICH), accordingly.

Apart from stability testing *per se*, the expertise of the graduate must first be directed at the establishment of suitable stability-indicating analytical methods, such that the appearance of degradation products of the drug can be mapped and quantified under real-time ambient or accelerated storage conditions. Similarly, the disappearance of the parent drug should be directly quantifiable. Such methods should use modern, fast techniques so that not only can they be used in the stability test programme, but also be translatable into quick, efficient quality-control tests to release batches of the resultant medicine for sale once it is in full production. Whether an analytical or formulation pharmacist, both will work together as a team along with other life science graduates to ensure the smooth development of new medicines and their efficient transfer from the laboratory and clinic environment into the pharmaceutical 'factory' to continuously provide the market with safe and effective, quality products.

### Clinical Supplies

Finally in this section, at the interface between pre-clinical and clinical development, sits the clinical supplies pharmacist whose role in the organisation is really quite unique. To many people, this is seen as a glorified community pharmacist role, dispensing product against prescriptions, except that in this case the patients might be 2000–3000 in number (especially during the later phase III stages of clinical development) in 20–30 centres around the world and being supplied with often a complex programme of cross-over, randomised (sometimes active versus placebo) medication against a protocol agreed by an independent research ethics committee.

Like their other pharmacist colleagues, working in formulation, analysis or production for example, they work according to a code of practice known as Good Manufacturing Practice and sometimes Good Laboratory Practice, where overlap with laboratory R&D areas such as toxicology or metabolism is necessary. Both codes provide guidelines and disciplines to steer scientists through the complicated array of activities such as good housekeeping, protocolling, conducting experiments, report writing, training, record keeping, standard operating procedures, hygiene, stock control, labelling and archiving. Responsibility is therefore understandably very high in this role and could make the difference between a successful, informative and well-executed study and one which is inherently defective, inaccurate, expensive and, of course, dangerous.

It is the one area of pharmaceutical R&D where the 'output' is actually directly administered to humans. In phases II and III, this predominantly means people exhibiting the disease state for which that medicine has been designed whereas, at the earlier phase I clinical pharmacology stage, smaller numbers (12–18) of healthy volunteers are recruited, often from a pool of willing company employees, to have the medicine administered to them for the first time in humans. Such studies are designed specifically to research tolerance, dose ranges, drug or food interaction, or to study the pharmacokinetics resulting from the specific absorption, distribution, metabolism and elimination (ADME) characteristics of that drug, often using radiolabelled forms to aid identity and quantification. Without question, pharmacists are involved in the provision of suitable formulations for this purpose.

## CAREER PATHWAYS

Earlier in this chapter, stress was given to the ways in which pharmacists could use their qualifications in the many directions which the profession offers and how this is reflected in the diverse ways in which the postgraduate, pre-registration training year may be structured.

Indeed, due to the understandable emphasis given to patient contact in the community, the latest suggestion (Anderson, 1993) is that the compulsory six-month minimum training in community pharmacy be extended to twelve months in order to underline the perceived importance of this aspect of the profession. Maybe then, rather like medics working in the pharmaceutical industry, pharmacists ought to be encouraged to spend an agreed proportion of their time in public-related activities in order to maintain their professional community health care image and avoid the pursuance of too narrow a sector of pharmacy generally. Quoting from the above literature reference, Stuart Anderson states: 'A single-minded approach in which we unambiguously train all pharmacy graduates to perform competently as community pharmacists—regardless of their future career aspirations—may well prove to be the best investment the profession can make for its own future'. Health care professionals and history will have to wait to see whether this is prospective wise advice or cautious overkill.

Whatever the final details of pharmacy training turn out to be, resultant career structures vary enormously, from the pharmacist running a single community pharmacy all his working life, to the individual who works his way up to a very senior position in the pharmaceutical industry.

Without wishing to show bias and realising that it is easily possible to extend the list many-fold, the first two names which spring to mind in this respect are Professor Trevor Jones (Wellcome) and Sir David Jack (ex Glaxo). Within the scope of this range of career aspirations, and concentrating particularly on the pharmaceutical industry now, one still sees tremendous scope for interesting and varied careers for the ambitious pharmacist. Earlier, it was stressed that a pharmacy graduate would probably enter the industry in a scientific role such as pharmaceutical development officer. Although typical, this would not deter a pharmacist from initiating his career in the industry as a registration officer, a medical information pharmacist or perhaps a clinical research associate, for example.

Just within Hoechst, it is possible to then see how the ambitions of the industrial pharmacist have been satisfied in many differing ways, either by choice or encouragement, so that pharmacists are presently found, or have been found, working as registration executive, adverse drug reactions monitor, medical information officer, commercial director, pharmaceutical representative, clinical research associate and personnel officer, as well as the more traditionally accepted scientific roles within drug development. It is because of their rather special broad skills that the industrial pharmacist has the ability to cross scientific and managerial boundaries with comparative ease and confidence. Not knowing exactly in which direction an individual's career may progress, it is very difficult to generalise about planned career structures in this way for the pharmacist, since so much relies on personal entrepreneurial spirit, opportunism and ambition, as well as proven ability.

Within the scientific community of the industry, however, a typical pharmacist would hold the basic pharmacist role, for example as a formulator, for a relatively short time, perhaps three to four years. During this period, he would receive on-the-job scientific training and off-the-job management/personal training to equip him as appropriate for future advancement. Due to the relatively small size of laboratory hierarchies, normal progression to section head is sometimes long awaited and the graduate may prefer to fill vacancies in other companies in order to speed up the process. This is often the case especially for ambitious characters, anxious to achieve their career maxima as quickly as possible, and results in a justifiably long curriculum vitae for future employers to ponder over regarding logical approach, common sense and evidence of real advancement, as opposed to merely job-hopping.

As section head, the pharmacist would lead a small team of graduates and technicians occupied in task-orientated scientific work such as formulation, manufacturing or analytical development, and the job itself would offer a mixture of scientific and management activity and responsibility.

Such a role naturally paves the way towards running an entire department, comprising typically three to four sections, along with a consequent swing in responsibilities to an even greater management and financial level. Scientific involvement would still remain very much in evidence, except that the individual would take on a more project administration task rather than bench-work orientation, and would be known for his scientific philosophies and opinions nationally and often internationally, usually by virtue of talks presented, publications and involvement in bodies which professionally represent the industry or the profession itself, e.g. Chemical Industries Association, Association of the British Pharmaceutical Industry or Royal Pharmaceutical Society of Great Britain.

The career pathway to department head would typically be expected to take 10–15 years, by which time the graduate would have reached his or her mid-thirties in age. Thereafter, armed hopefully with an impressive portfolio of qualifications, all-round scientific ability, successful track record and management skills, he or she could take any one of a number of career moves in the industry but, from there on, with little direct relevance to pharmacy, being of a more general scientific nature e.g. R&D director, or a totally different direction as previously mentioned. In large multinational companies, the prospect of transferring completely into another division such as fine chemicals, polymers or agrochemicals could also be a likelihood, based mainly on the management skills of the individual, whilst retaining some fringe scientific links.

## THE FUTURE

Finally, a word about the future of the pharmacist's role in industrial health care. For those pharmacists working in companies where the chief activity is that of drug discovery, the formulation and analytical skills of the pharmacist could unfairly be regarded as cosmetic and secondary to the perceived main job of designing new drug compounds. However, in more enlightened companies where the true potential of the pharmacist is fully recognised, and his or her broad knowledge base combined with specialist scientific skill is fully utilised, then tremendous added value can be gained from the natural synergies that pharmacists have with other science professionals in optimising drug development for the patient and maximising its value for the company. It is likely that pharmacy will continue to be used as a productive seed-bed for future industrial managers and, additionally, as the rate of discovery of new drug compounds inevitably and predictably falls, the importance of the pharmacist as an innovator, creator and problem-solver will increase still further to help meet the very latest challenges in the business of pharmaceutical medicine.

# Part III
# Careers in Clinical Research

# 10
# Career Opportunities for Physicians in the Pharmaceutical Industry

## Bert Spilker

Orphan Medical, Minnetonka, Minnesota, USA

The role of physicians in the pharmaceutical industry is not generally well understood by most physicians who work outside the industry. Reasons for this relate to a lack of knowledge about specific activities conducted by physicians working within the pharmaceutical industry and a lack of information about the processes and issues involved in drug discovery and development. Little information about potential careers in this industry is provided in medical schools, and most medical students do not have contact with industry physicians.

This chapter, which describes activities conducted by physicians within the pharmaceutical industry, is organised around a series of questions that physicians outside the industry might ask of physicians working within the industry.

## WHY DO PHYSICIANS JOIN A PHARMACEUTICAL COMPANY?

More physicians are applying to the pharmaceutical industry for positions because these careers offer meaningful challenges, and there is increasing competition for positions in patient care and in academia. The

*Discovering New Medicines: Careers in Pharmaceutical Research and Development.*
Edited by P.D. Stonier
© 1994 John Wiley & Sons Ltd

results of this situation is that the quality of physicians joining the pharmaceutical industry is increasing, as is the competition among physicians to obtain these positions.

The major reasons that a physician joins a pharmaceutical company are identical to the reasons a physician makes any career decision. Major ones include that the position seems challenging, offers opportunities for developing a meaningful career, provides generally adequate financial security, and provides other benefits. These factors provide physicians and their families the basis for a positive quality of life.

Numerous reasons for choosing a career within the pharmaceutical industry, as compared with other careers, relate to specific attributes of the position. These reasons often include the sense of personal satisfaction that evolves from participating in the development of important new drugs. These drugs offer increased benefits to patients in terms of enhanced survival, improved quality of life and a more productive life. Another reason is that many physicians have opportunities to be managers. Even for physicians who have little interest in management, administrative support and technical services are usually available to help them perform their job efficiently. This allows physicians to focus more of their attention on activities that require medical training. Other reasons for physicians to choose a pharmaceutical career are opportunities to travel, to attend medical and scientific meetings, to function as a member of a team in planning and implementing clinical studies, to interpret data, and to trouble-shoot and solve issues that arise.

Both clinical practice and academic life are viewed in a very positive way by the majority of physicians in those areas. However, some individuals join the pharmaceutical industry because of negative aspects (in their view) of responsibilities and the atmosphere in these or other careers. Some of the negative responsibilities might include long and often irregular hours on call, direct interactions with patients, teaching, and preparing grant proposals. Aspects of the negative atmosphere might relate to high malpractice insurance premiums, financial constraints on research, limited time available for research, or responsibilities viewed in a negative light.

For some industry physicians, a great proportion of their time is spent addressing clinical and scientific challenges. Clinical and scientific responsibilities include designing new studies, writing protocols, initiating and monitoring studies, interpreting data, preparing medical reports, extrapolating results, developing a clinical strategy to bring a new drug or new indication forward, and directing co-workers to help in these activities. These and many other activities will be discussed in more detail.

Administrative responsibilities may or may not differ for physicians within a pharmaceutical company as compared with physicians in other positions in academia. At some companies there may be specialists to help physicians with administrative tasks or to perform them (e.g. write final medical reports based on the physician's evaluation).

Individuals in numerous departments are available to help physicians perform their jobs more efficiently, thus enabling physicians to spend a greater proportion of their time on activities that require medical training.

## WHAT DO PHYSICIANS DO IN A PHARMACEUTICAL COMPANY?

Medical departments are the primary area in which physicians work. Companies organise medical departments in a variety of ways, and few standard positions exist that are quite similar among companies. Positions vary from the highly focused to the extremely broad. Focused positions may consist of a single role (e.g. set up clinical studies on drug A; consult on clinical studies in therapeutic area B). Broad positions usually consist of multiple roles, possibly involving multiple drugs. The majority of physicians in industry are closer to the multiple-role end of the spectrum, but for each person it depends to a large extent on their personality and whether they welcome or resist additional assignments and responsibilities. The nature of the company also plays a role, since some companies are more likely than others to assign multiple responsibilities to physicians. Common types of roles, activities, interactions and collaborations are described later.

### Roles

A number of roles require medical training, while other roles require scientific training. Physicians are generally challenged most and enjoy best those roles for which their training and experience has prepared them. Although a large number of roles are mentioned, physicians do not participate in all of them and most companies provide staff to help them conduct other roles.

The most common role of physicians in industry is to plan, initiate and monitor clinical studies (Spilker, 1991). After clinical studies are complete, some physicians edit data and supervise data processing. The next major step is to interpret the data. This process is either carried out directly or is reviewed by physicians.

An industry physician is also a consultant. Instead of conducting the activities mentioned above themselves, physicians often advise others on the medical perspective that must be considered on various points.

The consultant's role may be informal or it may be the central role assigned by the company.

Many physicians are managers who direct people, resources and activities, and are part of the line management (i.e. vertical hierarchy) of a company. Another aspect of a company's management refers to the matrix system, or horizontal organisation, in which each drug's development effort is referred to as a project. In a matrix management role, some physicians function as project leaders (Spilker, 1994). They are in charge of efforts to guide a drug's development from the preclinical stage to the stage of submitting one or more regulatory applications. To do this, they head a team of 6–20 people from various research, medical, marketing, and other departments that cuts across the organisation.

A physician also may collaborate with marketing staff to advise on design of appropriate market research studies, review advertising copy for appropriateness of medical content, and seek marketing product managers' views in designing marketing orientated clinical studies or quality-of-life studies.

A number of the roles described in this section are listed in Table 1. Four categories are used for ease of presentation.

**Interactions**

Collaborations with statisticians are important to virtually all physicians, and developing a good relationship with a competent statistician is an important goal for clinicians in industry. Statisticians give advice on the number of patients required for a clinical study, provide randomisation schedules for clinical studies, review clinical study protocols for content, determine which statistical analyses will be applied to study results, review the interpretation of data, and help write combined statistical and medical reports. Nonetheless, it is the clinician's responsibility to determine the clinical importance of the statistical findings.

Interactions with personnel working in drug regulatory affairs occur frequently. Companies generally use their drug regulatory affairs department as a funnel to enable written and verbal interactions from many groups within the company to present a common front to national regulatory agencies. All correspondence usually is officially transmitted through this group. Each physician who interacts with a regulatory agency is usually briefed by regulatory personnel prior to these meetings. If the physician is responsible for an investigational or marketed drug that has many regulatory issues associated with it, then a significant portion of his or her time may involve meetings with the regulatory agency and with other sections of the company. Depending

**Table 1.** Selected roles of physicians in the pharmaceutical industry.

*Clinical research roles and functions*

Identify, meet, interview and persuade clinicians outside the company to conduct clinical trials. Many of these clinicians are the most well-known experts in their field
Negotiate details of the protocol and budget with clinical investigators
Plan and write the clinical trial protocol
Lead round-table discussions with clinical investigators, monitors and consultants
Initiate clinical trials
Monitor clinical trials
Maintain contact with clinical investigators and deal with any problems or issues that arise
Assess adverse reactions that arise during clinical trials and discuss possible treatments with clinical investigators
Edit data collection forms
Interpret data obtained in clinical trials
Extrapolate data to new situations and develop new clinical hypotheses to test
Create clinical strategies for developing investigational drugs to the point of market approval
Create clinical strategies for post-marketing surveillance studies and new indications of marketed drugs
Collaborate with the medical team developing the drug
Collaborate with the company's project team developing the drug
Liaise with professionals in other divisions of the company as required
Order bulk drug and clinical trial drug supplies
Write periodic reports of project activities and other functions
Interact with other physicians, statisticians, pre-clinical scientists, information specialists, computer specialists and many others on an ongoing basis
Approve the supply of drug samples to outside academicians who wish to conduct animal studies. Approve the supply of formulated drug to outside clinicians who wish to conduct human studies
Critique potential licensing opportunities

*Marketing support roles and functions*

Review marketing advertisements and promotional materials
Telephone health care professionals to discuss and answer their questions

*Professional development and educational activities*

Teach university students
Conduct research or collaborate in research projects at universities
Lecture to different groups of company representatives
Discuss the process of drug development with civic groups
Attend seminars, courses and meetings within and outside the company. Present information when relevant
Read medical literature to maintain current awareness and knowledge
Advise company lawyers, marketers and non-medical scientists on medical perspectives
Improve expertise in one's specific area
Consult with other physicians

*Regulatory activities*

Generate regulatory submissions through written reports, summaries or evaluations
Report serious adverse reactions and deaths to regulatory authorities as prescribed by regulations or to regulatory personnel within the company
Participate at meetings with regulatory authorities

on the company, there may be a number of physicians within the regulatory affairs department. Even drugs with few regulatory issues involve various meetings, the preparation of applications, plus a number of data reviews (e.g. at end of phase II meetings). A knowledge of pharmaceutical regulations is generally acquired on the job, rather than in a training programme. Nonetheless, some individuals within a company develop interest and knowledge in regulations and transfer to the regulatory affairs department.

Physicians that head projects usually have a project coordinator or planner assigned to assist them. This individual provides many important services, such as planning the overall schedule and milestone dates for the group to achieve. This person also monitors the work being conducted in all departments to assess how well project members are adhering to their schedules. The coordinator acts to facilitate agreements and settle issues between departments, but does not get involved in issues within departments. This person often raises red flags for the project leader or others to address.

The scope of a physician's responsibilities is usually limited to either national or international activities. This factor depends primarily on the ownership of the company. It also depends on the organisational structure of the medical department. For instance, many US-based pharmaceutical companies have separate medical groups to conduct domestic and foreign studies. A number of companies are organised so that different medical groups conduct investigational drug studies and marketing-orientated studies. The latter group of physicians (and others) may report to either marketing or medical division managers.

## WHAT ARE THE AREAS IN WHICH PHYSICIANS WORK?

Areas in which physicians work that are outside the formal medical department investigating new drugs are mentioned briefly to provide a broad view of other areas in which many physicians work.

*Drug regulatory affairs*. Develops regulatory strategies, assembles regulatory applications and interacts with regulatory agencies via letters and at meetings. Serves as an interface for others within the company who interact with regulatory agencies.

*Drug information services*. Interacts with health professionals to provide information on the company's drugs regarding adverse reactions, treatment of overdose, various publications or other topics.

*Epidemiology*. Assembles adverse reaction information on the company's drugs. Designs, conducts and evaluates post-marketing surveillance studies. May interact directly with regulatory agencies.

*Statistics and data processing*. Involves numerous steps of editing data, entering them into computers, ensuring their quality, tabulating them, analysing them and preparing reports of the results. Statisticians have frequent interactions with clinicians and regulatory agencies.

*Pre-clinical sciences*. Some physicians join pre-clinical departments (e.g. pharmacology, microbiology, biochemistry, molecular biology) and conduct research relating to new drug discovery.

*Medical services*. This is a general term for a group that usually has a mixture of medical, marketing and administrative tasks. Its profile usually differs in each company. Physicians who prefer administrative, marketing and promotional activities may enjoy a position in this type of department.

*Project coordination*. This group oversees the project system and is the matrix arm of the company. Roles combine managerial and administrative responsibilities with scientific input into a wide variety of activities.

*Other areas*. These include patents, licensing, computers, education, training, commercial liaison and financial controller functions within the medical or R&D division. In addition, there are some physicians who become involved in pre-clinical sciences (e.g. pharmacology, biochemistry, toxicology) but these areas are not discussed in this chapter.

## WHAT ARE THE CHALLENGES AND OPPORTUNITIES FOR ADVANCEMENT?

Challenges come both from without and within an individual. Those from outside the person are provided primarily by the company. Other external opportunities for challenges include committee assignments for trade associations, professional societies associated with the pharmaceutical industry, professional societies independent of the industry, hospital work, research activities or teaching assignments at a medical school. Challenges from within individuals motivate them to work hard and achieve their goals. Challenges to excel are the same in individuals who join the pharmaceutical industry as in those based in academia or clinical practice.

Most medium and large pharmaceutical companies have a wide variety of positions that are available to experienced physicians who have demonstrated managerial and technical skills within the industry. These positions are often described as a 'dual ladder'. This refers to the fact that advancement may progress along either an administrative/ management or a clinical/scientific tract. Enlightened companies provide commensurate benefits to scientists and clinicians who become more experienced in their area but do not wish to give up their professional activities to take on purely administrative positions. Keeping creative scientists working in the laboratories and keeping productive clinicians working on developing drugs often provides greater benefits to a company than promoting these individuals outside their area of competence. Not all highly successful clinicians and scientists are competent and successful managers.

Specific positions that physicians may fill within the industry include:

- assistant medical director;
- associate medical director;
- medical director;
- medical division director;
- drug information services director;
- regulatory affairs director (plus assistant and associate directors);
- director of development;
- research and development director;
- project coordination director.

Exact titles often vary among companies and the relative rank, level and responsibilities are more important in judging a position than is the title. For example, a company may have two or three vice-presidents within R&D, whereas another company of equal size may have 10–15 vice-presidents in the same areas. Physicians with special interests in other areas (e.g. marketing, statistics) may seek and find positions in those areas. Also, depending on the company, numerous hybrid positions either exist or may be created to provide opportunities for physicians to develop their careers. The nature and responsibilities of these (and other) positions are described in more detail by Sampson (1984). Staff within medical departments may desire or be asked to focus their activities on one (or more) phase of clinical development.

## WHAT TYPES OF PHARMACEUTICAL COMPANIES EXIST?

This chapter describes the research-based company that is attempting to discover new drugs of benefit to humans, for instance. There are 40–60 such companies in the USA depending on how categories are defined and how companies are classified. Many small companies that are attempting to invent new drugs, particularly biotechnology companies, are not included in this category. A few biotechnology companies hire physicians to help with clinical development if they have products in (or near) the clinical research stage. On the other hand, many biotechnology companies either do not have drugs in clinical trials or they may have joint development or licensing arrangements with larger R&D companies. A few companies develop and then market drugs but do not seek to discover drugs. These companies also hire physicians. Companies that produce only generic drugs rarely hire physicians.

## WHAT CHARACTERISTICS DO PHARMACEUTICAL COMPANIES SEEK IN PHYSICIANS?

It is extremely beneficial, though not essential, for all physicians to have a period of clinical experience (after clinical training is complete) prior to joining a company. In the UK, for example, for membership of the Faculty of Pharmaceutical Medicine a period of at least two years post-registration general medical training is required. The ideal physician who joins a pharmaceutical company will be trained and board certified in the therapeutic area in which he or she will work. This usually involves internal medicine or one of its subspecialities, or another speciality (e.g. psychiatry, neurology, anaesthesiology, ophthalmology, paediatrics). Experience as a clinical investigator is extremely beneficial and worthwhile. Clinical pharmacology training and postdoctoral positions provide a good training for entering the industry. Physicians with training in a number of areas such as nuclear medicine or radiology may find that career opportunities are greater with diagnostic or medical device companies. On the other hand, pharmaceutical companies also hire many young physicians who are not specialists, but who have the personality to switch between fields, and are flexible in their approach. Therefore both medical specialists and generalists are desirable employees of a pharmaceutical company.

Two important characteristics that a company seeks in new physicians are a scientific orientation and the ability to work as a team player. Scientific ability is extremely important for physicians in industry because it is needed to design state-of-the-art clinical studies, develop clinical strategies, interpret data fully, prepare sound articles for publication, and develop drugs effectively and efficiently. A number of years ago most physicians who entered industry came from general practice. They generally had little or no training or experience in the science of medicine and were not orientated towards thinking as a scientist. Over the last 10–20 years there has been a steady increase in the number of physicians entering industry who have strong scientific backgrounds. In several cases, physicians also have earned PhD degrees prior to joining the industry.

Being a team player means that one operates as part of a group—not as an independent star. Teamwork is a comforting feeling to most people, because everyone on the team shares important goals and wants their project to succeed. The advantages for the physician using this approach are that ideas are constantly being discussed and debated among several (or many) people, and it is hopeful that good ideas and approaches become better ideas and approaches. On the other hand, the team approach may not favour the development of novel or risky ideas. Teams can be a conservative force, especially if a consensus is needed to make decisions.

Success is often defined as completing assignments on time and answering questions posed. Therefore, the team is judged on its ability to meet its goals, not on the outcome. Goals for a new drug should be to determine if it works, not to show that it works. Therefore, even if a new drug is found to be inactive or if unacceptable animal or human toxicity is found, the team would be judged successful if they determined that result rapidly and efficiently. Resources used by the terminated drug project would become available for other projects to use. This enables the new projects receiving resources to move ahead more rapidly.

## WHAT TYPES OF PHYSICIANS SHOULD NOT CONSIDER CAREERS IN THE PHARMACEUTICAL INDUSTRY?

Certain physicians, because of interests or temperament, probably should not seek a career in the pharmaceutical industry. The major characteristic that would raise a warning signal about entering the industry would be whether the physician enjoys clinical practice above all other professional activities. Other characteristics of those who would probably be unhappy in industry include wanting to be one's own boss, not particularly enjoying work with others on a collaborative team, or finding it difficult to be directed by non-physicians. Physicians who are not research orientated or do not enjoy research should not consider positions in clinical research.

Finally, some individuals do not like the idea that marketing considerations sometimes force compromises of clinical positions or even overrule clinical considerations. For example, a physician may believe it medically relevant and useful to test one of the company's drugs in a new indication, but marketing groups state that the eventual commercial return would be too small to justify the proposed clinical studies. Some companies are more willing to test new drugs in less commercially attractive disease areas than others. Nonetheless, a physician who is unable to accept the commercial influence on drug development decisions should carefully consider whether a career in industry represents the most appropriate choice.

## CONCLUSION

More and more physicians are finding that a career in the pharmaceutical industry is scientifically challenging, intellectually stimulating, and provides opportunities for personal and professional development that are outstanding. The wide variety of positions offers research, clinical, managerial and other focuses that are attracting an increasing number of physicians to the pharmaceutical industry.

## ACKNOWLEDGEMENT

This chapter was originally printed in the *Journal of Clinical Pharmacology* (1989, volume 29: 1069–1076) and is reprinted (with modifications) with permission.

# 11
# The Clinical Research Associate

Marian Saunders

SmithKline Beecham Pharmaceuticals, Epsom, UK

The role of the clinical research associate (CRA) within the pharmaceutical industry has evolved extensively over the past 20 years, paralleling the growing complexity of drug development over this period. In the early days, CRAs were employed very much as assistants, *helping* their medical adviser or medical director. Early medical departments were flat structures with a small number of CRAs often reporting direct to the medical director. The role of the CRA was restricted, with the company physician being the primary contact with the investigator, certainly for discussions on the study drug, the study design, or more importantly the study budget! I well recall a late-night discussion in the early 1980s between three (then) CRAs bemoaning the lack of career opportunities and the medical glass ceiling that appeared to be so close above our heads. Things changed very quickly for those three CRAs and the industry at large. As clinical trials became larger and more complex to manage, as drug programmes began to be coordinated on a global basis, as the number of Contract Research Organisations (CROs) proliferated, and as the full impact of Good Clinical Practice (GCP) began to dawn on the pharmaceutical industry outside the USA, the development opportunities for CRAs mushroomed, as did the numbers. It is difficult to gather accurate information on the numbers of CRAs/clinical scientists in the industry; suffice to say a major global pharmaceutical company is likely to employ hundreds worldwide. Taking the numbers

*Discovering New Medicines: Careers in Pharmaceutical Research and Development.*
Edited by P.D. Stonier
© 1994 John Wiley & Sons Ltd

of companies and CROs into account there would be thousands in the UK and major markets.

Confusingly, although the CRA job description evolved down many different paths, the job title often remained the same. There are CRAs who are still little more than couriers of drug supplies and Case Report Forms (CRFs), and CRAs who manage teams of other CRAs and physicians as the worldwide project leader for a drug development programme and/or therapeutic area. The term is almost generic for any non-medically qualified person working in a clinical research department. The majority of CRAs, though, fulfil the role of site monitor described in GCP guidelines (*Pharm. Ind.*, 1990). This chapter will consider the role of CRA as Site Monitor first, and then review the other roles under a general discussion of promotion/development opportunities.

## CLINICAL RESEARCH ASSOCIATE AS SITE MONITOR

The broad function of a site monitor is to be responsible for the initiation and monitoring of allocated clinical trials, validation of CRF data and reconciling study medication according to company Standard Operating Procedures (SOPs). The precise responsibilities would depend upon the individual company, the organisational structure and SOPs. The nature of the work will also vary subtly according to the investigational product (eg. drug, medical device or biotechnology product) and the stage of development. A fuller job description would probably include the following elements.

### Principal Responsibilities

1. Pre-study preparation:
   - review of draft protocol and CRFs;
   - feedback to study manager on issues that may impact the study, e.g. local medical practice, suitable comparative agents, local regulatory requirements.

2. To set up study sites:
   - identify and select potential investigators;
   - ensure the trial site has adequate space, facilities (including laboratories), equipment, staff and that an adequate number of trial subjects is likely to be available for the duration of the trial;
   - arrange outside contract laboratories as required;

- ensure investigator understands and follows correct procedures for obtaining informed consent and ethics committee approval;
- arrange indemnification as required according to local law;
- negotiate individual site budgets;
- ensure appropriate regulatory approval is obtained for the protocol, amendments and importation of clinical trial supplies.

3. To start up study sites:

- prepare study site initiation package and ensure necessary documentation is filed in the company operational files and in the investigator study file;
- conduct or assist with investigator's meeting;
- ensure that all staff assisting the investigator in the trial have been adequately informed about and comply with the details of the trial;
- ensure timely delivery of clinical trial supplies to study site.

4. To be responsible for all activities ongoing during the study:

- conduct regular monitoring visits to ensure adherence to the protocol and informed consent procedures;
- check that the storage, dispensing, return and documentation of the supply of investigational medicinal products are safe and appropriate and in accordance with local regulations;
- ensure investigator study file and company operational files are maintained appropriately;
- collect and review CRFs. Check all CRFs for completeness, legibility and plausibility, and compare data against source documentation. Query CRFs following review, resolve any queries received from the study manager or clinical data management, and track all CRFs collected;
- complete contact forms following monitoring visits or telephone contact with investigator;
- review patient recruitment at sites and take appropriate action to ensure recruitment of evaluable patients to plan;
- review CRFs for adverse events (AEs) and ensure all serious AEs are reported through the company serious AE procedure and to local regulatory agencies as appropriate;
- enable/ensure communication between the investigator and sponsor promptly at all times and provide the investigator with updated information regarding the drug and the status of the study on an ongoing basis;
- initiate, track and process study payments.

5. To be responsible for end-of-study activities:

- conduct end-of-study visit;
- discuss research report or publication with principal investigator and obtain signature where required;
- evaluate and document the suitability of investigator and site for future studies.

6. To keep up to date with relevant medical literature, developments in clinical research methodology, monitoring and local regulatory and ethical requirements.

## HOW TO BECOME A CLINICAL RESEARCH ASSOCIATE

### Qualifications

European Union GCP guidelines require that sponsors appoint a monitor who 'must have qualifications and experience to enable a knowledgeable supervision of a particular trial' (*Pharm. Ind.*, 1990). Most CRAs are graduates in a biological science subject such as pharmacology, biochemistry, physiology or pharmacy, and many have an MSc or PhD. A nursing background is also quite common, bringing additional skills and knowledge of the National Health Service (NHS) and medical profession. Given the increasing numbers of investigators who are employing nurses as study site coordinators to act as the primary contact between the industry and study site, this will presumably be an attractive source of new CRAs in the future. CRAs with medical degrees are rare in the UK or USA, although more common in some other European countries such as France. Some companies now encourage newly recruited physicians to work as CRAs for the first six months or so, to give them hands-on knowledge of the job before assuming the traditional management role.

### Personality Traits

Consider what a CRA is called upon to do on a daily basis. They have to manage a large, disparate group of people (the investigators), over whom they have no direct control, who often have a heightened sense of superiority over the CRA, and little natural inclination to pay quite the close attention to detail when conducting a clinical trial (particularly form-filling), that the pharmaceutical industry demands—matrix management at its most horrific. It is little wonder that a key personality trait is excellent interpersonal skills: a mixture of diplomacy, persuasion and threat! The job also requires close attention to detail, to be personally well organised and, dare I say it, a willingness to accept a measure of repetition. Designing studies, finding investigators and establishing a good working relationship with study site staff, and writing protocols and publications are the fun parts, but as with all jobs there is a significant routine component. CRFs have to be closely reviewed and the data contained within them compared with the source data in the patient notes or elsewhere. The ability to keep going at this task hour after hour, whilst often squashed into some cubby-hole in the corner of a hospital, calls for a special kind of person. Strange how one actually only remembers the nice sites where they ply you continuously with tea and excellent home-baked fruit-cake, and the investigator gives up his office to you.

Travel is a fact of life for CRAs. The extent of this, and its impact on home life, is somewhat determined by the organisation of the company. The extreme case would be a company that monitors a multinational study from its HQ base, necessitating extended trips to continental Europe, or even from the USA to Europe. Other companies monitor locally, and some even have regional-based field CRAs who work from home across a reasonably small area. Suffice it to say that travel would have to appeal strongly, be it by car or plane, and a fairly independent nature is called for to see one through nights alone in remote hotels and, even worse, the meals alone in remote hotel dining-rooms! For those CRAs monitoring international trials, linguistic skills would obviously be a benefit.

### How to Find a Job as a Clinical Research Associate

Many people become CRAs by moving from other departments within the pharmaceutical industry. People with experience of sales, regulatory, discovery research, medical information, clinical data management, medical writing or clinical safety all bring useful experience and knowledge of the drug development process. For people wishing to join the industry for the first time, CRA positions are advertised in the *New Scientist* and *Clinical Research Focus* (published by the Association of Clinical Research in the Pharmaceutical Industry), and many specialist recruitment agencies service the pharmaceutical industry. CROs often advertise short-term opportunities to gain experience of monitoring.

### What Sort of Clinical Research Associate to Become?

The role of the CRA as site monitor is quite standard across the industry, but a person considering becoming a CRA still has some choices to make. Firstly, CRAs are employed by both the pharmaceutical industry and CROs. The latter are service companies undertaking clinical studies on a contract basis on behalf of pharmaceutical companies. The advantages of starting with a major pharmaceutical company would be the likely existence of a training and induction programme, and the ability to focus and gain expertise in a specific therapeutic area or to follow the development of a drug from early clinical studies through to market. There would also probably be the opportunity to liaise with other departments in the company, such as regulatory affairs, clinical trial supplies, statistics, data management, toxicology, pharmacology, discovery research etc., giving a broader understanding of how drugs are discovered and brought to market. A CRO, on the other hand, is likely to provide you with exposure to many different types of drugs and/or therapeutic areas and an insight into the workings of many pharmaceutical companies.

Another decision facing the CRA aspirant is which phase of drug development to work in: the major choices being to specialise in early phase I volunteer studies, to work with investigational drugs that are not yet on the market (phases II–IIIb), or to work with marketed drugs (phase IV), where the aim is to develop and enhance the profile of the drug. At the risk of making sweeping generalisations, someone with a keen interest in the science of drug development might be more suited to the first two options, whereas people with more of an interest in marketing might find the phase IV support role more to their liking.

## Training

Training courses for CRAs have always been available, through the many independent companies offering professional training, the professional societies (ACRPI, Society for Pharmaceutical Medicine, BrAPP etc.) and specialist training functions within companies. However, a particular focus was placed on training in the early 1990s by the explicit statement in the European GCP guidelines that required the sponsor to 'appoint, and ensure the ongoing training of, suitable and appropriately trained monitors and their clinical research support personnel'. Many companies appointed specialist GCP/SOP trainers. Two reviews on training for CRAs and clinical research scientists (Mullinger, 1990; Maloney, 1990) provide an excellent overview of the training needs of new CRAs and how to deliver ongoing training to more experienced staff. More formal academic training is available through the Diploma in Clinical Science, initiated by the University of Wales and ACRPI, and an MSc in pharmaceutical medicine run by the University of Surrey.

## CAREER DEVELOPMENT

There is no set career structure for CRAs, and the potential for career development is very much dependent upon the individual company and its organisation. Within mainstream clinical research, there are two major routes to follow: therapeutic project management and CRA man management.

### Therapeutic Clinical Project Management

Owing to the ever-increasing cost of bringing a new drug to market, many companies now plan their clinical development programmes centrally, and implement these plans internationally. Few companies can afford to allow independent parallel development by local operating entities. There are opportunities for CRAs to move into roles managing the clinical project (i.e. clinical studies or programmes, as distinct from project management of the entire development process). This could be at the level of a study manager with responsibilities for coordinating one or more multicentre clinical trials, a drug manager with responsibilities for coordinating the clinical development programme for a specific drug or drug/indication, or responsibility for an entire therapeutic area with multiple drugs under investigation. Whilst it is true to say that many of the senior clinical project management positions are taken by physicians, this is not always the case. The management skills and therapeutic expertise developed by scientifically trained CRAs, if appropriately supported by medical advice for safety and regulatory purposes, provide an excellent background for a senior management position within a clinical research department. Sadly, in practice opportunities are limited, and high-potential CRAs with ambition are often forced to take sideways steps in their careers.

### General Management

Many companies have a hierarchical structure, with teams of CRAs being managed by a senior CRA or clinical trials manager, either on a project basis or providing general monitoring services to a number of projects. Growth opportunities are obviously limited by the number of levels of management, and with the ever-increasing trend towards flatter organisations and delayering it is difficult to progress too far on the basis of managing more and more CRAs, except perhaps in the largest of companies, or in smaller organisations where management positions are a luxury and allied disciplines are managed in unison by scientists with broad experience.

Although the most obvious route for advancement would seem to lie with therapeutic specialisation and project responsibilities, at some point all specialists do have to report to a generalist manager, even though it may be the chief executive officer! Again, in most companies the more generalist head of a clinical research department does tend to be medically qualified, although there are an increasing number of exceptions, particularly within CROs. Many high-calibre CRAs who attain senior management positions do so within contract research rather than a traditional pharmaceutical company.

## Other Opportunities Within the Pharmaceutical Industry

Depending upon the size of the organisation, many clinical departments do require support services, and these do offer career potential to CRAs. The administration surrounding clinical development is complex, and specialist knowledge and support can greatly facilitate the overall process. The sorts of services offered could include the following:

- clinical trials scheduling and manpower resourcing;
- clinical trials budgeting;
- clinical trials status tracking and reporting;
- clinical trials supplies ordering;
- management of CRO contracts;
- GCP and other training;
- internal quality control;
- SOPs development and maintenance;
- document management.

Opportunities obviously also exist in the pharmaceutical industry in departments other than clinical research, although initially such moves are likely to be sideways steps. Departments to consider are regulatory affairs, medical information, marketing (although sales representative experience is often considered mandatory), training, audit/quality assurance, or project management. CROs may also offer other career opportunities such as business development.

Many CRAs work on a freelance basis, either for themselves or for specialist independent companies. Part-time and flexible opportunities are becoming evident as companies rely increasingly on contract resource at the site monitor level.

## Opportunities Outside the Pharmaceutical Industry

As stated above, an experienced, successful CRA will have many marketable skills in matrix management, influencing people and project management. Such skills are presumably valued in other industries, and opportunities undoubtedly arise for moves to general management elsewhere. There are no obvious paths out of the industry, though. Career moves that I have known people make include:

- financial analyst specialising in pharmaceutics;
- recruitment for the industry;
- personnel management.
- pharmaceutical specialists in management consultancies.

## THE FUTURE ROLE OF THE CLINICAL RESEARCH ASSOCIATE

The role of the CRA has undergone a fairly speedy evolution over the past 20 years. Given the general pace of change in society generally, and the technological advances made, it is comparatively easy to speculate on the future role of the CRA. One senior industry manager even believes that the role will completely disappear over the next 10 years or so. He sees the increasing computerisation of medical practice and the greater emphasis being placed on pharmacoeconomic outcome measures, and postulates that all clinical trial data could be automatically downloaded from the patient notes, given the right information technology (IT) infrastructure. I still cannot help thinking that so much of CRA work is about communication and facilitation, and these skills would still be required to ensure rapid recruitment to *your* company's studies rather than others. Man's need to communicate with fellow man aside, the transcribing of data onto hand-written CRFs, which are validated against patient notes, and then entered into a computer database, would seem to be limited and perhaps we will need fewer CRAs.

Other possible changes in the role are that more and more clinical studies will be contracted out, and the site monitor responsibilities will be undertaken exclusively by CROs. Some people even speculate that the CRAs will be employed by, or at least based in, a given hospital or general practice, and will work on more than one company's projects. These two scenarios place even more emphasis on a skilled cadre of clinical research staff based within the pharmaceutical company who manage the project at the study, programme or therapeutic area level.

When all is said and done though, it is unlikely that the impact of IT on clinical research will be any greater than on the business world generally. After all, IT advances have the potential to dramatically change all aspects of our lives.

# 12
# A Career in Clinical Pharmacology

Nigel S. Baber

Glaxo Research & Development, West Uxbridge, UK

Clinical pharmacology is the scientific study of the actions of drugs in man. It is concerned with the safety, tolerability, pharmacokinetics and pharmacodynamics of new and established compounds, and the application of its principles leads to rational drug prescribing. Clinical pharmacologists occupy positions in academia, in the National Health Service (NHS), in regulatory authorities and in the pharmaceutical industry, and there is an increasing mobility between these areas of employment. In academia and hospital practice, clinical pharmacologists currently develop a specialist interest in one of the system-based specialities, such as cardiology or gastroenterology, take on responsibilities for hospital formularies, therapeutic drug monitoring or adverse event monitoring, or concentrate on developing links with or additional responsibilities for basic pharmacology in one or more therapeutic areas. Some serve as advisers on the Committee for Safety of Medicines.

In the practice of its discipline clinical pharmacology relies heavily on the controlled clinical trial, using a variety of designs, paying particular attention to hypothesis setting, critical end-point definition and sound statistical analysis. It seeks to understand how drugs work in producing both wanted and unwanted effects, and how dynamic effects are related to drug concentrations in biological fluids.

*Discovering New Medicines: Careers in Pharmaceutical Research and Development.*
Edited by P.D. Stonier
© 1994 John Wiley & Sons Ltd

Given this wide remit, clinical pharmacologists could, theoretically, be involved in virtually all aspects of drug evaluation, from first administration to man, through phases II to IV (see Box 1) into post-marketing surveillance. By their training and knowledge clinical pharmacologists are well placed to influence rational drug development well beyond

---

**Box 1. Definition of Phases**

In the text, the stages of clinical trials are referred to as phases I, IIa, IIb, III and IV. The generally accepted definition of these phases is as follows:

**Phase 1.** First administration studies to man. Single- and repeat-dose escalation studies usually in healthy volunteers to determine safety, tolerability, pharmacokinetics and dynamic responses, if measurable. Phase I studies usually include radiolabelled studies to determine metabolism and excretion of parent compound and metabolites, drug–drug interaction studies, and studies in patients with certain organ deficiencies, e.g. renal and hepatic. Bioequivalence and bioavailability studies are classed as phase I.

**Phase IIa.** First studies in the target patient population. Studies are either comparisons of one or more doses with placebo or active comparator, or dose-ranging with three to five different doses. Further kinetics may be undertaken in this population.

**Phase IIb.** Extension of IIa in larger numbers of patients, perhaps widening the entry criteria.

**Phase III.** Definitive long-term dose-ranging efficacy and safety studies to confirm doses for registration, and widen experience of safety. Population pharmacokinetics may be included.

**Phase IV.** Studies conducted after registration of the drug. Further comparisons with standard drugs and competitors; stress is on safety, patient acceptability and familiarisation in clinical use. Post-marketing surveillance studies may be required.

It should be noted that 'phase I' studies are not necessarily all conducted before phase II. More frequently they continue throughout the development programme.

the narrow range of phase I studies with which they are most frequently associated, and to provide a career path into other parts of the industry.

## POSITION AND RESPONSIBILITY WITHIN THE COMPANY

The precise position and responsibility of a department of clinical pharmacology vary from one company to another. Most frequently, it is part of the development operation. There are, however, some companies that locate the clinical pharmacology department within research, reporting to the research director. As clinical pharmacology forms a bridge between animals and man, this latter position may seem a logical one, but there can be disadvantages. Research directors may not fully appreciate the cautious approach that has to be taken when novel substances are given to man for the first time, compared with their speedier evaluation in animals. Ethics review procedures can be seen as an unnecessary hindrance and this may leave the clinical pharmacologist feeling somewhat isolated from his medical colleagues in phases III and IV.

This bridging function between animals and man is one of the key influences that clinical pharmacology has in rational drug design. Understanding the theoretical and practical aspects associated with taking new chemical substances into man is a challenging part of the clinical pharmacologist's job. The second and undisputed territory of clinical pharmacology is the planning, execution and reporting of the phase I programmes to evaluate safety, tolerability, kinetics and dynamics of new chemical substances. These studies are usually conducted in healthy volunteers from within the company, in purpose-built units either on the company premises or at a hospital site where volunteers from the general population are recruited. Phase I studies may also be conducted by academic or NHS clinical pharmacologists or within contract research organisations, under the sponsorship of the company.

Drug development responsibilities switch from clinical pharmacology to clinical research at a variable stage determined by the expertise within the two groups, and the resources available. However, clinical pharmacology has continuing influence and responsibilities up to issue of the international regulatory dossier (IRD), comprising the results of studies agreed in the clinical development plan. These studies will address such issues as drug–drug interaction studies in special populations, drug metabolism studies and studies designed to understand the mode of action of the drug. Clinical pharmacologists write the clinical pharmacology expert reports and summaries for their section of the regulatory dossier.

After the filing of a regulatory submission for a given compound, clinical pharmacology will have two specific responsibilities. First, it must respond to queries from the regulatory authorities, which are frequently directed at the pharmacokinetics and metabolism of the drug. Second, clinical pharmacology must play its part in defending the drug on the market, in developing new formulations and combinations, and in supporting local operating companies and marketing departments with product launches, symposia and publications (see Box 2).

---

**Box 2. Responsibilities of Clinical Pharmacology**

New chemical substance

↓

Animal studies

↓          ←    CP needs understanding and
                knowledge of these studies

Man (healthy volunteers)
Phase I          ←    Undisputed territory of CP

↓

Phases II and III    ←    CP contributes by conducting
                          studies such as drug interaction
↓                         and drug metabolism studies

Issue IRD

↓                         CP does studies to answer regu-
                          latory authority queries
                          regarding issues on
                          pharmacokinetics, drug metab-
                          olism etc.

Product licence and
marketing

↓

Post-marketing       ←    CP plays a part in defending the
surveillance              drug on the market, e.g.
                          developing line extensions

---

## COMPANY RESEARCH HEADQUARTERS VERSUS SUBSIDIARY

Research and development (R&D) is organised in a number of different ways in pharmaceutical companies. This has an impact on the siting and autonomy of the clinical pharmacology function. At company head-quarters, clinical pharmacology will have responsibilities for evaluating new chemical substances emanating from discovery research, and for coordinating the work of clinical pharmacology departments in the sub-sidiaries. The degree of 'control' as opposed to 'coordination and influence' that HQ clinical pharmacology can exert depends on the phil-osophy of the company and the reporting relationship between the boards of management. Many large companies establish some of their discovery research in countries away from HQ. These sites may specia-lise in drug discovery in selected therapeutic areas, and frequently have clinical pharmacology departments associated with them, in addition to that at HQ. A subsidiary clinical pharmacology department will also have the responsibility to support its own regulatory, clinical research and marketing functions for drugs undergoing registration, and those already on the market in that country. It is important, for the potential candidates interested in working in a subsidiary, to establish how much autonomy and authority this prospective group will have with respect to HQ. They may find themselves disappointed if they expected a fair degree of freedom but find all strategies are decided centrally, such that they cannot design or execute a study without HQ approval.

On the other hand, many large American companies have recognised that the Investigational New Drug (IND) procedure is cumbersome and bureaucratic, and that exploratory phase I programmes can be executed much more quickly in Europe. Added to this, the expertise of many European academic clinical pharmacologists is well recognised by American companies, who consequently encourage active clinical phar-macology departments to flourish in their European subsidiaries. This can give very considerable independence to these subsidiaries, and pro-vide opportunities for interesting jobs for clinical pharmacologists.

## HOW IS A CLINICAL PHARMACOLOGY DEPARTMENT ORGANISED?

The three basic elements that make up the discipline of clinical pharmacology—dynamics, pharmacokinetics and safety—are reflected to a greater or lesser extent in the size and organisation of the depart-ment. As mentioned before, phase I studies are conducted in clinical pharmacology units either on-site or within a hospital, in hospital departments or at contract research organisations. Many departments or divisions of clinical pharmacology have clinical pharmacokinetics within their structure. This is a great advantage because an under-standing of the dynamic–kinetic relations of drug action are critical to successful drug evaluation and are more effectively organised under one management.

Large departments of clinical pharmacology require an administrative function (referred to in Figure 2 as clinical pharmacology affairs) to plan study schedules, maintain standard operating procedures, aid in financial management and fulfil a quality-control function. Data management—the generation of case record forms, the entry of data from clinical trials, the production of safety and efficacy tables for study reports—may reside in the department of clinical pharmacology or be part of the data management group, which also manages the data from other departments. Statistics may or may not be within the clinical phar-macology department. Figure 1 shows the main departments with which Clinical Pharmacology interacts.

Figures 2 and 3 depict how a large department of clinical pharmacology might be organised. Figure 2 describes the classical two-dimensional line management structure, in which heads of subdepartments are responsible for functional and/or structural units. In practice, the running of such a department is more complex, and is better des-cribed by the three-dimensional model shown in Figure 3. The three dimensions are: (a) line management of each unit, as in Figure 2; (b) project management based on a new chemical substance or therapeutic

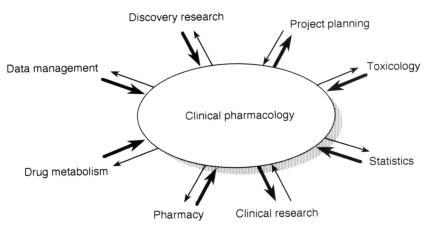

**Figure 1.** Departments interacting with clinical pharmacology. Heaviness of arrow indicates predominant direction of information flow.

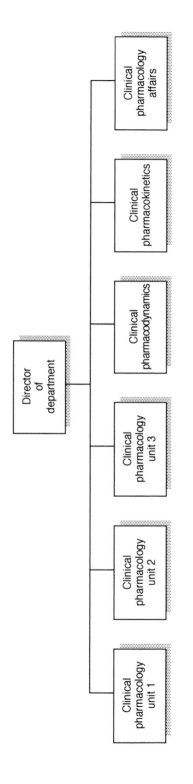

LINE MANAGEMENT STRUCTURE

**Figure 2.** Theoretical structure of a department of clinical pharmacology.

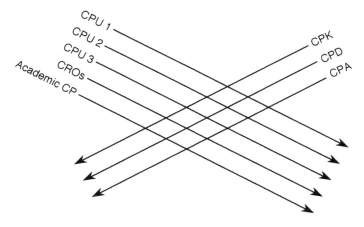

DIRECTOR OF DEPARTMENT

Study execution
(units)

Study and strategic
management (projects)

**Figure 3.** Matrix system management structure. Described here is a matrix system in which there is a mutual interdependence of the functions required to execute a series of tasks. CPU, clinical pharmacology unit (in-house); CRO, contract research organisation; Academic CP, academic clinical pharmacology departments; CPK, clinical pharmacokinetics; CPD, clinical pharmacodynamics; CPA, clinical pharmacology affairs.

area; and (c) speciality functions of dynamics, kinetics and clinical pharmacology affairs, cutting across the project and unit functions.

Such a matrix system requires a high degree of trust, and the ability to live with areas of some ambiguity where functions abut or overlap. It requires the need to work in multidisciplinary teams, which most physicians and scientists find very rewarding. It allows them to maintain their speciality expertise, experience project leadership, and gain some management expertise.

## WHAT ARE THE TASKS OF A CLINICAL PHARMACOLOGIST IN INDUSTRY?

The clinical pharmacologist in industry will work side by side with basic scientists, pharmacokineticists, nurses, data management scientists, statisticians and drug metabolism scientists. His or her interactions outside this immediate sphere will be with physicians and scientists working on phase III and IV programmes, with pharmacology, toxicology, the marketing department (to a lesser extent) and with discovery research scientists, as shown in Figure 1. Initially, this may seem a bewildering array of people to work with and it may be difficult for a physician, especially one coming directly from academia or the NHS, to understand precisely what the clinical pharmacologist's job entails.

Essentially, the tasks can be resolved into two major groups: project and unit. Project function involves the strategic planning of drug development to take it through all of its clinical pharmacological evaluation, supervising the execution of the studies to fulfil that plan, issuing the results from the studies and writing the clinical pharmacology sections of the regulatory dossiers. It requires a thorough understanding of the pharmacology and toxicology of the drug, a knowledge of the disease area in which the drug will be tested and a single-mindedness to champion the project. Unit function is orientated towards actually setting up and executing the studies that are required in the clinical plan and an interpretation of the safety and dynamic responses observed. Smaller departments of clinical pharmacology will combine these two functions so that an individual physician will both plan the strategy, write the protocols, execute the trials and write the reports. In both these functions, the safety aspects of volunteers or patients must be uppermost in the physician's mind. It is he who will make the judgements about the therapeutic ratio, the risk-to-benefit value of the new chemical substance and he will be responsible for the interpretation of adverse events.

Other tasks required of the clinical pharmacologist are responding to questions on the safety, dynamics and kinetics of the NCS (New Chemical Substance) for which he is responsible. These queries come from regulatory bodies, project teams within the organisation, medical sources outside the company and the marketing departments. He will be expected to be the resident expert in all aspects of the clinical pharmacology of the NCS, to keep abreast of the scientific literature in the area and to seek advice from experts in the field. Most companies encourage attendance at relevant scientific meetings and the publication of original work and of reviews.

## MANAGEMENT, ADMINISTRATION AND CLINICAL SCIENCE

Physicians who join a department of clinical pharmacology have a particular interest in how drugs can influence disease processes. They will wish to build on this foundation by increasing their knowledge of how current drugs work, what their strengths and weaknesses are and what opportunities exist for improving the design of new therapies. They will learn to do this, not in an academic environment, but in a commercial organisation, which is run on business principles and should thus be orientated towards making decisions and rewarding performance. Clinical pharmacologists are pragmatists; they like putting up and testing hypotheses by designing the experiments themselves by executing them and by scrutinising the data. They are, essentially 'hands-on' people. Whilst they must appreciate the commercial environment in which they work, and never lose the focus of getting a drug to market. The medico-marketing aspects of the business are not their primary interest, although this may well develop later.

The practical aspects of the job, as indicated above, are most easily satisfied by working within a clinical pharmacology unit, and some physicians will find job satisfaction in executing phase I trials, trying out new equipment and developing novel methodologies to test new potential drugs. Project-orientated physicians tend to be more interested in achieving their goal through others, by influencing the progress of compounds through interdisciplinary project teams and by taking on more administrative responsibilities. As in all organisations the clinical pharmacologist will, sooner or later, have to decide if he wishes to remain directly involved with his technical discipline, or take on a more managerial role, both of projects and/or people. Most clinical pharmacologists feel most comfortable when they retain a strong technical base to their job, but a complete change to full-time management is perfectly possible, dependent on the usual factors of skills, opportunities, training and good fortune.

## REQUIREMENTS FOR ENTERING A DEPARTMENT OF CLINICAL PHARMACOLOGY

The personal characteristics desirable in a physician who is considering a career in clinical pharmacology include curiosity, a desire to understand the pathophysiology of disease, the ability to assimilate information from several different disciplines and to be able to reduce it to a few key questions from which hypotheses can be formed. The individual will be questioning, laterally thinking, yet focused. He will need to feel confident in dealing with experts in other disciplines, such as chemists, pharmacologists and toxicologists, who may not fully appreciate the limitations of taking novel substances into man for the first time.

It is possible, though unusual, for a senior clinical pharmacologist at Reader or Professorial level to come into a department as its head. Senior academics contemplating such a move need to be very certain that they can manage the different pressures and responsibilities of working in a commercial environment. More frequently, a physician will enter a department of clinical pharmacology between senior house officer and senior registrar grade. A higher qualification is required for most good posts—either the MRCP (UK), an MD or PhD. Many physicians have both the membership and research degree. A postgraduate research degree or intercalated BSc or BMedSci is a distinct advantage, as it indicates to the prospective employer that the candidate has an aptitude for research, and may have publications already. Candidates may come from academic departments of clinical pharmacology, in which case they will frequently have had some training in clinical trial design, report writing and statistical analysis, and usually have a rudimentary knowledge of pharmacokinetics. Most frequently their training in clinical pharmacology is based in one of the therapeutic specialities which is practised in the department from which they have come. There are no rules as to which is the better speciality. If the requirement is for a clinical pharmacologist with a particular speciality interest, then obviously the candidate offering the best match is likely to succeed. However, a general clinical pharmacologist may well be able to train in any or a number of therapeutic subspecialities after employment, in which case the candidate's personal attributes may be more important in a successful application than specialist knowledge.

Many physicians entering clinical pharmacology in industry do not come from academic departments of clinical pharmacology. Again, if a therapeutic match is required then it will be sought from that speciality. Experience indicates that cardiology, gastroenterology and endocrinology give the right kind of training, not only in technical and trial design methodology but also in the way physicians think about early drug development problems. Anaesthetics is also a valuable speciality, particularly for those physicians who work in the clinical pharmacology units.

Many physicians who enter industry today have had some involvement in running a clinical trial, frequently for a pharmaceutical company. Clinical pharmacology trials have several features which make them different from Phase III and IV studies. They are usually single centre and smaller in size (tens of subjects rather than hundreds). The trials require more intensive monitoring and close adherence to the protocol, as a small number of missing data points—such as blood sample times—can ruin a clinical pharmacology trial. Clinical pharmacologists often analyse their own data, before handing it over to a statistician, and have good opportunities to present and publish their own work. Thus, inherent in the differences between a physician interested in clinical pharmacology studies compared with phase III and IV trials is the fact that he or she will be closer to the execution of the trial, to the handling of the data, and interpreting the results for decision-making purposes. Phase III and IV physicians tend to be more interested in the strategic organisation of clinical trials and in coordinating a team of clinical research associates to monitor the trials on a national or multinational basis.

## CAREER DEVELOPMENT FOR CLINICAL PHARMACOLOGISTS

Major pharmaceutical companies will want their clinical pharmacologists to keep up to date with theoretical and practical aspects of their job. Training will be undertaken within the department by senior staff, by attendance at specialist courses in pharmacodynamics and kinetics and by taking part in pharmacology society meetings. Regular attendance and membership of a national clinical pharmacology society is a distinct advantage and an opportunity for academic contact. Those physicians with a therapeutic speciality should be encouraged to have membership of their respective societies. As many companies work on a multidisciplinary project team system, they will provide project management training at more senior levels. Computer training is now routine for data management and analysis. Clinical pharmacologists in industry need to be flexible and robust, because well over 50% of novel substances fail to reach full development, and they may need to change therapeutic area. This is not as horrendous as it sounds, as the basic principles of pharmacology and toxicology of drugs, and developing a phase I programme for any novel chemical substance, is common to most drug developments. In addition, a change of drug area gives a richness and variety which may not be available to phase III and IV physicians.

## CAREER OPPORTUNITIES FOR CLINICAL PHARMACOLOGISTS

The training and experience gained in a good department of clinical pharmacology is an excellent preparation for moves into most other parts of a pharmaceutical company.

Individuals come into contact with most other departments and will soon come to appreciate what suits their talents, expertise and ambitions. Clinical pharmacologists, both medically qualified and basic scientists, who have spent several years in clinical departments can move into all of the areas shown in Figure 4.

The most frequent move is into clinical research, to gain experience in phase IIb, III and IV studies. This often occurs when the individual

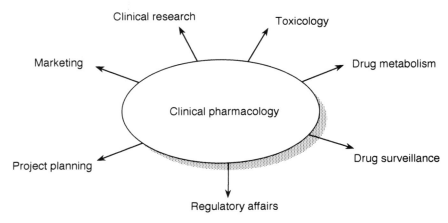

**Figure 4.** Possible career moves for clinical pharmacologists within the industry.

'follows' his or her drug into the later stages of development. Some companies have a career development policy of moving physicians through different departments, to give them a 'balanced' education. In other instances, career moves are more haphazard, and are a combination of desire for a change, aspiration towards management of staff and interest in working abroad. Some companies encourage secondments to subsidiaries, or into other departments at HQ. Most of these opportunities have to be sought positively by the individual.

Career opportunities in discovery research are less frequent, and unless clinical pharmacologists have a very strong research track record and can 'hold their own' with their basic science colleagues, this should not be contemplated. However, there is more than one major company that has a clinical pharmacologist as its R&D director, so a successful career in research is quite possible.

Many physicians in pharmaceutical industries have, as their ultimate goal, the medical directorship of a company. There is no reason at all why clinical pharmacologists should not attain this position. However, in order to gain the necessary experience, it is likely that the individual will have to leave clinical pharmacology and spend time in clinical research, possibly working in or running the medical department of a subsidiary company. Moves, both lateral and upward, between companies are now as frequent as staying within a company to gain experience, and to prove to the individual and potential future employers that the prospective candidate has 'got what it takes' to manage a multidisciplinary department.

There are excellent career opportunities for clinical pharmacologists starting out in the speciality, in a number of limited programmes with academic departments. Some companies will fund jointly or in toto a two- or three-year training programme such that the individual will spend a period in the company's clinical pharmacology department, and the rest of the time in academia. This arrangement may well lead to the gaining of an MSc, MD or PhD, and the incumbent can experience working in a commercial environment before making a permanent commitment.

At later stages in their careers, clinical pharmacologists may choose to work in the regulatory authorities where their knowledge and experience are particularly welcome, or in rarer instances move into academic positions. The current programmes leading to the awarding of the Diploma of Pharmaceutical Medicine and admission to the Faculty of Pharmaceutical Medicine have major clinical pharmacology components to their courses, and there will be much greater mobility between academia, industry and regulatory authorities in the future (Baber, 1991; Turner, 1993).

## THE FUTURE OF CLINICAL PHARMACOLOGY IN INDUSTRY

The pressures and constraints which are bearing down on all pharmaceutical companies, because of competition, rising research and development costs, governmental pricing policies and the complexity of drug discovery and evaluation in multifactorial diseases, will undoubtedly have a major impact on the numbers and kinds of physicians who will enter and be retained in pharmaceutical companies. The impact of major mergers, strategic alliances and licensing agreements is already having its effect on the structure and function of medical departments. Clinical pharmacologists—both medically qualified and those with appropriate specialist qualifications—will be in an excellent position to take command of some strategic positions, and to have satisfying and challenging careers. Four examples of future developments are :

1. *Pharmacodynamic and pharmacokinetic relations, dose–response and surrogate markers.* There is an internal company desire and a regulatory pressure to generate the maximal amount of useful information from phase I and II studies, so that correct doses are selected for phase III programmes; the relation between kinetics and dynamics is exploited to justify dose regimen and to investigate cause-and-effect relationships between surrogate markers and therapeutic response. It is thus hoped that the clinical development programmes can be shortened, with fewer patients exposed overall and fewer regulatory

questions to be answered. Clinical pharmacologists—dynamicists and kineticists—are at the heart of this debate.

2. *Generic prescribing and inter-company competition with drugs of the same class coming off patent.* The battle to demonstrate superiority between two products which have the same dynamic effects but may have real or marginal kinetic or pharmaceutical differences is becoming increasingly common (e.g. $\beta$-blockers, $H_2$-antagonists, non-steroidal anti-inflammatories). The prizes will go to those companies that can demonstrate clinically relevant differences in tightly controlled, imaginatively designed trials, with dynamic, kinetic and biopharmaceutic components. Again, this is the role which clinical pharmacologists must fill.

3. *Biotechnology and gene (or gene product) therapy.* The promise of these approaches to pharmacotherapy is only just being explored. It is quite uncertain what kind of toxicological studies will be needed or relevant to man, what the challenges of novel delivery systems will have for pharmacokinetics, and how short- and medium-term efficacy will be judged. Again, clinical pharmacology must remain at the forefront of these developments, representing the interests of patients and volunteers who will be exposed to these novel therapies.

4. *Pharmacoeconomics and pharmacotherapy in primary care.* A number of initiatives in the UK have come together at about the same time. Foremost among these are the establishment of a Minister of Science and Technology, the publication of the 'Health of the Nation' White Paper resulting, as one of its recommendations, in the decision to spend 1.5% of the NHS budget on R&D managed through a central and regional committees, and the perception, rightly or wrongly, that pharmaceutical companies are making large profits which are adding substantially to health service costs. Obtaining 'value for money' and being able to demonstrate that value has been obtained is a priority for the Department of Health. Working this through to drug development has highlighted the emerging discipline of 'pharmacoeconomics', which is regarded in some quarters as a 'soft social science', which cannot usefully contribute to judging the value of drugs based on the traditional measures of efficacy and safety. Be that as it may, pharmacoeconomics is here to stay, and unless physicians show an interest in it and how objective measures of treatment 'outcome' can be explored, then it may become the realm of the economist to advise politicians on the value of therapeutic interventions. There is a real opportunity for clinical pharmacologists, both in industry and academia, to be at the centre of this debate, and to align it with the rational teaching of therapeutics in primary care.

## CONCLUSION

Clinical pharmacology in the pharmaceutical industry has firmly established itself as the guardian of phase I studies. It acts as a bridging discipline between research development to man, and integrates knowledge from a number of pre-clinical disciplines for the safe and timely exploratory evaluation of novel substances. At the other end of drug development, it has to help defend the marketed drugs against competition from generic compounds and devise novel methods to test new formulations and combinations. Current and future challenges of using pharmacokinetics/pharmacodynamics modelling population kinetics and dynamics for defining dose response and therapeutic ratio must be taken up by departments of clinical pharmacology. Emerging disciplines of biotechnology and pharmacoeconomics are other areas where clinical pharmacology can play a central role. The flexibility of the discipline and its strong ties with research, academia and regulatory authorities will continue to make it an attractive career option for creative and imaginative physicians and scientists.

# 13
# The Pharmaceutical Physician in Clinical Research

## Karen Summers

Syntex Pharmaceuticals Ltd, Maidenhead, UK

Pharmaceutical companies develop drugs in the hope that they will be used by physicians as medicines to treat patients. The process of drug development is a long one involving chemical synthesis and screening of candidate compounds for pharmacological activity and then extensive animal pharmacology and animal toxicology testing. The next step is the determination of the kinetics of the compound in healthy human volunteers, and, if the results are favourable, the scaling up of synthetic methods from the laboratory to the factory. Finally clinical trials are carried out to show that the product is safe and efficacious to use as a medicine—the process of clinical research.

If the last part of this process is completed successfully and documented adequately the company can then submit the results of the whole body of pre-clinical and clinical research to the various national drug-licensing authorities and apply for licences to market the product as a medicine.

It follows that the clinical research part of this process is the one on which the success of all of the stages of development depend. As a result the carrying out of clinical research and clinical trials are the most important parts of any drug development. It is because this all-important last step is one of showing that a drug can be used safely by physicians as

*Discovering New Medicines: Careers in Pharmaceutical Research and Development.*
Edited by P.D. Stonier
© 1994 John Wiley & Sons Ltd

a medicine that pharmaceutical companies employ their own physicians to advise on, and to supervise the conduct of, clinical trials of the company's products.

## THE PHYSICIAN IN INDUSTRY

Pharmaceutical companies are large and complex organisations, and the clinical stage of drug development is a large and complex undertaking. The jobs done and the parts played by a pharmaceutical company physician in this process are many and varied. They range from that of an international medical research director working from the company head office with responsibility for the whole of the international development of all of the company's drugs, to the junior medical adviser in a subsidiary company with the job of managing the clinical research projects delegated to the local research department in which he or she works.

However, no two pharmaceutical companies are identical and companies do not have the same patterns of working or the same sorts of management structures or even the same titles for the same functions. Therefore the uses companies make of the physicians they employ are surprisingly varied, ranging from the pharmaceutical physician acting exclusively as a source of medical information and advice (hence the title 'medical adviser') to the pharmaceutical physician acting as a line manager with a work-load more administrative than medical in nature. The similarities between this latter role and the increasingly administrative function of senior doctors in the British National Health Service (NHS) are striking. Nevertheless there is much to be said for line managers understanding the process they are asked to manage.

In practice a career in pharmaceutical medicine often sees a physician joining a company because he or she has specialist medical knowledge needed by the company to develop a particular drug in a particular indication. Later, when he or she has developed a thorough working knowledge of the practice of pharmaceutical medicine and understands the business of designing, organising and completing clinical trials, these skills may be employed for the purposes of project design and project management at an international level. Alternatively the experienced pharmaceutical physician may be employed as the line management of a team of medical advisers, study monitors, clinical research associates (CRAs) and other support staff involved in running clinical trials.

These roles of the pharmaceutical physician are not limited to pharmaceutical companies themselves. Because drug development is a race against the clock to get a drug developed before its patent life has expired, many companies farm out parts of a drug development plan to independent contractors, or clinical research organisations (CROs), which provide the company with an experienced temporary work-force to put a particular project into practice rapidly. This allows the drug company to complete its development on time. The temporary work-force may include not only CRAs but also pharmaceutical physicians.

It is clear that the pharmaceutical physician may play a part at many different points in the clinical development process, from the planning stage, through the pilot studies (phase II) and proving trials (phase III), through the stage of preparation of study reports for use in product licence applications, to an active involvement in the further investigation of the safety (post-marketing surveillance) and efficacy in new indications of drugs already on the market.

It is not possible to describe all of the jobs pharmaceutical physicians undertake. The following sections give brief overviews of what some of the jobs entail.

## THE MEDICAL ADVISER IN THE SUBSIDIARY COMPANY

The most common position for a pharmaceutical physician to occupy as his or her first post in a pharmaceutical company is that of medical adviser in a subsidiary company. Pharmaceutical companies are multinational corporations and have significant subsidiaries, or daughter companies, in most countries around the world. The medical adviser will probably have been working in the hospital service prior to taking up his or her appointment. Most often new medical advisers have made their career move from an NHS training post as a registrar, research fellow or a senior registrar. He or she will often have obtained a higher medical qualification (e.g. MRCP) or will have completed his or her specialist training. It is also not uncommon for such individuals to have obtained a research degree such as an MD or a PhD as a result of a period of laboratory-based research.

The company the new medical adviser has joined will probably be in the process of developing a compound with an indication in the same field of medicine in which the medical adviser was previously practising. However, this is not always the case, and some companies set considerable store by other aspects of the candidate's CV such as evidence of organisational or communications skills, and ability to speak one or more European foreign languages.

The medical adviser in the subsidiary company will be involved in the practical organisation of clinical trials. These will form part of an internationally coordinated clinical development plan with the aim of producing a programme of studies to make up the file needed to get product licences to market the compound as a medicine. He or she will of course report to the medical director of the local subsidiary, but in practice there will be more day-to-day contact with the international project manager for the drug under development.

If the clinical trials programme is in the 'set up' stage the medical adviser will be involved in the review and fine tuning of the centrally planned study protocols he or she will later put into practice. This will mean attending planning meetings at the parent company's headquarters. He or she will also be expected to make contact with appropriate British specialists to obtain their advice on trial methodology and on suitable specialists to invite to take part in the development. The protocols for the studies may be modified in the light of these discussions and ideas for locally initiated research projects may be formulated.

Following on from this the medical adviser, perhaps assisted by a CRA, will contact and interview suitable specialists and agree terms for their participation in the research project as principal investigators. Questions such as how many patients will be enrolled, what funding will be required, what documents the local ethics committee will wish to see, what arrangements need to be made with local or central laboratories for blood testing, and who to contact in the hospital pharmacy to arrange for the storage and dispensing of clinical trial supplies will all need to be considered.

To assist him or her in this task the company will have a set of standard operating procedures (SOPs) which lay down the steps to be taken and the documents to be collected as part of the process of initiating a clinical trial. These are often quite detailed and exhaustive. The purpose of having them is to ensure that the company's research projects comply with the American and European regulations governing Good Clinical Research Practice (GCP).

At an early stage in the 'set up' phase the company may organise a meeting of the principal investigators to brief them in detail about the drug to be studied and the protocol to be followed. The medical adviser will attend to ensure that there is at least one familiar face to welcome the local investigator, especially if the meeting is an international one, and to ensure that all of his or her national concerns are taken into account.

The medical adviser may find that instead of setting up clinical trials as part of a drug development his or her first task is to take over the local management of a project which is already up and running. It is then necessary for the progress of clinical trials to be monitored, and this is done by making regular visits to each of the study centres to check the data for obvious errors and for completeness. These monitoring visits are also used to overcome any administrative problems and to sort out any misunderstandings which are affecting the smooth progress of the study. Here again the company will have SOPs which will help the medical adviser and the CRA to do the job properly.

During the monitoring stage of the running of a clinical trial the medical adviser may find that much travelling is needed, unless he or she is lucky enough to have a good team of CRAs allocated to the project. If the monitoring is done thoroughly and a medical eye is kept on the abnormal laboratory test results and the side-effect reports as they come in, many problems can be prevented. In addition the analysing and reporting of the clinical trial will proceed rapidly if the study has been properly monitored. At this stage in the project there may also be meetings of the company personnel from the countries participating in the project. These are often held at the headquarters. Their purpose is to review progress and to allow the study monitors to swap notes on problems encountered and solutions found.

The final stage in the process of running a clinical trial will see the medical adviser supervising the closing down of the study and taking part in the preparation of the data for analysis. A final meeting of the investigators may be held at which the results are presented. A paper may need to be prepared for publication or a poster may need to be produced for presentation at a conference. The medical adviser may have an active part to play in the preparation of the study report, although this is often done centrally at the company headquarters. Certainly it is important for the contact with the investigators to be maintained since the company may wish to involve them in presenting the study findings to a wider audience at a later date.

It will be seen from this that the role of the medical adviser in the subsidiary company is a challenging one calling upon both medical and organisational skills. It is also a highly enjoyable one, bringing with it contact with leading figures in medical research and no small amount of international and domestic travelling.

What else will the medical adviser spend his or her time doing? Further training is always an important part of any job. It is likely that a new medical adviser will be sent on courses to learn about clinical research methods, and to prepare him or her to sit the membership examination of the Faculty of Pharmaceutical Medicine of the Royal Colleges of Physicians. Companies may also provide specific clinical or therapeutic area training, especially if a medical adviser is asked to take on a project in a new therapeutic area in which he or she has no previous practical experience. This is a frequent occurrence as companies bring new drugs into clinical development but do not usually change their medical advisers once they have recruited and trained them. Companies with non-English-speaking head offices may provide language training and most companies will offer promising candidates the opportunity to be seconded to the head office for a period of further training.

The likely career progression from the post of medical adviser is either in the direction of international project management and the company head office, or alternatively in the direction of man management and regulatory affairs, with the aim of becoming the medical director of a subsidiary company in due course.

In conclusion, the medical adviser in the subsidiary company faces a challenging task of using his or her medical and administrative skills to ensure that clinical trials designed by the parent company or initiated locally are performed to the highest standards and are completed in time to permit the company to use them to gain product licences for new medicines.

## THE MEDICAL ADVISER IN THE COMPANY HEADQUARTERS

Pharmaceutical physicians who start their careers in a company's headquarters will find themselves doing a very different job from their colleagues who have joined a subsidiary company. New pharmaceutical physicians in a headquarters company are likely to be employed either on the clinical development of new drugs or on the revamping of old drugs. This involves work on research projects designed either to get new drugs onto the market or to extend the active life of products already launched and marketed. It is not uncommon for companies to have two central research groups: one for new products and one for marketed products.

The type of activities the two sorts of jobs entail could not be more different. The primary goal of the one is to produce information of a type needed for gaining product licences, and the goal of the other is to produce clinical research of use in marketing a drug.

In the pre-marketing research group everything is very scientific and structured. Each medical adviser is assigned to a project and will find himself or herself responsible for the development of a protocol or family of protocols which may be put into practice in any of a number of countries where there are subsidiaries with medical research groups. The protocol will be developed to a strict timetable, and the medical adviser will be responsible for planning and running the research project to time and to budget. He or she will be able to call upon a wide range of resources both within and outside the company for medical advice (expert panels) and for the preparation of case record books, clinical trial supplies and other essentials for setting up a clinical trial.

He or she will have to visit the countries in which the study will take place and will have to attend the investigator meetings organised to ensure that the study runs smoothly. The aim of the job is to ensure that each part of the development plan delegated to a subsidiary is completed on time.

Later, in the running of the trial, the medical adviser will have to monitor the rate of recruitment and the data quality, and will have to be available to solve problems for the medical advisers in the subsidiaries. The organisation of the regular project progress meetings will also be the responsibility of the head office medical adviser. However, the real charm of the job comes at the end of the project when the data are all in and it is time to analyse, interpret and report it. Here a good medical mind and an inquiring scientific approach can tease much interesting and sometimes unexpected information out of the data. The final investigator meeting will be the highlight of several years of careful planning and scrupulous monitoring, culminating in the successful outcome of the project.

The medical adviser in the marketing support group will have a rather different time. There will still be an international role to play but the aim will be to commission and facilitate research which results in publications which can be used to advertise the drug, or to organise studies intended to extend the licence and confirm the safety of the drug now that it is on the market.

The nature of pharmaceutical marketing activity is such that it is important for the marketing group of any pharmaceutical company to have good relations with the specialists who use and endorse its products. Medical research into those products forms a good bridge between the company and the key opinion makers. It can be very stimulating to set up exploratory studies in collaboration with leading specialists, but care has to be taken to ensure that the data are of such a quality that the company can use the results for product licence purposes as well as for publication. The company SOPs and the rules of GCP must still be applied, and the medical adviser has a very important role to play in moderating the desires of the marketing people, and maintaining proper medical ethical standards.

Another aspect of research with marketed products is the setting up and running of post-marketing surveillance studies. These are designed to obtain large bodies of information about the side-effects and about the efficacy of marketed drugs in routine use. The inevitable consequence of any research activity is that a drug gets talked about and used. Great care has to be taken to ensure that research of this type is not subverted for the purposes of promoting sales rather than answering scientific questions. This is where the medical adviser has such an important part to play. By safeguarding the medical ethics and scientific integrity of the study he or she automatically safeguards the company from charges of malpractice. The design and execution of such studies is therefore a very important job. Nevertheless other qualities are also needed to make a successful phase IV pharmaceutical physician.

Whereas the early stages of drug development require the strict application of scientific method, the later stages of a drug's evolution in the market-place call for creative and imaginative application of scientific information. It was such an imaginative leap that turned the unwanted side-effect of hirsuitism in the antihypertensive drug minoxidil into a treatment for male-pattern baldness. This niche in clinical research is certainly not to everyone's taste, but it can be a fertile ground for career development for the medical adviser with an outgoing personality and an enthusiasm for making things happen.

Both types of head office medical advisers have the same training needs as the subsidiary company medical adviser, and the career paths open to them are probably not very different either.

## THE PHARMACEUTICAL PHYSICIAN AS INTERNATIONAL PROJECT MANAGER

A pivotal post in the middle orders of the head office clinical research group is that of international project manager. The individual in this post is responsible for steering a particular compound through the various stages of its clinical development and for seeing it over the registration hurdles and into the market-place.

The key task is the writing and managing of the clinical development plan for the new compound. This is an interactive process which involves gathering information from a wide variety of sources both within and outside the company. The plan is drafted, discussed, redrafted, reviewed, rewritten and rediscussed until a final version is arrived at which gives the company the best chance of achieving its goal of obtaining a product licence and so bringing the new compound to the market-place. The final version of the plan will define the types of pilot studies needed in phase II to determine if the drug is effective in treating the target disease. The plan will define the stopping points and the decision points for cancelling or scaling up the development. It will outline the range of phase III studies needed to confirm efficacy and to show superiority over marketed competitors. It will define the clinical data which will be needed to gain the granting of a product licence.

From the development plan the project manager and his or her team will be able to draw up a timetable for the drug development and will be able to plan the logistics required in support of it. How much drug will need to have been synthesised at what stage in the development? How much manpower will be needed in the subsidiaries to run the clinical trials? What level of funding will be needed? These data will also allow the medical advisers working on the project to plan their individual protocols.

The international project manager therefore needs to have regular meetings with the director of international clinical research in order to ensure that the plans for the product fit in with the rest of the company's research strategy, and above all that the planned work can be afforded. The international project manager also needs to maintain close contacts with the medical departments in the subsidiaries where the trials are being run, and to maintain good relations with the international opinion makers in the relevant therapeutic areas.

This is a very challenging and highly demanding job, calling not only for medical skills but also for great management, planning and diplomatic skills. It is an interesting and absorbing job in itself as well as being an essential staging post on the journey to the top of the research and development tree.

## THE PHARMACEUTICAL PHYSICIAN AS INTERNATIONAL MEDICAL RESEARCH DIRECTOR

Probably the most interesting post in a pharmaceutical company's research and development (R&D) hierarchy is that of international medical research director. This job entails directing the entire clinical research programme of the company and coordinating and balancing the demands of the various drug development projects. It is a job which requires great skill and which draws on years of practical experience in international project management.

The international medical research director has to compete in the internal company battles for an appropriate share of the R&D budget, as well as keeping a close eye on all the different drugs in clinical development. Plans for individual drug developments need to be reviewed and their progress monitored. Decisions need to be made about which projects to push and which to abandon.

A company which has an international medical research director with a good supporting team will succeed where other less well-organised businesses fail.

## CONCLUSION

Pharmaceutical physicians are employed in a wide variety of jobs in the clinical development of drugs. All of the posts require a high level of medical knowledge, and most also call for good organisational and interpersonal skills. The more senior posts require knowledge and expertise which can only be gained by working in more junior posts, since there is no substitute for practical experience.

In the end the business of developing drugs into medicines is a medical matter and it is only right that pharmaceutical physicians should be the most influential employees involved in this process.

# 14

# Statisticians in the Pharmaceutical Industry

Trevor Lewis

Pfizer Central Research, Sandwich, UK

The primary aim of a medicinal drug development project in the pharmaceutical industry is to produce a dossier of information which satisfies regulatory authorities that a particular medicine is suitable for marketing. The information in the dossier is derived from data which have arisen from experimental work in the laboratory and in the clinic. Thus the design of experiments capable of producing useful information and the analysis of the resulting data are central to achieving this primary aim. Since the design and analysis of experiments are areas of primary activity for the statistician, it follows that the statistician has an important and central role to play in the process of pharmaceutical R&D.

In the context of clinical research, this central role is clearly recognised by the regulatory authorities. The recent EC Note for Guidance on Good Clinical Practice for Trials on Medicinal Products in the European Community (CPMP Working Party, 1990) emphasises the importance of a statistical contribution in the areas of experimental design, randomisation and blinding, and statistical analysis. More specifically the guidelines state: 'These procedures also include good statistical design as an essential prerequisite for credibility of data and moreover, it is unethical to enlist the co-operation of human subjects in trials which are not adequately designed ...'. Furthermore, the guidelines indicate that 'Access

*Discovering New Medicines: Careers in Pharmaceutical Research and Development.*
Edited by P.D. Stonier
© 1994 John Wiley & Sons Ltd

to biostatistical expertise is necessary before and throughout the entire trial procedure, commencing with designing of the protocol and ending with completion of the Final Report ...'.

It is this *enlightened* view of the regulators, exemplified by the EC GCP guidelines mentioned above and the history of thorough statistical evaluation of dossiers by the Food and Drug Administration (FDA) in the USA, that has encouraged the pharmaceutical industry to become one of the major employers of medical statisticians. In the UK alone there are over 500 qualified statisticians working in the industry, employed by a variety of companies from large multinational research-based organisations to smaller domestic manufacturers of generic products, and also biostatistical contract research organisations which are playing an increasingly important role. The vast majority of these UK-based statisticians are members of PSI (Statisticians in the Pharmaceutical Industry), an independent association formed in 1977 to promote professional standards of statistics in matters pertinent to the pharmaceutical industry. In 1992, PSI and other similar associations in Europe collaborated to form the European Federation of Statisticians in the Pharmaceutical Industry to provide a European perspective on statistical issues in the industry.

In this chapter I will attempt to describe the range of methodological challenges facing the statistician working in the pharmaceutical industry, the skills required by the statistician to succeed in this environment and the potential scope of the statistician's role (see also PSI, 1989). Purely for convenience in this chapter I will refer to the statistician as 'he', although it should be recognised that approximately 50% of statisticians in the industry are female.

## THE VARIETY OF METHODOLOGICAL CHALLENGES

One of the fascinating aspects of statistics as a subject is that the most fundamental concepts are the most difficult to grasp and explain. These concepts, such as the nature of variation and the role of randomisation and blocking, guide the approach to experimental design, whilst the meaning of interval estimates and $p$-values guide the interpretation of the results of statistical analyses.

Thus, the first challenge facing the statistician embarking on a career in the pharmaceutical industry, as indeed in any industry, is to convert his theoretical knowledge about these concepts into the practicalities of the experimental setting in which he finds himself. He then has to move quickly to a position where he can guide the scientist or physician to understand not only how these basic concepts influence their experimental work, but also how to interpret the results of more advanced techniques based on mathematical models. These models make further assumptions about normality, homogeneity of variance, proportional hazards, and the like. The mistake often made is to focus on explaining the intricacies of the mathematical models, rather than ensuring that the data are viewed and summarised appropriately, and that the fundamental concepts which enable one to extrapolate from sample to underlying population are well understood.

A further important adjustment that the statistician needs to make in order for his contribution to be relevant to the experimental work is to appreciate the experimental constraints within which he is working and the nature of the measurements that are being made. Thus many textbook criteria for optimal design and analysis will need to be adapted to the real-life situation. For example, although it may be theoretically optimal to design a study so that all sequences of three treatments (ABC, BCA, CAB, BAC, ACB, CBA) are used, ethical constraints may dictate that treatment B must occur before treatment C, and so only the sequences (ABC, BCA, BAC) can be administered. Additionally, optimality criteria of minimum variance and unbiasedness for estimates in practice may take second place to robustness in the presence of missing observations or outlying values.

It is these considerations that make each experimental situation and each data set a unique challenge to the applied statistician, ensuring a stimulating and invigorating environment in which to work.

The pharmaceutical industry is of course a regulated industry, which places a further framework within which those involved in experimental design and analysis need to work. This framework of regulatory guidelines is sometimes seen as a further set of constraints which limit the scope of the statistician to use his technical insight to most appropriately extract information from the data. In fact this is becoming less of an issue, as the guidance given by the regulators on statistically related topics is becoming more mature. Rather than prescribing specific approaches to use, most guidelines seek to outline principles to follow, define conventions to adopt (where the choice is otherwise arbitrary) and on the basis of the regulator's experience of previous licence applications, proscribe against using inappropriate approaches. Thus well-thought-out guidelines are helpful to the industry statistician, rather than constraining. Of course the guidelines are written from the regulator's perspective, and so are often cautionary, advocating approaches which may help the regulator confirm the robustness of the findings presented by the pharmaceutical company. As an example, the regulators may wish to see an intent-to-treat analysis derived from all the data collected on all the patients. I do not believe this is because the regulators feel that such an analysis is ideal, rather that they want to confirm that the findings presented in the dossier are not dependent on some rather arbitrary criteria chosen by the pharmaceutical company for selecting analysable data and evaluable patients.

So what is the range of techniques used by statisticians working in the pharmaceutical industry? Well, it is wide and varied, reflecting the intrinsic interest of the process by which new medicines are discovered, developed, manufactured and marketed.

The modern discovery chemist has access to a database of information on tens, if not hundreds, of thousands of compounds. In order to efficiently select from this database, multivariate techniques of classification, clustering and discrimination clearly have a role to play. Quantitative structure–activity relationships (QSAR) have been utilised by discovery scientists for many years as part of the process of linking chemical properties to biological activity. These relationships rely on multiple regression and a variety of multivariate techniques which still require considerable refinement to fully address the problems posed in this area of application.

The discovery biologist typically works with scarce experimental material (tissues or animals) in a well-controlled laboratory setting. It is in this area of work that principles of experimental design can accrue great benefit in terms of efficient (and hence ethical) use of resources and optimising the precision of treatment comparisons. Experiments range from primary screens which typically focus on one primary endpoint per experimental unit (tissue/animal) to more complex experiments on promising compounds, with extensive measurement over the time-course of treatment effect.

A part of the development process which is well regulated is that of animal toxicology, with regulatory authorities laying down the broad requirements of experimental design in order to determine the toxicological profile and therapeutic index for the compound in prescribed species of animals. Although designs may be standard, this area of work throws up interesting problems in the analysis of the time-course and distribution of events.

The production of the compound on a small scale to support the research effort, the development of a pure and stable formulation with appropriate release properties to support clinical research, and subsequent scale-up of production for the commercial formulation present the pharmaceutical scientist with many interesting challenges, some of which benefit from a statistical contribution. For example, response surface methodology assists in determining the optimum formulation, mathematical modelling is used to assess drug action (metabolism and pharmacokinetics), and sampling inspection and quality-control methods are applied to large-scale production to guarantee the quality of the pharmaceutical product.

It is in clinical research (phases I–III) where the majority of statisticians in the industry provide their contribution, dealing with trials carried out on healthy human volunteers and patients. This is a fascinating area of research owing to the range of experimental situations. At one extreme small, short-term, well-controlled trials are carried out in specialist clinics with intensive measurement of volunteers on a second-by-second basis. At the other extreme large multicentre multinational trials are carried out, treating hundreds of patients for several years with infrequent visits to the clinic to assess the progress of patients who are otherwise going about their normal daily life.

A clinical development programme may take around five years, during which the statistical challenges evolve as progress is made from exploratory trials to confirmatory trials, as appropriate measures of drug effect are developed, as the safety profile of the drug is understood, and as the advantages over existing therapies are confirmed. It is important to recognise that each clinical trial is not an isolated experiment, rather a contribution to a full clinical development programme. Thus the advice given by the statistician on experimental design and statistical analysis of a particular clinical trial needs to recognise the trial's role within the total programme, the specific objectives of the trial and the overall objectives of the programme.

The specific statistical methodology used in clinical research is obviously dependent on the disease area under study. Because of the nature of most clinical trials, being carried out on out-patients, designs need to be simple in terms of structure in order to ensure compliance with the protocol of assessments. Thus the main issues of design relate to the nature and timing of measurements in order to achieve the trial objectives.

In fact clinical trials typically generate large quantities of data as the safety of the patient is carefully monitored throughout the trial, and as the patient's response to treatment is assessed over time. A major analysis challenge is therefore one of data reduction, with the aim of deriving summary measures of effect for each patient which are clinically relevant and so can be analysed in order to give a meaningful comparison of the experimental drug and positive/negative controls. Additionally, in order that valid conclusions can be drawn from the trial, the analyses need to account for the effect of missing data, early withdrawals from the trial and patients who violate the protocol. It is these practical issues of data analysis that provide a similar level of intellectual challenge for the statistician working with clinical trials data, as do the methodological issues for the statistician working with data from laboratory experiments.

As well as including analyses of data from each individual clinical trial, the regulatory dossier will also contain meta-analyses, pooling data from several studies. Some of these analyses will be prospectively defined in the clinical development plan, others will be post hoc to address questions that have arisen during the course of the development programme or that have arisen from the review of the dossier by the regulatory authority.

Finally, once the drug is marketed further data are collected from clinical trials, post-marketing surveillance studies and market research. Here again statistical methods have a role to play in extracting information to support the effective commercialisation of the pharmaceutical product which has resulted from many man-years of research investment.

## SKILLS AND KNOWLEDGE REQUIRED BY THE STATISTICIAN

In the previous section I have outlined some of the technical statistical challenges that are presented to the pharmaceutical statistician. However, the ability to apply statistical methodology to well-formulated problems is only the foundation on which the statistician must build other skills and knowledge in order to develop a rewarding and influential career in the pharmaceutical industry. The broader set of attributes that I believe are required are summarised in Table 1, and discussed in more detail below.

### Technical Foundation

The statistician is always working with someone else's data, whether it be assisting the biologist with an experimental design or analysing the results of a clinical trial. In either case, when the research scientist (i.e. the client) comes to the statistician for input the starting point is invariably for the statistician to understand the experimental situation and its objectives. This discussion, as a minimum, will lead to the formulation of the problem to be addressed in statistical terms, but more often than not will also refine, and make more specific, the client's view of what is required. It is this process of problem formulation which is fundamental to the impact that a statistician can make to the research project.

Having correctly formulated the problem, then it is the application of statistical methodology, which is at the centre of the statistician's education, that will enable progress to be made towards solving the problem.

**Table 1.** Skills and knowledge required by an effective pharmaceutical statistician

---

*Technical foundation*
Problem formulation/solving
Statistical methodology
Statistical computing/packages

*Knowledge of the context*
Scientific background
Drug development process
Regulatory guidelines/company SOPs

*Communication skills*
Report writing
Oral presentation
Consultancy

*Project management skills*
Task/resource planning
Process engineering
Managing change

---

Thus a thorough understanding of statistical principles and methods and the ability to apply them to real-life situations is the basic technical contribution required of the statistician.

The application of methods is typically achieved through the use of statistical computer software. Packages are now available which facilitate the processing of large databases of information, the exploration of datasets, the presentation of summaries and the carrying out of formal inferential statistical analyses. Long gone are the days when limitations in computer power and suitable software inhibited the statistician's ability to complete an appropriate data analysis. The challenge of today is to understand the structure and conventions of the clinical database, and maintain an awareness of the full scope of analysis and reporting functionality that is available in extensive software products such as SAS.

## Knowledge of the Context

For the advice given by the statistician to be relevant to the work of the research scientist, the statistician needs to understand the context of the experimental work. This can be split into three main areas, namely the scientific background of the project, the drug development process and the framework of regulatory guidelines and requirements.

The scientific background includes the disease area being addressed, the measurement of disease and therapeutic benefit, and the mode of action of both the experimental drug and existing marketed products. Knowledge of the drug development process helps position the current experimental situation and understand how the results will be used to aid management decision-making or establish claims for the profile of the drug. An understanding of regulatory guidelines, and their reflection in the form of company SOPs, clarifies the requirements for quality processes, the extent of the information expected by the regulators and the format in which they expect it to be presented.

Most major pharmaceutical companies recognise the benefits of ensuring that employees have this knowledge and so are prepared to invest in developing a broad understanding in their staff through extensive training programmes. The aim is not, for example, to make the statistician an expert cardiologist, rather to ensure that in consultation the cardiologist and statistician can design experiments to most effectively and efficiently deliver information to answer well-defined, relevant questions.

## Communication Skills

This is an area in which most statisticians do not have a natural gift when starting a career in the pharmaceutical industry. This could be a reflection of the attributes of the type of person who has a flair for mathematical, logical and analytical subjects, or simply that communication skills are not developed and exploited as part of a mathematical/ statistical education. Whichever is the case, communication skills are of paramount importance to the pharmaceutical statistician and need to be developed at an early stage of the statistician's career.

To emphasise this point I would like to take two quotes from an excellent paper (ASA Committee on Training of Statisticians for Industry, 1980) entitled *Preparing Statisticians for Careers in Industry*. Although nearly 15 years old, and not directed specifically at the pharmaceutical industry, much of what is covered in this paper is very relevant to the subject of this chapter. The quotes are as follows:

> Industrial statisticians gain *recognition* through the quantity, quality, timeliness and *impact* of their work: do it, do it well, do it now, *see that it is used*.

> Statistical results are of little value if the client doesn't *understand* them and *put them to work*. The success of an industrial statistician is a direct function of the *impact* of his or her work on company business.

The parts of the quotes in italics emphasise where communication skills come into play. The statistician cannot expect his contribution to be adopted simply because it is logically sound, he needs to be prepared to represent it through formal presentations (written or oral) and persuasive argument in informal discussions. It is through these skills that the statistician and his subject have the appropriate level of impact and influence on the projects in which he is working.

The comments made above about the value of communication skills are, of course, appropriate to colleagues of all disciplines working in a multidisciplinary research environment. The reason to emphasise their value for the statistician goes back to a previous point; namely that the statistician is always working with someone else's data. Thus inevitably the statistician is part of a customer–supplier chain, in which he is both customer (at the problem formulation stage) and supplier (when delivering the results of analyses). Thus acquisition of knowledge and understanding, and dissemination of information, are critical to the statistician's ability to make a useful contribution.

Statistical consultancy in the industry takes on a number of forms, depending on the individuals involved, the organisation of the company and the culture within the company. The latter two points are mentioned as they strongly influence the expectation of the role that the statistician should play. Inevitably that role is part of a matrix organisational structure with function and project forming the two dimensions. Simplistically, the statistician's influence in the projects is easier to achieve in an organisation with a strong project emphasis which recognises the statistician as a key project team member. In many large pharmaceutical companies this is the case in clinical development project teams. However for the quality of the statistical contribution to be maintained at a high level, then this strong project emphasis must be reinforced by a strong functional structure. The reason for this is that it is the latter which guarantees the career development of the staff and advances the nature and quality of the statistical contribution over time. This is particularly important during a period of growth in the organisation and rapid change resulting from technical advances and process improvements.

The consultancy role for the statistician falls into two broad categories: *advisory* (providing the client with statistical guidance) and *collaborative* (participating as a member of a multidisciplinary research team).

In the advisory role, strong communication skills are required to work with the client to define the problem in a manner which empathises with the client in addressing the practical constraints which inevitably influence his experimental work. Wherever possible, the aim should be to provide the client with his own statistical tools and the knowledge of how to use them.

In the collaborative role, the statistician will not only bring his technical expertise to the work of the project team, but will also contribute to broader activities of the team, playing a part in processes of planning, problem solving and decision making. It is in these areas that the logical and analytical skills often possessed by the statistician prove to be of considerable value.

### Project Management Skills

As alluded to in the previous section, the experienced statistician can play a full part in the management of a multidisciplinary project team. For example, clinical development project teams for major phase III drug candidates are often quite large, and the data processing and reporting may involve several data managers and statisticians. The data managers are responsible for the preparation of the database from which the statisticians and data managers generate material for the final report which forms part of the regulatory dossier. The coordination of this activity often falls to an experienced statistician and its efficient conduct is often critical to the timely preparation of the dossier. This intensive involvement in the *end-game* of putting together the dossier, and subsequently responding to regulatory questions prior to gaining approval to market the medicinal product, is both invigorating and challenging.

The pharmaceutical industry is becoming an increasingly competitive industry. One aspect of maintaining a competitive edge is to develop medicinal products in a shorter period of time, despite the increasing demands of the regulatory agencies. This is in part addressed by pharmaceutical companies refining the complex process of drug development and taking advantage of technological advances in the collection, processing and presentation of data. As contributors to this process, experienced statisticians will often take part in initiatives to re-engineer the process or introduce new technology to provide improvements in quality and timeliness.

## CONCLUDING COMMENTS

In describing the skills and knowledge required by the statistician I have hopefully conveyed some idea of the scope of the statistician's role in the pharmaceutical industry. It is a role that is based on the technical foundation given by a statistical education, which has the potential to extend to a fulfilling and influential role, provided these technical skills are allied with an understanding of the pharmaceutical industry and the development of project management and interpersonal skills.

I have now worked in the industry for nearly 12 years, having previously spent eight years as an academic, lecturing mathematics and statistics at university. I have found the industry an exciting area in which to develop a career, in part because of the intrinsic interest of the drug development process and also because of the growth and change that have taken place in the industry over the last decade. It is an industry which provides the statistician with a broad range of data analysis applications in which to bring alive the statistical methods he has been taught. I would strongly recommend the industry to anyone embarking on a career as an applied statistician, as the challenges of the next decade are likely to present even more opportunities than those of the past decade.

# 15
# Careers in Data Management

## Sheila Varley[1] and Colin Webb[2]

[1]ClinTrials Research Ltd, Maidenhead, UK and [2]Amgen Ltd, Cambridge, UK

Over the last 20 years, data management has become increasingly important to clinical development. There has also been an increase in regulatory requirements for establishing the efficacy and safety of new drugs, and therefore corresponding increases in both the quantity and quality of the required supporting data. Increasing computerisation and improved technological support within the pharmaceutical industry over this time, not only in study analysis but also in the planning, implementation and operation of clinical studies, have enabled review and registration to occur within realistic time limits. In this regard data management has made a significant contribution.

## FUNCTIONS OF DATA MANAGEMENT

Data management is concerned with all aspects relating to data processing and analysis. Data management has a multifunctional role within the various stages of clinical development, including some if not all of the following.

### Review

Data management plays a role in protocol review. Data management reviews tables and listings to assist in clearing the data together with

*Discovering New Medicines: Careers in Pharmaceutical Research and Development.*
Edited by P.D. Stonier
© 1994 John Wiley & Sons Ltd

assisting statistical groups to categorise the data and assess patient outcomes.

In addition, data management plays an important role in review of the clinical study report, ensuring consistency and accuracy in study results and conclusions.

## Design

Data management plays a key role in the design of the database and case record forms (CRFs) for the clinical study. In association with the quality assurance group, data management is responsible for ensuring consistency between the protocol and CRF, and confirming all matters relating to data format and entry. Data management may also be responsible for organisation of the final printed CRF, ensuring that this is attractive and in logical order for the investigator.

## Data Processing and Analysis

All aspects relating to processing and analysis of the clinical study data are the province of data management. These include data coding, entry, validation and verification, transfer of data, programming and statistics.

More recently, data management has become linked with quality assurance. The database is the fundamental clinical data source for registration of a new drug. Therefore, a crucial role for data management is to establish and maintain accurate computer databases for clinical studies, essential to the preparation of final study reports and data summaries for regulatory purposes.

## Project Management

Project management attempts to minimise any conflict of interests and to achieve reporting of the clinical studies within realistic time limits. Data management plays a key role in coordinating the requirements and priorities of different projects within and between each therapeutic group.

## RANGE OF CAREERS

Data management offers a range of important roles in clinical development and, as a consequence, attracts people from varied backgrounds and with different levels of qualifications. Data management may also offer an attractive alternative for personnel with experience in research, clinical research, quality assurance and auditing, regulatory affairs and information technology who may be looking for a career change. The growing importance of data management within the research and development structure has encouraged movement of personnel with a range of backgrounds.

Careers may range from that of data entry clerk to head or director of data management. For the majority of positions some medical and/or computing experience is required; often a degree in life sciences, nursing qualifications or a B-TECH are a prerequisite. In addition, the individual needs to show an aptitude for computer work, to be very methodical and accurate, and to be able to work well both on his or her own and as part of a team involving clinical and statistical personnel.

Considering the different levels at which individuals may become involved in data management gives some idea of the range of careers available. Of course, as with other disciplines within the industry, there is some variation between companies in the job descriptions and responsibilities associated with the different titles.

Individuals with data entry experience and some medical background, such as that provided by nursing experience, and with proven initiative and attention to detail, may consider a position in data entry, as for example a *data entry clerk*. In this position, the individual would work on his or her own with minimum supervision, entering data rapidly and accurately via a keyboard onto the computer, checking the data and editing any errors.

Those who have achieved GCSEs and have an aptitude for creative design and computer work may consider a role in CRF design, as a *CRF designer*. Here, the individual would gain experience in desktop publishing software used to design CRF pages, developing a library of standard CRFs to streamline CRF production. The person would need to be able to prioritise work in line with project management decisions within data management. The CRF designer may also be responsible for preparation of the final printed CRFs via liaison with external personnel.

Individuals with a degree or equivalent qualifications in the life sciences, and with an aptitude for computer work and attention to detail, may consider a position as a *clinical data coordinator/manager*. In this position, the individual would be responsible for the creation, updating, maintenance and validation of clinical study databases and for the provision of computerised reports of these data. Thus the clinical data coordinator is a key member of the clinical project team, and should be able to prioritise work in line with project management decisions. Proven aptitude for this work may lead to career possibilities within quality assurance or within an IT group.

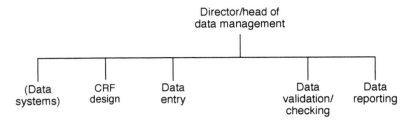

**Figure 1.** Reporting structure within data management: flat management structure.

Finally, those with a degree or equivalent computing qualifications may consider a position as a *programmer*. In this position, the individual would be responsible for setting up and maintaining a secure database, and for analysing and reporting the data to specific deadlines. As a prerequisite, the individual would need to be able to work well as part of team involving both computing and non-computing specialists.

An essential component of the majority of positions within data management is the ability to work effectively as part of a multidisciplinary team, involving liaison between data management and clinical research and regulatory personnel. The individual must be able to ensure that other members of the team are able to recognise realistic time constraints involved in his work and to plan for these within the different projects. Thus, assertiveness is a very important characteristic for many of these positions.

Figures 1 and 2 indicate the interrelationships between these positions. Ultimately, all personnel working within data management will report to the director or head of data management. Depending on the size of the company or the contract research organisation (CRO), there may be either a flat management structure, in which each group reports directly to the head of data management (Figure 1), or a more hierarchical structure, in which personnel report to the manager for each group, who in turn reports to the head of data management (Figure 2), with the sub-groups organised along therapeutic lines.

## TRAINING

As with other disciplines within the industry, training is essential for any data management position. Training is needed to ensure consistency with standard operating procedures, to provide an appropriate understanding of the relevant therapeutic areas, and to provide education in new technologies and various aspects of data management.

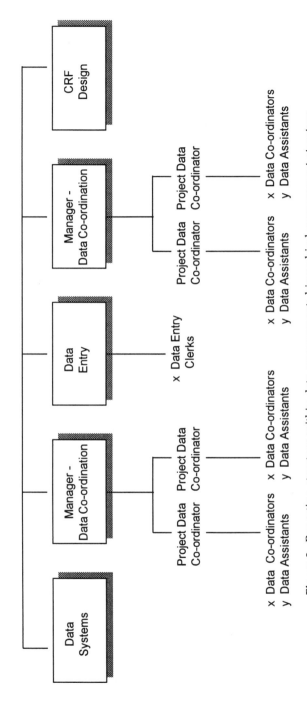

**Figure 2.** Reporting structure within data management: hierarchical management structure.

Training is given on the job and in external and in-house seminars, courses and meetings. On-the-job training is an essential part of the training process. The individual needs to become familiar with internal operating procedures for coding, review and cleaning of data, and with the required software packages. It is usual for the clinical data coordinator or equivalent positions to play a key role in on-the-job training of new data management personnel.

The individual also needs to gain experience in a range of other subjects. All individuals require understanding of the different functions of data management and of clinical development as a whole entity. A basic understanding of Good Clinical Research Practice, the rules governing the conduct of clinical trials, and of quality assurance and audit are also required. In addition, for the majority of positions at least a basic understanding of the therapeutic areas is required. This training may be provided by external courses or by in-house seminars and workshops.

Furthermore, graduate staff may be offered training courses in personnel development, such as project and time management, presentation skills, problem solving and negotiation skills, to further career development.

## CAREER DEVELOPMENT

Experience in data management can offer a range of possibilities for career progression within the pharmaceutical industry.

Within data management, many companies offer, or are working towards, parallel career progression. A new graduate may work for two to five years as a data coordinator/monitor/analyst and then may take on additional project and management responsibilities for up to five members of staff. Training in management skills such as interviewing, counselling, coaching, delegation or people management would enable the individual to advance to a first-line management position at a relatively young age.

Alternatively, staff may decide to specialise in one of the many areas of data management, thereby progressing to a senior level as a sole contributor and being acknowledged for individual technological knowledge.

However, progression within data management is not the only career option. Other possibilities include the following:

1. *Clinical research*. Transfer to clinical research, initially as a field monitor, is a popular option. One move which may be particularly successful is from the position of data coordinator to that of field

monitor. An aptitude for attention to detail and previous nursing experience are very important attributes for both positions. Prior experience of the problems associated with data collation may also be useful in minimising the volume of data queries during secondary and tertiary monitoring stages in-house.

2. *Medical writing/regulatory.* Preparation of clinical reports, which involves good writing skills and the ability to interact with others in the team may make medical writing an attractive option for data management staff. Alternatively, the qualities needed in data management would enable staff to work in a Regulatory affairs group where attention to detail is vital.

3. *Quality assurance.* With changes in European regulations governing the conduct and reporting of clinical studies, quality assurance has become a rapidly growing area within the industry. Individuals who have shown an aptitude for attention to detail within data management may consider a move to quality assurance.

Characteristics necessary for positions in data management, i.e. an aptitude for attention to detail, accuracy, the ability to work as part of a team with varying experiences, assertiveness and the ability to organise work in accordance with various time schedules, are very much sought after in the range of disciplines within clinical development. Experience in data management therefore provides the individual with considerable flexibility in career progression.

## THE FUTURE OF DATA MANAGEMENT

Data management has evolved as an integral and important part of the clinical development structure. Evidence of the dramatic growth in career development in data management is seen by the phenomenal growth of the Association for Clinical Data Management (ACDM), which has expanded from a membership of 120 in its first year 1987 to over 750 in 1993.

The growing importance of data management in clinical development has also been reflected in the changing patterns of reporting within companies. In the past data management had usually reported to the head of clinical research, in some cases via statistical groups. However, with recognition of the integral role of data management within clinical development, there has been a trend for a change in reporting structures to allow a direct reporting of the group to the medical director.

There would appear to be considerable expansion of the role of data management in clinical development. Technological advances in computerisation, such as optical imaging, object-orientated databases, distributed databases, electronic data transfer from source, and voice and character recognition, mean that future prospects for careers in data management will be particularly bright and offer exciting opportunities. Added to this increased recognition of the importance of data management to the registration process. A career in data management can offer the individual a range of benefits that other disciplines within the industry may not or cannot match.

# 16
# A Career in Clinical Quality Assurance

## Richard K. Rondel

Oxford Workshops, Woking, UK

Describing the prospects for a career in clinical quality assurance (CQA) is hampered by the fact that the discipline is young, poorly defined and, as yet, not universally recognised by the pharmaceutical industry. There is thus little yet in the way of 'track record' on which to base assessments.

The nature of the job, the requirements for performing it well, and the career prospects for those entering CQA will be assessed against that background. The information provided, though largely subjective, should be sufficient to allow a prospective entrant to ask sufficient questions, at interview, for him or her to sensibly assess the job prospects in any given company.

## WHAT IS CLINICAL QUALITY ASSURANCE?

The description of career prospects in many sectors of the pharmaceutical industry is made easier by the fact that the activities described are, in general, well established and well understood. This is not the case for quality assurance in the clinical setting, however, and it may thus be helpful to explain what quality assurance is, how it has developed, and how it is practised (see Box 1).

*Discovering New Medicines: Careers in Pharmaceutical Research and Development.*
Edited by P.D. Stonier
© 1994 John Wiley & Sons Ltd

---

**Box 1.  Definitions**

**Clinical quality assurance**. The application of quality assurance to the conduct of clinical research. In the pharmaceutical industry setting this means, essentially, the conduct of clinical trials. These trials can be for the evaluation of any treatment modality, be it drugs, devices, vaccines or biologicals.

**Quality assurance**. The systems and processes established to ensure that a clinical trial is performed and the data are generated in compliance with GCP requirements. Quality assurance is validated through in-process quality control and in-process and post-process audit.

**Quality control**. The operational techniques and activities undertaken to verify that the requirements for quality of the trial have been fulfilled.

**Audit**. A comparison of raw data (more commonly referred to as source data) with data on case record forms (CRFs) and interim and final reports. This would include validation of data both pre- and post-computer entry.

**Inspections**. It should be noted that when audits are performed by government agencies (e.g. the American Food and Drug Administration (FDA)) they are usually referred to as inspections.

---

## ORIGINS

The origins of CQA can be traced back to the time when government controls were introduced for the production of drug substance. These were intended to ensure that the methods by which drugs were manufactured, including the quality of both plant and ingredients, met certain pre-established standards which could be checked by inspection. In this way the purity of the final substance could be ensured, the identity and proportion of any impurities rigidly controlled and batch-to-batch consistency maintained. These regulations for Good Manufacturing Practice (GMP) were introduced, first, in the USA in

1973, and subsequently recognised and implemented in pharmaceutical manufacturing plants worldwide.

One major result of this development is that any drug not manufactured to GMP standards will not be accepted by any health authority for registration in that country. Thus compliance with GMP regulations is an essential prerequisite for the registration and subsequent marketing of a drug anywhere in the developed world.

Following this, regulations were developed—again in the USA—to govern the conduct of certain aspects of the pre-clinical evaluation of drugs in laboratory animals. These were introduced in 1976 under the title of Good Laboratory Practice (GLP). As with GMP, these became rapidly accepted and implemented worldwide.

Thus, regulations covering the production of drug substance and its testing in animals have been available for the past 20 years or more, and now operate on an international scale with (mutually recognised) standards of operation and inspection.

Against this background, it is interesting to reflect on the fact that for the conduct of the clinical testing of drugs—which many would argue is the most critical part of the drug development programme—it has taken so long for similar standards to be introduced. In fact, it was not until July 1991 that regulations governing Good Clinical Practice (GCP) were produced in final form within the (then) European Community (EC). (It is worth noting that these guidelines were drafted and produced by the EC's Committee on Proprietary Medicinal Products (CPMP). They are therefore commonly referred to as 'the CPMP guidelines on GCP'.)

They were subsequently incorporated into Commission Directive 91/507/EEC, which came into force on 1 January 1992. In association with this process the Clinical Expert Report, which is now a standard part of regulatory submissions to the health authorities of EC (now European Union (EU)) member nations, is required to include a statement by the expert, confirming that the trials contained in the submission have been conducted to the GCP standards laid down in the CPMP guidelines.

## LEGISLATION GOVERNING THE APPLICATION OF CLINICAL QUALITY ASSURANCE

As described above there is, therefore, a clear obligation on sponsors of clinical trials intended for inclusion in regulatory submissions to conduct those studies according to the prevailing GCP guidelines. This obligation covers all the activities described in the GCP guidelines; the reader is advised to procure a copy of these guidelines and to become fully conversant with the contents.

One complete section of the guidelines (Part 5) is devoted to quality assurance; this consists of six clauses, as follows:

1. A system of Quality Assurance, including all the elements described in this chapter and the relevant parts of the Glossary, must be employed and implemented by the sponsor.
2. All observations and findings should be verifiable. This is particularly important for the credibility of data and to assure that the conclusions presented are correctly derived from the raw data. Verification processes must, therefore, be specified and justified. Statistically controlled sampling may be an acceptable method of data verification in each trial.
3. Quality control must be applied to each stage of data handling to ensure that all data are reliable and have been processed correctly.
4. Sponsor audit must be conducted by persons/facilities independent of those responsible for the trial.
5. Any or all of the recommendations, requests or documents addressed in this Guideline may be subject to, and must be available for, an audit through the sponsor or a nominated independent organisation and/or competent authorities (inspection).
6. Investigational sites, facilities and laboratories, and all data (including source data) and documentation must be available for inspection by competent member state authorities. These may be seen as having their equivalent in the inspectors used by FDA.

Some comments on these clauses may be appropriate at this stage:

1. The system is composed, basically of:
   (a) staff,
   (b) facilities, and
   (c) documentation.
   These items will be discussed in a later part of this chapter.
2. This requirement is potentially rather demanding. One has only to think of the size, scope and geographical distribution of the clinical research programmes in most companies today to realise that its application would require a substantial CQA resource.
3. Applying quality assurance to the various stages of data handling represents a specialised area of CQA and specific comments on this are not appropriate in this chapter. For a detailed review interested readers are referred to Chapter 14 of the textbook entitled *Clinical Data Management*: Eds. Rondel RK, Varley S, Webb C (1993) John Wiley.
4. The interpretation of what is implied by the word 'independent' is somewhat subjective. The situation is in some ways easier when, as

is often the case at present, the company does not have its own clinical quality assurance function. In this case an outside contractor is normally used. This is comparable to the year-end audit of a company's financial statement which, conventionally, is carried out by an external accountant or firm of accountants.)

5. The term 'competent authorities', though not further defined here, is taken to mean audit by members of a government health authority. At present, few EU member states are actively involved in this process though, doubtless, the situation will change (see also clause 6).

6. The material that must be available for inspection is extensive. It is perhaps worth noting as an example that, up to now, FDA (Food and Drug Administration) inspections carried out in Europe have normally been targeted on pre-selected investigational sites.

## THE PURPOSE AND FUNCTION OF CLINICAL QUALITY ASSURANCE—AN OVERVIEW

The prime purpose of CQA is to ensure that GCP, as defined in the official EU or other national guidelines, is complied with fully. This is achieved, first by identifying the activities which constitute a clinical trial and formulating rules which, if followed, will ensure that GCP requirements are met for all of these. These rules are conventionally set out in the form of standard operating procedures (SOPs). As defined in the EU guidelines on GCP, the SOPs must cover every stated requirement of GCP that governs the design and conduct of a clinical trial. It logically follows that GCP cannot be implemented in the absence of a comprehensive set of SOPs.

SOPs are rules for the conduct of a procedure. As such they are not immutable but organic and should be changed when necessary. They should therefore be regularly reviewed and updated by the various operating groups. The CQA function, which is independent of the operating groups, is usually responsible for seeing that this happens and for maintaining the appropriate records.

CQA functions, second, by establishing systems to check how thoroughly the rules are being and have been followed. These systems comprise quality control—are the rules being followed?—and audit—were the rules followed? Audit can be applied at various stages of the clinical trial process. Thus at the pre-trial stage, for example, audit will check that protocol design is congruent with the relevant SOPs and has appropriate input from all relevant operating functions, including statistics and clinical data management.

During the on-study stage, audit can also perform data validation at the level of the trial monitor and of clinical data management (pre- and post-computer entry).

Post trial, audit can examine the manipulation of data for analysis, the computer outputs and the presentation of the raw data. Lastly, the report itself will be audited, first for compliance with the relevant SOP(s) and then for content.

It is interesting to note that there has been a gradual change in approach where audit is concerned. At one time CQA audit tended to be applied at the stage of the production of the clinical trial report. The clinical trial process being the lengthy and slow-moving business that it often is, this led to a situation where, by the time audit was performed, the trial may have finished many months, or even sometimes years, previously. This in turn meant that the investigator may have moved, retired or even died, patients may have left the area, hospital departments closed and hospital records been either destroyed or lost. In these circumstances, problems uncovered by the auditor may thus become incapable of resolution.

The current practice, reflected in the official EU guidelines, is to perform 'in-process and post-process' audit. Thus auditors now operate on a through-trial basis so that the risk of uncovering irretrievable problems is obviated or substantially diminished.

In-life audit of trials does mean that investigators and company staff must get used to being visited, during the course of the trial, by members of the CQA group. This in turn requires careful explanation of what is involved. Time spent in a full and sensitive briefing of those concerned prior to an auditor's visit is time well spent.

Finally, in defining the purpose of CQA we have to consider the question of bias. Everyone involved in a clinical trial has, to a greater or lesser degree, to control and, in effect, to 'audit' their own activities. Nevertheless, human nature being what it is, some degree of bias is inevitable. The tendency to become fond of 'my' compound is well known and can lead to bias in a number of ways. A properly constituted quality assurance function will provide a clear, balanced and unbiased view of what is going on. It follows that this function can only be properly performed by people who are truly independent of the day-to-day running of clinical trials.

## THE CONDUCT OF CLINICAL QUALITY ASSURANCE

### What Facilities are Needed?

As already defined, quality assurance consists of systems and processes. To establish these, certain elements are required, namely:

1. *Staff*. The staffing structure of the CQA department depends very much on the attitudes of the company's senior management. In some companies the need for competent, wide-ranging CQA is recognised, and will be reflected in the creation of a group whose size is sensibly related to the clinic research work-load. Other companies may still see CQA as a 'necessary evil' requiring the smallest possible investment, while yet others may decide not to have an internal CQA function at all.
2. *Facilities*. These broadly consist of offices, computer systems and filing cabinets. The proper application of CQA also requires the use of appropriate archiving facilities. Ideally, these should provide a dedicated storage area with limited access governed by suitable security measures. The creation of a custom-built archive can be an expensive activity.
3. *Documentation*. The foundation of all CQA systems is the provision of an appropriate range of SOPs covering all the activities involved in conducting a clinical trial to GCP standards. Other SOPS are usually added which relate to other (non-GCP) aspects of the medical/clinical research group's activities and which may regulate various administrative, logistic and financial activities. (The story of one major US multinational company, which is reputed to have an SOP for the use of the middle management toilets, is probably apocryphal! It does, however, illustrate the ever-present danger of excessive recourse to SOPs.)

### How Should it be Performed?

The operation of CQA is applied in two main areas: in-house, and at the investigational site.

*In-house*

Here, the main responsibilities of the CQA function relate to:

1. *Standard operating procedures*. The CQA function operates as follows:
   (a) To create (or supervise, and/or coordinate the creation of) those SOPs required for the proper functioning of the clinical trial process.

(b) To ensure that all SOPs, once created, are evaluated and updated on a continuing basis at regular, pre-set intervals, so that each remains totally relevant to the requirements of the function it governs.

(c) To see that all staff using the SOPs either have their own complete, up-to-date set of SOPs or have proper access to them if they are to be provided on a shared basis.

(d) To ensure that all staff are familiar with the SOPs, usually through the provision of appropriate training systems.

2. *Equipment*. To arrange for the provision of the filing and communication systems needed to fully implement the operation of the company's SOPs. This includes the creation of an appropriate archive.

### At the Investigational Site

This usually refers to the unit within which the clinical trial is performed. If the study is in phase I, this may be performed on company premises if the company has its own phase I unit, or externally at either an off-site company unit or by an external contractor. The last is the most common situation these days. If the study is in phase II or III, the site is most likely to be in the setting of a hospital or major clinic. Studies in phase IV will often be conducted by general practitioners.

Wherever the trial site is located, the CQA function must ensure by means of appropriate audits that the standards of conduct of the study (e.g. compliance with the protocol, proper supplies accountability, etc.) and the quality and recording of the data generated meet the required standards and that the quality control systems (of which monitoring of the study by CRA is by far the most important element) are functioning effectively.

Additionally, in cases where ancillary specialised tests are being performed (e.g. in haematology, biochemistry, cardiovascular or respiratory laboratories) these also will need to be subjected to appropriate CQA assessment. (This may sometimes involve interfacing with the GLP control systems.)

### How is Clinical Quality Assurance Implemented?

Quality assurance has been practised at the pre-clinical level for many years, under the requirements of both GMP and GLP. CQA is, by contrast, a relatively new discipline and, as yet, there is little or no written guidance on how it should be implemented. While the GCP Directive makes official statements on what CQA should achieve, it does not pronounce on how this should be done.

As a result, those wishing to establish a CQA function do not, up to now, have any authoritative documents to which they can refer and which will give them clear guidance in this area. However, certain general statements can be made, based on experience to date, which can serve as a framework on which to build. These fall under four headings.

*Staff Selection*

Clinical research is very different from its pre-clinical counterpart, and with the possible exception of phase I studies it is subject to an almost infinite variety of ways in which things can go wrong, ranging from erratic investigator performance, through the inherent biological variability encountered in dealing with patients, to other factors such as the impact on trials of political decisions (sudden closure of hospital wards), industrial action (sudden withdrawal of one or other essential services) even down to considerations of the seasons (availability of suitable patients with, say, winter bronchitis; patient dropouts due to summer holidays etc.).

Against this background there is a rapidly developing consensus that personnel involved in CQA must, or should ideally, have a good grounding in clinical research. This is reflected in the increasing tendency of companies to employ both medically and non-medically qualified personnel in CQA who have been engaged in the supervision and/or monitoring of clinical trials for periods of time sufficient to give them a full understanding of the variables in clinical research that need to be considered in applying the quality assurance process. Such considerations may explain why the practice of transferring people from the GLP field into CQA is diminishing, in favour of taking on staff with clinical research and/or data-handling backgrounds.

CQA management is responsible for ensuring that quality control is exercised by the operational groups. As part of this, they will ensure that the SOPs contain adequate mechanisms for these quality control checks to be made. They must also ensure that the SOPs are being followed. In summary, they are responsible for ensuring that SOPs, suitable in scope and content, exist and for providing audit to ensure that these are being followed by all those involved in the trial process.

*Reporting Relationships*

Within the CQA system quality control, as it applies to clinical trials, is part of the day-to-day responsibility of the members of the operating groups. These will report in the normal way through line (or matrix) management. The auditor's reporting line must be independent of this process, though the degree of such independence is nowhere defined.

In practice, the CQA reporting relationship varies widely from company to company, in some cases being to the chairman or managing director, while in others it is to the medical or clinical research director.

As a general rule, the higher the position to which CQA reports, the better. This will help to ensure that the CQA process is seen to be truly independent of those actually conducting the work, with the associated confidence that this will bring in the unbiased nature of the CQA findings. It will also help to ensure that recommendations made by CQA have the necessary 'clout' to be implemented in a prompt and thorough way. This latter consideration is particularly important if the company wishes to practise 'rate-limiting' CQA—a process where each new stage in the trial can only begin once the previous stage has satisfied all CQA requirements.

## Status

The extent to which companies believe in the importance of CQA as opposed to merely paying lip service to the need is reflected by the status they award the person in charge of the function. In many cases the quality assurance manager is an ex-CRA (clinical research associate) who retains the same status in the organigram. The ability of such a person, in such a position, to bring any real influence to bear in the introduction and implementation of CQA can easily be imagined. Other companies with perhaps more sense of commitment will award their CQA manager a status equivalent to the medical or clinical research director. Clearly, there are factors of both a political and an economic nature to be considered here. Each company will have to make its own decisions in the absence of any official guidance.

## Contractors

While CQA must be established as an intrinsic part of the company's clinical research systems, its implementation can be taken care of to a greater or lesser extent by outside contractors. This applies not only to quality control through contract monitoring, but also, and more especially, to contract audit. In fact attractive arguments can be advanced for utilising external contractors in this field, who can be seen to be neutral and free of any internal bias. The situation is analogous to the world of business generally, where financial auditors are brought in at the end of each year to examine the company's accounts. There is the further advantage that contractors can be 'picked up and put down' and thus do not affect head counts and staff budgets.

Lastly, properly established contract research organisations (CROs), especially those doing phase I studies, will have their own quality assurance function, these days, to guarantee the standards of their work; they should be borne in mind, along with conventional pharmaceutical companies, when looking at career prospects.

## CAREER PROSPECTS IN CLINICAL QUALITY ASSURANCE

Against this background the following points need to be considered by those thinking of entering a career in CQA.

### The Job Description

The essential activities involved in CQA have already been described, and will operate in whatever area the job holder wishes to work, be it the EU or the USA. (Where the latter is concerned, however, application of quality assurance at the company level is not a stated requirement—unlike the situation now in the EU.)

Thus the job description may encompass all, or only some, of the activities described, depending on whether the job holder is an 'indian' or a 'chief'. In many companies at the present time—even quite large ones—there is only one person doing CQA—sometimes without dedicated secretarial services.

### Size of the Clinical Quality Assurance Department

As stated this may be and often is small—sometimes to the point of inadequacy. However as the significance, and the value, of CQA becomes more apparent it is likely that CQA departments will grow to dimensions more appropriate to their required objectives.

### The Job Content

This ranges from the creation and implementation of the required systems, through in-house and field-site auditing, to the creation and maintenance of archives. Each of these fields of activity can be a major job in its own right and will have its appeal depending on the character and qualifications of the job applicant.

Similarly, each requires an extremely detailed knowledge of every aspect of that particular part of the clinical research process. In this sense the job content is intellectually challenging and requires not only substantial experience but also a genuine interest in the conduct of clinical research. The commonly held idea that quality assurance is a bureaucratic paper-shuffling activity could not be further from the truth. For those entering CQA with the correct motivation the job is fascinating and provides a unique opportunity to be constructively involved in every stage of the clinical trial.

Indeed, to do the job properly, it can be argued that those in CQA need to know more about what is going on than the people actually responsible for a given operation. A good CQA person can, in that sense, become a 'guru' to whom operational staff can refer for authoritative advice on the problems they may encounter in doing their job.

Where audit in particular is concerned, this will involve the CQA job holder in assessment of the conduct of trials in a wide range of disease states and provides challenges that are both intellectually and emotionally stimulating.

## Qualifications and Personality Characteristics

In the absence of any published guidelines, comments on these can only be subjective, though taking account, nevertheless, of current practices.

From the author's personal experience, the principal qualification for practising CQA is to have a solid grounding in pharmaceutical industry clinical research. It is hard to believe that this can be acquired in much under three years and longer experience—say up to five years—would be better.

Beyond this, other biomedical qualifications, such as BScs, PhDs, degrees in pharmacy etc., can be helpful in determining the scope (and seniority) of the job. A nursing qualification should be included in this list. Because of their training, nurses may make valuable members of the CQA team.

The extent to which a medical qualification is desirable is debatable. The potential advantages of having a medically qualified person in the CQA group will usually be balanced against organisational considerations of both a financial and a hierarchical nature.

It is unlikely that the job holder will perform successfully without the following personality characteristics:

1. A genuine liking for people: CQA is *not*, contrary to some views, a job for introverts or 'loners'.
2. A mellow and mature personality: the operation of CQA can sometimes lead to alarmed, resentful or angry reactions from company

staff or clinical investigation team members—often through misunderstandings of what CQA is trying to achieve. The CQA job holder must be able to meet these without confrontation and resolve them in a constructive way. He or she must work with, and carry along with him or her, staff who often (wrongly) perceive the job as being that of a 'policeman'.

3. Well-developed diplomatic skills: this goes with (2) above.
4. An interest in dealing with things in detail, and in understanding exactly what is going on. This needs the twin abilities of competent digestion of paper-work, allied to determining what is *really* being done through discreet and, if necessary, persistent questions.
5. A methodical and meticulous approach to the work: this is especially true where auditing is concerned.

From all of this it could be said that the ideal CQA person is a paragon of virtue! A summary of the required character would be one who can perform a detailed job quietly and effectively and who can also soothe the ruffled feathers that inevitably occur when CQA is in full operation.

### Training and Education for and on the Job

The training and education required for entry to the CQA field have already been described. Extension of these activities while on the job will largely consist of acquiring experience through performance.

There are currently very few training courses on offer specifically for CQA personnel, though this will certainly change. This present state of affairs simply reflects the relative 'newness' of the discipline.

### Career Course: Routes Upward and Routes Out

Where the CQA department is composed of one or two people, the route upward is limited to gradual expansion of the department, with the associated possibility of the job holder rising 'up the pyramid'.

Where the company has a large CQA group with associated recognition of its importance, the head of the group (manager/director) is well placed, through his extensive knowledge of all aspects of the clinical research and allied processes (e.g. clinical trial supplies), to move into other senior management positions in the R&D division. Project management might be one example of this. Because of his or her knowledge of the strengths and weaknesses of the company's research operations senior positions in company general management are also a possible route upwards.

For those in less exalted positions who seek a route out the picture is not so clear. Much will depend on the situation in the company concerned, in terms of the size, importance and influence of the CQA group in relation to other operating units. The discipline has not yet existed for long enough to provide examples in this respect.

As the various UC member states develop their own governmental CQA and audit activities reciprocal movement between industry and government appointments may become a possibility. Similarly, it seems likely that academic units may need to develop quality assurance functions as they come to work increasingly closely with industry. Exchange possibilities might also exist here, though the financial aspects could be less attractive to those accustomed to industry pay scales.

## THE FUTURE FOR CLINICAL QUALITY ASSURANCE

In general, at least within the EU, the future for CQA is bright. The legislation developing in the whole area of GCP governing the quality of clinical research will certainly progress. Companies will be faced with the associated need to achieve these standards as part of a successful registration dossier. This should result in increased appreciation of the role of CQA in achieving these standards ('do it once and do it right') and the economic returns that come from timely registration. Indeed, the point at which company management can see the operation of CQA in terms of improved financial performance may be the point at which CQA will assume its rightful place and role within the company.

Those either entering or already practising CQA may consider that conveying this message effectively to their senior managements should be one of their prime considerations, if they wish to see their chosen career flourishing.

## CONCLUSION

Clinical quality assurance is undoubtedly interesting, intellectually challenging and worthwhile. Furthermore, on present evidence the CQA function is certain to grow in scope and importance.

# 17
# Careers in Contract Clinical Research (I—Europe)

## Malcolm J. VandenBurg and Ian Dews

MCRC, Romford, UK

Contract research organisations (CROs) are an exciting development of the last decade which began in the USA and subsequently spread to Europe. They grew out of the realisation that it was scientifically and commercially sensible for pharmaceutical companies to bring in expert consultants in areas in which they lacked in-house resources or specialised experience.

CROs function in a similar way to firms of solicitors or accountants in that they act under contract on behalf of their clients to perform specialist tasks. They vary enormously in size, activities and organisation.

Virtually all CROs start as 'one-man bands' and many continue to be very small. The one man (or woman) is usually a professional with long experience in the pharmaceutical industry who tires of the corporate life and decides to offer his or her services on a consultancy basis. At this stage the employment opportunities offered by the fledgling CRO are limited to secretaries.

If the consultant survives the difficult early months and decides to expand the organisation, the next generation of professional staff is likely to be recruited from the founder's contacts within the industry. The newcomers will almost certainly be experienced people brought in to develop a specific area on the strength of their track record and may

*Discovering New Medicines: Careers in Pharmaceutical Research and Development.*
Edited by P.D. Stonier
© 1994 John Wiley & Sons Ltd

well enter the organisation as risk-sharing partners rather than employees.

Many CROs develop no further than this. A few, however, will acquire the resources from accumulated profit or outside investment to become comparatively large companies with a complex hierarchy of staff, perhaps located in several countries. The largest CROs are as big as, and often bigger than, the corresponding departments of major pharmaceutical companies.

Most of the small CROs (and some of the larger ones) work only in particular areas such as data processing or regulatory affairs. The choice usually reflects the professional background of the founder. Larger organisations are more likely to offer the complete range of services necessary to carry a drug from initial design of the clinical operation plan all the way to registration and on into post-marketing surveillance. A few are also able to provide related services such as training and hospital research unit management.

Although CROs are open to as many organisational possibilities as any other company, most perceive their ability to respond quickly and with minimal bureaucracy as an important selling point. Various forms of matrix system are therefore popular and, as a rule, communication between disciplines is freer than in other parts of the industry.

## WHO DO CONTRACT RESEARCH ORGANISATIONS EMPLOY?

The staff profile of a CRO hinges on its size and its range of services. A lone consultant selling only medical writing will need one secretary, or may even do his own word processing; a leading multinational will need the complete range of professional disciplines at all levels of seniority in a number of countries.

The obvious corollary is that anyone seeking a career in contract research will need to pitch themselves at the right organisations.

Highly experienced people, with good contacts throughout the industry, are likely to know the proprietors of very small CROs and invitations to join one will inevitably come by word of mouth rather than by formal advertisement.

The next size up has a lot to offer to the middle-ranking professional who has learned the basics of his or her job and is now seeking greater responsibility and variety. As a small CRO grows to medium size, it must recruit competent physicians, clinical research associates (CRAs), data managers, statisticians and regulatory personnel. Each of these is likely to join a team of no more than two or three in each discipline and will undoubtedly carry a wider work-load and a greater degree of responsibility than would go with the equivalent job in a drug company.

For the newcomer to the industry, however, the largest CROs are the best. Only they have the resources to support training programmes for entry-level staff together with the strength in depth to offer an 'apprenticeship' style of teaching. As there are only a few very large CROs, entry-level opportunities in this sector of the industry are inevitably limited but they have a great deal to offer if they can be found. The range of projects, therapeutic areas and client companies encountered in a large CRO provide a breadth of experience unmatched elsewhere, while the ongoing need to convince clients of the quality of a CRO's staff means that formal training is taken very seriously.

## WHAT DOES THE WORK CONSIST OF?

The very nature of contract research is that one never knows for whom or on what one will be working next. Active projects being undertaken by the authors' company at the time of writing include:

- designing the clinical development plan for a heart failure drug;
- planning a cost–benefit study in the gastrointestinal field;
- reviewing the safety database of a haematological product;
- setting up a programme of antibiotic studies across Europe;
- combining American and European data to compile a UK licence application for a psychotropic agent;
- setting up an epidemiological study;
- compiling a licence application in angina and hypertension for submission to all four Scandinavian authorities;
- updating the syllabus for a series of Good Clinical Practice (GCP) courses;
- assisting a hospital research unit through the changeover from health authority to trust;
- a monitor training exercise based on role-playing the part of the difficult investigator;
- monitoring adverse events in a major post-marketing surveillance project.

## WHAT SORT OF PERSON DOES WELL IN A CONTRACT RESEARCH ORGANISATION?

Obviously, to cope with the role described above, one needs a broadly based professional background together with basic pharmaceutical skills. Even more important is the right personality. A successful professional in contract research needs the right balance between self-confidence and willingness to learn. He or she will need to be self-motivated and resourceful and to have the interpersonal skills necessary for working closely with fellow professionals from several different disciplines. The ability to project courtesy and competence is an enormous asset in dealing with clients.

## WHAT ARE THE ADVANTAGES OF A CONTRACT RESEARCH ORGANISATION?

More than anything, a unique level of job satisfaction. In no other aspect of the industry can a professional contribute in so many ways to so many interesting projects.

Closely linked to this is the outstanding on-the-job training that comes from handling literally dozens of major projects each year in a wide range of therapeutic areas for a large number of European, American and Japanese companies. This is supplemented by the opportunity to attend outside courses. It is perhaps not surprising that a serious problem faced by leading CROs is head-hunting of their staff by pharmaceutical companies.

Another attraction for many of us is the friendly working atmosphere that is usually found in a CRO: first names and good communication between departments are common; office politics and plastic coffee-machine beakers are rare.

In the longer term, a talented and hard-working member of a CRO team is likely to find fewer obstacles to development and promotion than in a mainstream company. All directors of function in the authors' company were recruited by internal promotion.

## WHAT ARE THE DISADVANTAGES?

Nothing is perfect and CROs, like other companies, have their downside. It always used to be said that one great disadvantage was the lack of job security compared with mainstream pharmaceutical companies. While it is certainly true that CROs cannot fall back on the reliable income from a well-established drug, the recent history of the pharmaceutical industry suggests that the swallowing of one drug company by another is at least as real a threat to jobs.

A more genuine problem stems from the inability of even the largest

CROs to match the resources devoted to creature comforts by multi-national corporations. If your dream in life involves elegant offices in manicured parkland, contract research is not for you. A taste for subsidised cordon bleu dining-rooms or club-class travel would be similarly misplaced.

On a subtler level one must remember that the high visibility which allows the talented worker to rise rapidly through the organisation can be disastrous to the time-marker. Few CROs can afford passengers.

# 18
# Careers in Contract Clinical Research (II—USA)

## Jan I. Drayer

G. H. Besselaar Associates, Princeton, New Jersey, USA

Contract clinical research organisations (CROs) have gained recognition as a much needed resource for the pharmaceutical industry. CROs have been around for about 20 years, and their acceptance has ranged over time from 'never used' to 'using them all the time'.

Currently, there are probably more than 300 CROs in the USA and an equal number in Europe. Because of differences in regulations guiding clinical research, the number of CROs in Japan is small. It is likely that this number will increase once Good Clinical Practice (GCP) for clinical research has been universally accepted. This could occur as soon as 1995 following the third International Conference on Harmonization (ICH).

In a recent survey, an increase in the use of CROs is projected for virtually all clinical research services. Within the USA these services will emphasise phases IIIa, IIIb, IV and pharmacoeconomic studies (Vogel, 1993). Others have projected annual growth at 20% for an estimated total market size of $1.8 billion in 1996 (Lightfoot, 1992).

It seems evident that job opportunities in clinical research in CROs will increase, while those in the pharmaceutical companies may remain stable or decrease due to pressures to become more cost-efficient in the changing health care system.

Before addressing specific job opportunities and career paths within

*Discovering New Medicines: Careers in Pharmaceutical Research and Development.*
Edited by P.D. Stonier
© 1994 John Wiley & Sons Ltd

CROs it is important to recognise the differences among CROs and differences between CROs and pharmaceutical companies.

## CONTRACT CLINICAL RESEARCH ORGANISATIONS

CROs can be divided arbitrarily into three categories (Table 1). Some CROs, mostly the larger organisations with more than 500 employees, provide full services in all areas of clinical drug development, from consultation to pharmacoeconomic studies, including phase I through IV clinical research, data management and biostatistics and regulatory affairs services, and typically all of that on a worldwide basis. A few of these companies have linked with sister organisations to provide non-clinical and laboratory services as well as clinical drug development. In particular, such linkages provide better and more timely interactions

**Table 1.**   Types of clinical CROs

1. Full service
   Consulting on drug development
   Data management and statistics
   Regulatory affairs and
   Clinical research, phases I–IV

2. Full service, specialised
   Local/national
   Phase I only
   Phase IV only
   Pharmacoeconomics

3. Specialised, not full service
   Consulting, e.g., on
   ● Drug development
   ● Regulatory affairs
   ● Statistics
   ● Project management

   Stand-alone services, e.g.
   ● Data management
   ● Medical writing
   ● Study site monitoring
   ● Investigator databanks

   Special testings, e.g.
   ● Cognitive function testing
   ● Ambulatory blood pressure monitoring
   ● Holter monitoring

non-clinical (e.g. toxicology) and clinical services needed for the approval of a new compound, thereby gaining time and reducing spending.

A second category of CROs include those that provide full services but focus on specific areas. The number of such CROs is relatively small, with in-house staff ranging from 20 to several hundred employees. This category includes CROs that work within one geographical area (e.g. UK, Europe or the USA), in a specific phase of clinical drug development, or in areas of new interest such as pharmacoeconomic studies. They provide all services needed (e.g. regulatory affairs, statistics) to provide a complete end-product such as a clinical trial report.

A third category includes CROs that provide specialised services only (e.g. phase I clinical research or phase IV and other periapproval studies). The majority of CROs fit this category. The size of these organisations is usually small, from a single individual to fewer than 100 employees. Most specialised CROs provide consulting services only in well-defined areas of expertise (e.g. regulatory affairs, statistics, project management, professional training of clinical research staff); others perform services on a stand-alone basis (e.g. data management and statistics, medical writing) or services in the actual conduct of clinical trials (e.g. field monitoring, investigator databanks). Again, other examples of specialised CROs include those that provide special testing services for clinical trials (e.g. cognitive function testing, ambulatory blood pressure monitoring, Holter monitoring). The list of specialised CROs is endless and is likely to increase when new niches become apparent. It is noteworthy that a number of CROs are forming international or transatlantic alliances to serve the pharmaceutical industry.

Full service CROs actually fit all three categories listed in Table 1. It seems obvious that job opportunities and career development are more widely available in full service organisations than in specialised CROs. This chapter will focus on the first two categories of CROs.

## WORKING IN A PHARMACEUTICAL COMPANY OR A CONTRACT RESEARCH ORGANISATION

The work environment is quite different between pharmaceutical companies and CROs, although the services and standards for such services are similar (Table 2). The ultimate goal for both organisations is to perform parts or all aspects of drug development according to adequate standards that lead to market approval for and successful marketing of the new pharmaceutical compound in a timely and cost-efficient manner. Preferably, this goal is reached in the spirit of full partnership.

**Table 2.** Differences between pharmaceutical companies and full service clinical CROs

| Pharmaceutical company | Full service clinical CRO |
|---|---|
| *Services* | |
| Regulatory affairs | Same |
| Data management/statistics | |
| Clinical research | |
| *Standards* | |
| Set by regulatory agencies | Same |
| Local legislation | Same |
| Company-specific SOPs | Company- or CRO-specific SOPs |
| *Organisation* | |
| Around medical disciplines | General |
| *Projects* | |
| From IND through NDA | Mostly small or large parts of clinical drug development projects |
| *Project management* | |
| *(manpower/cost)* | |
| Long-term planning | Short notice |
| Annual budget | Project-specific contract with detailed, aggressive time lines |
| | Tight cost control |
| *Expertise* | |
| Focus on selected therapeutic areas | All therapeutic areas |
| *Number of MDs* | |
| Many | Few |

The standards for the services are set by the regulatory authorities (e.g. Good Laboratory Practice, Good Manufacturing Practice and Good Clinical Practice), local legislation and by supporting standard operating procedures established by the pharmaceutical company or the CRO. However, in contrast to CROs, most clinical research departments in the industry are organised around medical disciplines (e.g. cardiovascular drug development, gastrointestinal clinical research). Projects performed by CROs are usually smaller and of shorter duration than those done within the companies. CROs most frequently are asked to perform large clinical trials with electronic databases or clinical trial reports as end-points, while pharmaceutical companies are involved in the entire process from Investigational New Drug (IND) through New Drug Application (NDA) and beyond. Consequently, the clinical research staff in pharmaceutical companies will gain significant expertise in a single area of medicine or on a single new compound, while those working in CROs will become experts in how to conduct and report on clinical studies for a great variety of compounds. While clinical research activities in large pharmaceutical companies may include five to ten different products at the same time, CROs may work on a larger number of pharmaceuticals during a single year. In larger CROs, this number may reach 100. Therefore, in-depth knowledge on each drug can be expected within a pharmaceutical company, while it is virtually impossible for a CRO to carry in-house scientific expertise for all compounds they work on and in all areas of medicine. The CROs will provide such expertise in a few areas of medicine through their own staff and in the other areas by working with outside scientific consultants. Consequently, physicians for example employed by pharmaceutical companies are more often hired because of their knowledge in a medical speciality, while those in CROs are hired because of their interest in the clinical research process and in a broader medical exposure.

This difference is further emphasised by the often vigorous demands put upon CROs with a focus on tight (at times too tight) time lines and budgets. It is not unusual that the pharmaceutical company demands services to be provided in a time-frame that cannot be met by themselves, while CROs tend to be optimistic in the time lines and budgets they present. Therefore, the CRO will have to focus constantly on process improvements, cost reductions and increased efficiency, while maintaining the highest standards of quality.

To assure adequate medical input in each project, increasingly demanded by pharmaceutical companies, some CROs have created separate scientific affairs groups of full-time employees and consultants in key areas of medicine who will provide input on drug development plans, protocols, case report forms, adverse experiences and clinical trial reports as project team members without necessarily assuming the role of project managers.

In contrast to most pharmaceutical companies, many of the project management tasks in CROs are being delegated to non-physicians. Since the number of physicians employed by the industry is much greater than the number of full-time physicians in CROs (with equally large clinical research departments) it has been said that, in the area of the central nervous system, drug development is held back by a shortage of suitably qualified physicians working in the industry. This is due to the existence of an educational system which places enormous emphasis on academic achievement and appears to regard a move to the industry as a defection (Darbourne, 1993). It is worthwhile to extend this observation by adding that, in general, the pharmaceutical industry and academic institutions have been inadequate in providing training to physicians in clinical research and drug development. Physicians in clinical research obtain their expertise in a pharmaceutical company by working on one drug, one indication for a drug, or even on just one clinical trial over a long period of time. The physician generally will be regarded as experienced in clinical research when the drug they worked on has been approved by the regulatory authorities and brought to market.

However, it should be recognised that this experience is based only on an '*n* equals 1 trial' and may not guarantee success in the development of the next compound. Moreover, this educational process is not helped by the fact that less than 20% of the compounds that reach phase I testing will continue on to phase II and reach the stage of marketing approval, and that the duration of employment of many physicians in a specific clinical research department in the industry is often less than the time it takes to bring a compound from IND to NDA approval. If indeed, as has been suggested, pharmaceutical companies would focus on the early critical phase of clinical drug development and leave the late phase of development to CROs, this picture could change significantly.

The early phase of drug development (from IND filing to completion of early phase II studies which establish preliminary safety and efficacy of the drug) is usually of short duration (one to two years) and requires input from specialists in the area of medicine concerned. Therefore, in a reasonably short period of time, a physician could gain expertise in this phase of development by working on a variety of compounds. The late-phase development (from late phase II through NDA) would be conducted by specialists in the clinical research process (CROs), and because of the exposure of physicians working for CROs to a multitude of projects at each moment in time they would soon gain significant expertise in this area.

The various tasks requested from physicians employed by CROs are listed in Table 3. They are arbitrarily divided into those related to the clinical research process (operations), into those related to the preparation of documents requiring professional scientific input, and interactions with partners required for both tasks (operations and document preparation).

As discussed, all of the tasks listed may not necessarily be performed by one and the same physician, and the list of duties for a particular physician may change as rapidly as new projects arrive at the CRO's doorstep.

**Table 3.** Tasks frequently performed by physicians in clinical research

---

1. *Clinical research operation*
   Personnel assignment to projects
   Training of staff
   Supervision of study management, including
   - Investigator selection
   - Review of completed case report forms
   - Review of enrolment in clinical trials
   - Contract management; on time and on budget performance

2. *Document preparation*
   - Clinical drug development plans
   - Investigator's drug brochures
   - Clinical trial protocols
   - Case report forms
   - Adverse event reports
   - Clinical trial reports
   - Regulatory submissions

3. *Interaction with partners*
   - Colleagues in the sponsoring pharmaceutical company
   - Outside consultants
   - Investigators
   - Regulatory authorities

---

Some of the tasks or functions that are commonly available in a pharmaceutical company and not in a clinical CRO include involvement in non-clinical drug development, the evaluation of licensing candidates, interactions with the legal department related to product liability, review of advertisements and promotional campaigns for pharmaceutical compounds and training of marketing and sales representatives.

Qualifications for physicians who would like to be employed by the full service CROs described in this chapter include any or all of the following: being service (client) orientated, ability to work in teams, having strong project management skills, being goal orientated, being interested in clinical research and the drug development process, and having an ability to work according to tight budgets and time lines for multiple clients at the same time, while maintaining the high standards common in clinical research. Physicians employed by CROs usually have had experience in pharmaceutical companies in clinical research or related areas such as medical affairs or drug safety. They maintain and grow their skills through on-the-job training, interactions with colleagues within the organisation, with outside consultants and with the multitude of partners in the pharmaceutical companies that they work with.

Recently, disturbing perceptions and facts related to differences in interactions between pharmaceutical companies and CROs and clinical study investigators and their study staff have been reported. Specifically, problem areas have been identified such as timely payment for services provided, demands on study staff on completeness and accuracy of case report forms and speed of enrolment, and professionalism of the monitoring staff (LoVerde *et al.*, 1993). It was felt that, in contrast to pharmaceutical companies, at least some CROs did not adequately consider the need of investigators and study staff for timely funding to allow them to employ all study staff needed throughout the duration of the trial. Some monitors from CROs also were perceived as unreasonably demanding and requesting immediate resolution of 'irrelevant' issues related to completed case report forms and not accepting the high ethical standards and scientific input from investigators.

These observations point to significant communication gaps between study staff and CROs and the need to foster a true team spirit in the completion of the clinical trials (Drayer and Newman, 1993). This is probably related to the time and cost pressures put upon the CROs by the pharmaceutical companies, and the changing environment at investigator sites. At least in the USA, the conduct of clinical trials is now more frequently implemented by study coordinators with consultative help from investigators. Groups of study coordinators have formed successful organisations that deal directly with the pharmaceutical industry to acquire new projects. At a time where interactions between pharmaceutical companies and CROs are at the highest level seen so far, as is evident from the many conferences and symposia on 'Working or Partnering with CROs' that are being held and the fact that some companies actually are using the largest CROs as a bench-mark of performance, interactions between CROs and investigators/study staff are just beginning. The physicians within CROs could play a key role in improving the communication with the study staff and come to a better understanding of each other's needs and expectations. In this light, it is important to remember that the goal, services and standards to be provided by the pharmaceutical industry, CROs and investigators/study staff are quite similar: to conduct quality clinical research that leads to timely and cost-efficient evaluation of the safety and efficacy of new pharmaceuticals which fill an unmet need from the medical profession and patients.

Career development opportunities within a CRO are fewer than in a pharmaceutical company, usually directed towards increased responsibilities (from more diverse services to more projects) and potentially culminating in becoming an executive of the organisation. Opportunities for general management experience are greater in CROs than in pharmaceutical companies. Because of the differences in work environment between pharmaceutical companies and CROs, some physicians find relatively soon that they prefer a more hands-on environment such as is found in a pharmaceutical company, while others with even greater entrepreneurial spirits start their own consultant firms, a new specialised non-full service CRO. The CRO world also offers a unique opportunity for pharmaceutical physicians to look at companies from the outside and to decide which might be good to work for.

Currently, pharmaceutical companies most frequently turn to CROs at times of increased work-load, reduction in personnel available within the company or, for smaller companies, joint ventures, or subsidiaries of larger companies, the lack of local expertise and manpower. In addition, companies partner with CROs to conduct international or national mega-projects. In some of these projects, services for one project are requested from two CROs. This creates a new dimension, where professional staff of 'competing' CROs have to join forces to complete an often complex project for the same pharmaceutical company.

The increasing complexity and size of clinical research projects for new compounds, the disappearance of development of 'me-too' compounds, and the down-sizing of pharmaceutical companies will bring increasing demands for operational and scientific input on clinical research from CROs without reducing the pressure to perform on time and on budget. As within the pharmaceutical companies, this is likely to lead to more mergers and acquisitions by the larger CROs, broadening of the service package to include non-clinical and laboratory testing (among others) and to more failures of smaller, less experienced CROs.

The future of CROs ultimately depends on the future of the pharmaceutical industry. To paraphrase a quote of John F. Douglas: They (pharmaceutical companies and CROs) must get it (drug development) right first time with zero defects (Douglas, 1993).

## Part IV

# General Careers in Pharmaceutical Medicine

# 19

# A Career in Product Registration and Regulatory Affairs

Pat Turmer

Hoechst Roussel Ltd, Denham, UK

In almost all countries there is some form of governmental control before medicines for human and veterinary use can be sold or supplied. In its modern form this was probably encouraged in Europe by the thalidomide problem in the early 1960s. However, even before this event controls like the Therapeutic Substances Act in the Poisons Laws in the UK gave a legal structure to the sale of medicines and in the USA the Food and Drugs Acts of 1906 and 1912. Now with ever-increasing new chemical, biological and bioengineered drugs formalistic controls exist almost everywhere.

The pharmaceutical industry, which produces these new drugs, is a high-risk industry in which long development times are usual. The process of 'drug registration' is the last step in the long process of introducing a new drug. This is the formal submission of documents to a regulatory agency in order to get approval to market. The regulatory process starts much earlier and should be seen right the way through the development process and must continue once the drug is marketed.

The aim of this chapter is a brief overview of product registration and regulatory affairs.

*Discovering New Medicines: Careers in Pharmaceutical Research and Development.*
Edited by P.D. Stonier
© 1994 John Wiley & Sons Ltd

## JOB DESCRIPTION

The 'job' of product registration in its simplest aspect may be described as obtaining and maintaining authorisations to market medicinal products in as many countries worldwide as necessary. Within this all-encompassing statement lie a wide variety of actual jobs dependent on the geographical area, size and structure of company, type of product, head office or subsidiary section, size of department and structure of department.

Most major pharmaceutical companies are located in Europe, the USA or Japan, and these areas are where most regulatory positions are to be found. Other significant countries are Canada, South Africa, Australia and New Zealand.

To understand the job description it is necessary to know something about the general system of obtaining licences to market medicines. A certain amount of product development is described in other chapters of this book so a brief summary is all that will be given here relating to the various stages of development to the regulatory process.

Drug development starts with the synthesis of a chemical compound which is tested pharmacologically to determine its activity. It is also tested toxicologically to determine its possible unwanted effects and to estimate a therapeutic index or a ratio of activity to toxicity. At some point in this development a decision has to be made whether or not to progress to tests in humans. This is when the first formal regulatory activity becomes necessary, although it is hoped that there has been regulatory input in the preceding development phases.

In most countries there is some approval or registration procedure needed before potential drugs can be tested in humans. The degree of regulation varies considerably but in all cases a minimum level of toxicology is required, together with varying amounts of pharmacology, chemistry and pharmacy. A clinical protocol describing the study to be carried out is also required. This information has to be assembled and presented in the appropriate form to the concerned regulatory body. Any necessary updates, amendments and renewals have to be carried out.

During or following clinical trials a decision has to be made concerning the suitability of the trial drug for marketing. Many factors will influence this decision. If marketing is appropriate an application to obtain approval must be made in those countries in which it is planned to sell the product. This requires a marketing authorisation (MA) application. This varies in format and detail from country to country but the core data content is similar for most countries worldwide. There are three main parts describing chemistry and pharmacy (or technical aspects): experimental, biological and toxicological aspects, and clinical details. These three parts are accompanied by administrative details which will vary from country to country.

This registration application is presented to the regulatory authorities of the appropriate countries, whose professional staff will review the content. If it is acceptable, permission to market the product will be given. This may take several years in some countries and involve much dialogue with the regulations and often amendments to the data. Once on the market a product now enters another phase in its life cycle. It is now necessary to keep the various authorities updated with new findings or developments, obtain approval for any changes in manufacture, apply for new indications or additional pharmaceutical formulations, and keep the product information up to date. At pre-defined intervals, which may vary according to country but which are usually every five years, the authorisation has to be renewed. The procedure to be followed varies according to country.

## NUMBERS AND DISTRIBUTION

It is difficult to assess with any accuracy the total number and distribution of regulatory personnel. There is no formal register or exclusive qualification. Some estimate may be obtained from membership of institutions or societies restricted to regulatory affairs professionals such as the British Institute of Regulatory Affairs (BIRA), the European Society of Regulatory Affairs (ESRA) and the Regulatory Affairs Professional Society (RAPS), and often more recent national bodies such as the French (AFAR), Italian (BRAS), German (MEGRA) and Belgian regulatory affairs societies.

BIRA, the first of these bodies, is restricted to persons working full or part time in regulatory affairs. It is not limited to British members, as can be seen by its membership distribution. In 1992 it had 99 fellows (persons with over 10 years' experience and having made a contribution to regulatory affairs), 806 members (greater than two years in full-time regulatory affairs) and 385 associate members (less than two years in full-time regulatory work or in a post only partly concerned with regulatory affairs). Of this membership the geographical distribution was as follows: UK 977, Europe 261, rest of the world 52 (*BIRA Journal* 1994, 13/1, AGM Supplement).

ESRA has a membership of 204, of whom 97 also have BIRA membership (*BIRA Journal* 1994, 13/1, AGM Supplement).

## JOB CONTENT

The job content is as varied as the industry itself. Regulatory input is required at all levels of the pharmaceutical industry, from the smallest company marketing and selling one medicinal product to the largest multinational. The involvement may vary from a purely organisational role, with the main work being done by contract agencies, to an entire department of regulatory affairs with a staff of maybe up to 100 reporting at board level.

The variety in the job may come from several sources, as indicated in the job description. The organisational set-up of companies varies and the regulatory aspects may be stratified by therapeutic group with responsibility for 'cardiovascular' or 'respiratory' or 'dermatological' products, for example, depending on company interests. This is most likely in companies with a wide range of interests. The responsibilities may be geographical, with regional groupings such as Europe, the USA, Japan, South America, Africa, the Middle East and the Far East.

A division may be made between research compounds and marketed products, with separate sections responsible for clinical trial approvals, marketing authorisation applications and the maintenance of marketed products. Another option is to divide responsibility according to discipline, with separate groups responsible for the technical, experimental/ toxicological and clinical aspects of a registration file. Often a combination of the above groupings occurs in practice. The location in 'head office' or in a subsidiary will play a major role in defining job content. Multinational companies have their head office location where most of the information will be assembled and collated and a 'basic documentation set' compiled. This 'basic documentation' must then be adapted according to the authority to which it will be submitted. This may also be done at 'head office' or it may be done locally. It may be a major undertaking, with significant additional items to be written or parts to be translated, or it may only require the addition of a local application form. This will vary according to the nature and structure of the 'basic documentation set', which may be very basic, consisting of reports and technical details and hence requiring considerable additional work or, as is more usual, a file based on either the European or American preferred format, in which a certain level of structure is imposed and detailed summary documents are included. The transposition of an American format file or New Drug Application (NDA) to a European file (EC file) or vice versa can involve a considerable amount of restructuring, although the basic information content is very similar. The process of international harmonisation is now well under way with regard to the actual data but the format aspects are still very varied.

Regulatory involvement may include considerable writing, particularly summarising of experimental, toxicological or clinical tests and detailed indexing and cross-referencing of files. It will certainly require the ability to handle large volumes of paperwork and to be able to extract quickly and accurately the key information from a document.

The ability to communicate, either with other regulatory specialists or with pharmaceutical, pharmacological, toxicological and clinical experts in the company, is also an essential requirement.

Depending on company structure, regulatory personnel may communicate entirely within the company, liaising with research and development staff and with other regulatory personnel, or they may communicate with professional experts from the national regulatory bodies. In all cases an ability to express oneself clearly and concisely is essential.

In some countries the pricing of a drug is part of, and closely allied to, the registration process; in others there is an environmental assessment needed and increasingly now a pharmacoeconomic consideration. These aspects may come into the regulatory portfolio.

## QUALIFICATIONS AND PERSONALITY CHARACTERISTICS

As can be seen from the job content a good basic life sciences background is an almost essential prerequisite for a job in regulatory affairs. It is possible to enter regulatory affairs from many directions as there is no primary qualification directly relating to the area. For a direct entry into regulatory affairs as a first job after graduation a pharmacy degree would seem one of the most appropriate, as it will have covered, if albeit only briefly in some cases, most of the aspects of drug registration. However, new graduates entering industry, particularly into such a general or wide-ranging area as regulatory affairs, may find it difficult to appreciate all the aspects of the job. There can be advantages in gaining industrial experience in a more specialised area before moving into regulatory affairs. Thus as well as pharmacists, pharmacologists, toxicologists, microbiologists, clinical research scientists or information specialists may all find their previous experience helpful and their specialist knowledge of value to the regulatory affairs department.

In positions where there is extensive writing or summarising involved, medical writing experience could be advantageous.

In a large multinational company with widespread interests, opportunities will exist for personnel with a wide range of qualifications, but many companies are small and specialised and here specific qualifications may be more important. Examples of these are companies specialising in ophthalmic products or in vaccines, blood or immunological products. Here the regulatory requirements are of a more specialised nature although the same general procedures apply.

There is no ideal or typical regulatory affairs character. There are, however, certain characteristics which are helpful. Capacity to work under pressure is advantageous, if not essential, because the submission of a marketing authorisation application comes at the end of a long development process and often the time needed for this process is underestimated. When the clinical work is finished it is a commonly held view that marketing should follow soon after. Another useful skill is the ability to handle large amounts of paperwork. Regulatory work is long term: it can take six to twelve months to complete and file an application and then anything from six months to four years or more to complete the assessment procedure, thus the ability for long-range planning, good work scheduling and a retentive memory are advantages. Communication skills have been mentioned earlier and cannot be over-emphasised.

## TRAINING AND EDUCATION FOR AND ON THE JOB

As stated previously, there is no specific first qualification for regulatory affairs. However, it is now a complex and wide-ranging area of work. The main training is 'on the job'. This may involve, in a large department, rotation around several job areas or in a small unit, gaining general experience by the necessity of attending to all aspects of the job. In both cases it is very much a learning-by-experience situation.

Coming from another branch of industry may bring with it a knowledge of some aspects of regulatory affairs; for example, a clinical research scientist could have an awareness of the regulations applying to clinical trials, or a medical information officer might have useful product knowledge for handling post-licensing activities such as product information updates and labelling information, as well as information-handling skills which could be useful in preparing a variety of regulatory documents.

As well as 'on-the-job' training there are a variety of commercially run training courses, meetings and seminars. Courses specific to regulatory affairs are run by BIRA, ESRA and RAPS, while many other organisations include meetings on regulatory affairs in their programmes.

Specifically educational are the BIRA Introductory Course and the Diploma in Regulatory Affairs run by BIRA in association with the University of Wales at Cardiff.

In some countries the regulatory authorities run occasional information meetings or seminars on topics of current importance.

Many national authorities issue news-letters or information sheets which contain detailed changes in legislation, new regulations or updates on items of regulatory importance. Some journals include material, the *Regulatory Affairs Journal* being one which contains entirely matters of regulatory interest.

## CAREER COURSE

Entry into regulatory affairs may be as a junior member of the team, with upward progress by specialisation in one area of regulatory affairs in management. Clearly a large multinational company will be able to offer more in terms of career development than a smaller or more specialised company. However, the latter can often offer more scope for development in specific areas of expertise.

It is important at an early stage in a career to acquire as wide a range of experience as possible before either specialising in a specific area or moving to a more managerial role or specialising in regulatory affairs in terms of general regulatory strategy, input into research and development (R&D) and legal aspects. It is very rarely as clear cut as this and often senior regulatory positions involve all these aspects to a greater or lesser extent.

## ROLES AND RESPONSIBILITIES IN MEDICINES RESEARCH AND DEVELOPMENT

Roles and responsibilities are largely determined by what the company will allow and what the individual will or can respond to. Regulatory affairs ideally should be involved from the start to the end of the drug development, but whether this is active or passive involvement depends on the personalities involved. Does participation at a meeting mean sitting and listening or does it mean contributing to the discussion?

It is my belief that a well-informed, competent regulatory executive can contribute significantly to the drug development programme. There is a need for the contribution to be positive. Too often it seems that regulatory input is seen in a negative light, always putting difficulties in the way of progress. This should not be the case since appropriate input may enable time to be saved.

So what is the role of regulatory affairs in medicines R&D? To be taken seriously and given the opportunity to participate in drug development the regulatory contribution must be able to provide accurate information on current guidelines, guidelines in development, current regulatory thinking, international requirements and local/national differences. Using this knowledge a regulatory strategy applicable to the product in question can be determined.

Much will depend on what responsibilities are given to the regulatory area. Speed in development is essential and often, once the experimental and clinical work is complete, it is expected that dossier submission will follow very rapidly. What opportunities are there for the regulatory department to facilitate preparation of reports? Delegation of work, organisation of resources, use of external consultants and contract houses should all be part of the strategic plan.

In order to fulfil this full and demanding role it is necessary to have the background and confidence to interact with scientists and clinicians at all levels of development. It is not, however, necessary to have the in-depth expertise; the essential is a sound scientific background and the overall concept of the registration file which is often not available to the specialists. This overall view can sometimes be the most important contribution of the regulatory area to development, ensuring that there are not major inconsistencies between the various sections of the registration file.

In some cases, the regulatory department is only brought into the picture at the end of the development. At this stage the contribution is smaller but nonetheless important; the file still has to be put together and submitted. It needs to be checked for completeness and inconstancies overall. It must, however, be said that if a development is to be successful there has to have been someone taking the overall view as described earlier even if it has not been the regulatory department.

## ROUTES UPWARD

The routes upward will depend on where one wants to go. The obvious career development is from junior of the department to senior and manager. Along the path there will be many diversions, possibly to section head or responsibility for a geographical area or therapeutic area or for chemical/pharmaceutical, toxicological or clinical aspects. Specialisation at this level often means continuing to play an active part in the day-to-day regulatory process, whereas at managerial level in a large department the emphasis will probably swing to strategic and personnel aspects rather than routine regulatory activities.

Here again company structure will play a part. Does the regulatory department play a role in strategic planning or is the role limited to dossier submission with strategy determined elsewhere? This might determine whether the upward route is also possibly the outward route, although regulatory strategy in this instance should be considered as the final goal in the regulatory career.

A problem with progressing upward in this manner is that the decision-making process could become divorced from the regulatory process. Good communications and information networks are necessary to keep optimum efficiency.

What can be an interesting career development is responsibility for a local development such as a line extension in one country which may, if successful, be utilised more widely. Here experience can be gained in strategy and planning without the pressures inevitable with a large international project. Thus, career moves within the industry could progress from a position in a subsidiary with major activities on a national level to a major European responsibility through to an international role.

Once again the scope and responsibilities of the role will depend largely on the type of company and its internal structure. There are, however, sufficient companies and structures to offer considerable scope to the variety of ambitions that are found.

It must not be forgotten that there are other regulatory opportunities besides direct employment in the pharmaceutical industry. Many senior regulatory personnel are now setting themselves up as consultants to the industry and it is in areas like this that experience gained from a career in regulatory affairs can be put to good use. It also offers the opportunity to continue to utilise such skills rather than take on greater managerial responsibility associated with or employed by a contract house.

Finally, and not to be forgotten, are careers within the regulatory agencies.

## ROUTES OUT

Career development outward from regulatory affairs is more difficult to summarise. In theory there are many opportunities. In practice it may not be so easy. The obvious routes outward are into the legal area, particularly that concerned with labelling, product information and advertising approval. In some organisations these items may be covered by the regulatory affairs department. The commercial licensing department which handles the licensing of products from or to other companies is another possibility.

Patients, particularly with the introduction of the Supplementary Protection Certificate Scheme in Europe, could be an appropriate move.
With the increasing legislation, health and safety is another area worth
considering.

At a higher level a move into corporate or strategic planning could be
considered but company structures vary considerably, so it is difficult to
be precise about opportunities. Being in the right place at the right time
is often the most important factor.

If a complete change of direction is sought a training period may be
required. For example, moving into marketing often requires a period
to be spent 'in the field' as a representative. Advertising, where a
knowledge of both products and the legal requirements is required, is
a thought worth pursuing; however, the caution and understatement of
the regulatory affairs world might not be an ideal background for this
area.

With the increasing dependency on electronic means of data handling
and the prospect in the not too distant future of electronic submission
of regulatory data there should be opportunities for regulatory personnel in information technology/systems.

If all these ideas fail to satisfy it is always worth considering going
back to the laboratory and finding out first hand why all the things that
seem so obvious to the regulatory people just don't happen in practice!

## EXPANDING THE SCOPE OF THE JOB

If this suggestion was put to most regulatory affairs managers they
would look at you with amazement and say they had quite enough to
cope with as it is. This is probably true. But for those who do find the
horizons limited the answer probably lies in a closer involvement in the
drug development programme, either overall or in a particular area, e.g.
clinical trials or toxicology, such that the provision of regulatory advice
could be related more closely to the R&D need. Alternatively a move to
specialise in, for example, biotechnology products could be the answer.

Does expanding the scope of a job mean encompassing more aspects
or does it mean becoming more specialised? Both approaches could be
appropriate. Where a new requirement comes into being and there is an
option of forming a new organisation to take it on or including it into
the existing structure, opportunities for job expansion or enrichment
may occur. Thus in recent years growth areas have been patient information, health and safety at work, particularly safety (COSHH) data
sheets, electronic submission of regulatory data, Good Laboratory/

Manufacturing/Clinical Practice, standard operating procedures, and quality assurance/auditing.

All these infringe to a greater or lesser extent on the activities of the regulatory department and could offer possibilities for job enrichment or, relating back to the previous subject, a change of direction.

## THE FUTURE FOR THIS JOB ROLE

The future could see some significant changes. This particularly applies in the European region, where the European Medicines Assessment Agency comes into operation on 1 January 1995. It is difficult to predict just what effect this will have in the short term, but long term it should simplify procedures in Europe and by offering a unified system reduce the duplication of effort that currently exists. Whether this will mean a reduction in personnel or whether, as requirements and standards expand, it will merely mean a relocation from small national units into large pan-European units is hard to foretell.

When and if everything that can be regulated has been regulated, Europe has become fully harmonised and closer regulatory relations have been established between Europe, USA and Japan then job opportunities may decrease. At present, however, there are no signs of this happening.

# 20
# Pharmacoepidemiology and the Pharmaceutical Industry

Ronald D. Mann

Drug Safety Research Unit, Southampton, UK

The job description of today's pharmacoepidemiologist is likely to change quickly. Pharmacoepidemiology is a new and emerging science that involves segments of the traditional disciplines of pharmacology, public health, statistics and epidemiology. Its practitioners come into it from any one of those disciplines and those with formal training in more than one of them are at an advantage.

It has been recognised for many years that we cannot, except by good fortune, detect rare type B adverse reactions before a new drug is marketed. The shadow of the thalidomide children falls over this subject—for it tries to address the fact that another thalidomide-like disaster can be minimised, but not totally prevented, only by diligent post-marketing drug safety surveillance. The reason is not far to seek: very few applications for permission to market a new drug contain data on more than 3000 patients. A new drug, if given to the more than 300 000 000 patient-population of the European Union would, if it penetrated 1% of that market, be given to 3 000 000 people. It it had a very rare but fatal adverse effect in one in 30 000 patients who received it, then it would kill 100 people, and these would be scattered in haphazard order across Europe. The need is to spot what is happening and the problem will have to be detected *after* marketing, simply because there is no real

*Discovering New Medicines: Careers in Pharmaceutical Research and Development.*
Edited by P.D. Stonier
© 1994 John Wiley & Sons Ltd

possibility of discovering something that happens in only one in 30 000 subjects from data on only 3000 patients.

## PUBLIC HEALTH

Post-marketing surveillance (PMS), or drug safety monitoring, is part of the business of pharmacoepidemiology—and this part is dominated by the various systems of spontaneous adverse reaction reporting which are used in different countries around the world. The most well known of these schemes are the Yellow Card reporting scheme of the Committee on Safety of Medicines in the UK, the somewhat similar scheme of the Food and Drug Administration in the USA and the central compilation of these types of data undertaken by the World Health Organization in Uppsala, Sweden. The most interesting of these schemes is that of the pharmacovigilance operation in France: this has shown that establishing well-organised regional centres of pharmacovigilance improves adverse drug reaction (ADR) reporting when the centres are staffed by clinical pharmacologists able to give advice to prescribers and linked into a national network controlled by a national reporting centre.

Work of this type—PMS, pharmacovigilance, drug safety monitoring (for these terms are synonymous)—is akin to the surveillance methods traditional in public health medicine, but applied to data on marketed drugs. Many of the practitioners of this branch of pharmacoepidemiology are medical people, for the diagnostic skills and understanding of the clinician are needed if sense is to be made out of individual case reports of suspected ADRs; they are, however, doctors with an interest in public health, for it is the skills of that discipline and of epidemiology which become relevant when the data have to be applied to large populations and whole communities.

## PHARMACOLOGY

Pharmacoepidemiology, as a science, places great emphasis on the pharmacological segment of its name and many of its practitioners are pharmacists or clinical pharmacologists by way of formal training. The work is always concerned with drugs and a knowledge of pharmaceutical products is of great relevance.

In many units pharmacists work alongside medical people in the creation and use of drug and disease dictionaries for these are essential tools in the process of computerisation. Global awareness is needed not only because patients travel, taking drugs from country to country, but also because we need to work towards a single set of dictionaries that all workers can use, and these need to be associated with definitions of ADR reporting terms so that the data are not corrupted by misunderstandings and misclassifications.

## STATISTICS

Many of the best studies in pharmacoepidemiology are observational in nature. There is a lot to be said for the type of PMS study in which nothing is done that interferes with the decision of the prescriber regarding which drug to prescribe for his individual patient. The data are gathered after the prescribing decision has been implemented—and this avoids the manifold biases that creep into non-observational studies.

The observational method does, however, pose great challenges to the statistician, many of whose most familiar methods are suspect or inappropriate when the treatments have not been allocated in random order. Care also needs to be taken in PMS studies to link outcomes with exposure within understood time windows; much attention has to be paid to exploring possible biases and confounders and to validating clinical events and confirming initial diagnoses.

Thus, the statistician working as part of a pharmacoepidemiological team finds the work challenging and interesting for it offers many emphases which are different from those that arise in the randomised clinical trial (RCT), itself highly resistant to bias and much used in demonstrating efficacy. Drug safety work raises different challenges and requires computational facilities and methods that can handle huge quantities of data.

## EPIDEMIOLOGY

The methods used in hypothesis-testing pharmacoepidemiological studies (as distinct from the hypothesis-generating methods, such as spontaneous ADR reporting) are essentially those of the epidemiologist—the case–control and cohort techniques that have formed the cornerstone of traditional epidemiology. Thus, many workers in this field have originally been trained as epidemiologists and it is certain that no unit can operate without advice from those with training and experience in this subject.

## SPECIAL ISSUES

Pharmacoepidemiology in the pharmaceutical industry is much bound up with drug safety; new emphases, which are expanding these units rapidly in some companies and university or other research centres, are concerned with drug utilisation and cost-effectiveness. Pharmaco-economic studies are readily seen by the pharmaceutical industry to be in its own interest, whereas there is reason to think that the industry will, by and large, study drug safety only when it is made to.

The pharmacoepidemiologist studies the real world of drug usage: the randomised clinical trial, despite its vast strengths, has real weaknesses. The worst of these is that it usually excludes the type of elderly patient with more than one disease, who is taking more than one drug at a time, and who presents the most common and difficult clinical problem in everyday practice. The pharmacoepidemiologist, especially if he or she has worked, or is working, on one of the large multi-purpose databases, uses methods which observe these patients treated as their doctors, wisely or unwisely, choose to treat them. Some of this work is also being undertaken, under difficult conditions, in Third World and emerging countries and it is encouraging to see some of this work appearing in the relevant journals.

There is also an increased interest in studying diseases, and disease/drug interactions, rather than just drugs alone, and this can be informative. A recent pilot, unconfirmed study from my own unit (Mann *et al.*, 1993) has suggested that the benefit of hormone replacement therapy (HRT) in protecting against myocardial infarction in women may be confined to non-smokers. Few things can be more important than confirming or refuting this finding for it seems possible that smoking lessens this protective effect—and, therefore, perhaps, other protective effects—and this is a matter of public health importance to large populations. Challenges appear and need to be sorted out and an example has recently occurred with triazolam: our study (Mann *et al.*, 1992) on the VAMP multi-purpose database in the UK shows little difference between this drug, temazepam and nitrazepam in people who have received one or other of these agents and no other benzodiazepine—this finding contrasts starkly with the data shown by the spontaneous ADR reporting schemes and it would seem to be of obvious importance to know why this is.

The first book-length study of this subject is *Pharmacoepidemiology* by Strom (1989); the first journals totally devoted to it include *Pharmacoepidemiology and Drug Safety*, of which the present writer is editor-in-chief, and *Post-Marketing Surveillance*, edited by Professor Chris van Boxtell. As the science has become established societies devoted to it have appeared; principally these are the *International Society of Pharmacoepidemiology* (executive director Professor Stan Edlavitch, University of Kansas Medical Center, Department of Preventive Medicine, 3901 Rainbow Boulevard, Robinson 4004, Kansas City, KS 66160-7313, USA) and the *European Society of Pharmacovigilance* (honorary secretary Professor M. Ollagnier, Hôpital de Bellevue, 42055 St Etienne, Cedex 2, France.

The science-based task of the industry in developing new and increasingly safe remedies for disease brings scientists and medical people together in partnerships which aim to improve the sciences that are used and the products that are available. Pharmacoepidemiology offers a similar challenge and a new set of opportunities—for new people, new methods and a new internationalism is needed and these things beckon those choosing or developing their careers.

# 21
# Careers in Medical Information

Janet Taylor

Shire Pharmaceutical Development, Andover, UK

The medical information department of any pharmaceutical company is one of its key resources. For many doctors, pharmacists and other health care professionals, the medical information department is the first point of contact when they need help with information about a company's products. Often, the information required is complex and is frequently required quickly in order for important decisions to be made about patient management. The customer therefore expects the medical information officer to be helpful, confident and professional. The information officer must be knowledgeable about the company's products and be able to provide the required information in a timely and appropriate manner, ensuring that it is precise and accurate. The customer also expects to be treated with respect, in keeping with his or her professional standing.

Similarly, the company's own field-based sales representatives may be looking for somebody to help them provide that essential support to satisfy a health professional's request for more information.

Therefore, within the company, the medical information department has a key professional relations role. Its staff must be appropriately educated, well trained and fully equipped to fulfil this vital technical *and* ambassadorial role on behalf of the company—a very special person indeed.

*Discovering New Medicines: Careers in Pharmaceutical Research and Development.*
Edited by P.D. Stonier
© 1994 John Wiley & Sons Ltd

## THE ROLE OF A MEDICAL INFORMATION OFFICER

The role of the medical information officer (the job title may vary, e.g. medical information executive, information pharmacist) can vary greatly between companies, depending on the size of the company, whether it is research based or a generic manufacturer, whether it is a head office or subsidiary site, and other issues relating to company culture or history.

Within the UK it is a requirement for all ABPI (Association of the British Pharmaceutical Industry) member companies to have a scientific service that is responsible for information about the medicines which they market. This is also part of a European Council Directive (92/28/EEC, 1992).

Therefore, in the majority of cases in the UK, the key role of medical information officers is connected with providing this scientific service. The role could probably best be summarised thus: to answer technical inquiries about the company's medicines from members of the medical, pharmaceutical and other health care professionals in support of the safe and effective use of the company's medicines.

In the UK, research-based companies would have at least one person responsible for this function, with the medical information officer being responsible for the whole inquiry process. Generic manufacturers may have a more limited service. In Europe the role is somewhat less developed, with the probable exception of companies whose headquarters are in Europe. This is probably just a question of size. However, in some companies in Europe, inquiries from the medical profession are often dealt with by pharmaceutical physicians or clinical research associates (CRAs), with a librarian or information specialist providing the necessary information.

In the USA, company headquarters usually have large medical information or professional service departments with similar roles to those found in the UK.

The majority of UK medical information departments in research-based companies report to a medical director or other medically qualified person.

Besides offering a technical information service to the medical and allied professionals, most information officers will be heavily involved in providing information support to all areas of its own company—to both clinical, research and commercial departments. Further details of these roles are discussed under 'Job content'.

## NUMBERS AND DISTRIBUTION

Every pharmaceutical company in the UK would be expected to have at least one member of staff responsible for medical information, although generic manufacturers may have minimal resources. However, in smaller companies or subsidiaries, it may be necessary to combine this role with another function such as regulatory affairs, drug safety or clinical research.

In total, there are probably approximately 300 graduates plus a further 150 support staff involved in the provision of medical information within pharmaceutical companies in the UK. In addition to this, there are a further number of individuals who provide a service to companies on a freelance or locum basis.

Department size varies from one part-time medical information officer to 20-plus personnel in some of the larger international headquarter sites. However, in some headquarters sites, the role may differ in that contacts may be internal (e.g. overseas subsidiaries) rather than external. An average-sized department for a medium-sized UK operation of a research-based company would be four to six medical information officers plus support secretarial/clerical staff.

As mentioned before, the number of medical information officers elsewhere in Europe is somewhat smaller.

## JOB CONTENT

This will depend on the exact role of the site (subsidiary or headquarters). However, it can generally be expected to include at least the following roles:

1. Answering technical inquiries from the medical and pharmaceutical profession, by phone and in writing. Customers may include doctors, pharmacists, nurses, other health care professionals, research workers, students and members of the public. The exact nature of inquiries will depend on the product range, e.g. prescription-only products or over-the-counter products.
2. Provision of technical information to:
   (a) company sales representatives;
   (b) marketing;
   (c) clinical research;
   (d) regulatory affairs;
   (e) other company staff.

3. Current awareness services to company staff.
4. Product safety, including adverse reaction monitoring.
5. Creation/maintenance of a company product publication database such that information can be rapidly and easily retrieved.
6. Review of the company's promotional material to ensure that it is technically accurate and conforms to the necessary codes of practice and legislation.
7. Involvement in project teams developing new products.
8. Announcement of new product/product changes; liaison with journal editorial staff.

In addition, a number of individuals may be involved in a number of other areas, such as:

- representative training;
- product complaints;
- creation of prescribing information for health professionals, e.g. data sheets;
- product leaflet creation, for health professionals and the public;
- labelling/packaging text;
- writing, e.g. product monographs, training manuals, reviews, journal publications;
- editing a company's clinical trial reports for publication;
- provision of an inquiry service to overseas subsidiaries;
- management of a company's library;
- management of a company's archives or records.

An insight into some of the key roles is described below.

### Answering Technical Inquiries

This will involve talking to a customer (or receiving a written request), assessing their needs, searching the literature, evaluating information, summarising the information and presenting the facts in a clear and balanced written or verbal reply within the time-frame the customer needs (this may often be minutes, not days).

### Provision of Information to Company Staff

This may be a reactive service, with an inquirer requesting information on the company's own products, those of competitors or on a particular therapeutic area, or a proactive service.

Information required by clinical research staff may need to be particularly complex or exhaustive. Often, this may require searching commercial literature-orientated medical databases such as Medline.

### Proactive Current Awareness

An important competitive advantage of companies is to ensure relevant staff are kept up to date with new information from the literature. This is usually the role of the medical information department, who would scan journals, set up specialised profiles on commercial databases, review the data, extensively evaluate it, select relevant information and deliver it to customers in a timely and concise way.

Information needs to be tailored to each individual customer's needs and therefore medical information staff will work closely with the customer to establish their requirements.

### Product Safety

Although some companies may well have a separate group for this function (often called pharmacovigilance, drug safety, product safety or drug surveillance), this may well be handled by the medical information department.

Companies have to fulfil a legal obligation regarding the reporting of adverse reactions to worldwide regulatory authorities and also need to ensure that they are fully up to date with the safety profile of their products.

Therefore, staff will have an important role in identifying potential reactions from the literature and as a result of inquiries or spontaneous reports of adverse reactions from members of the medical profession. They may also be involved with following up these reports and maintaining a database of adverse events relating to company products.

### Product Publication Database

All companies, whether a subsidiary or a headquarters site, will tend to have access to their own product database giving details of key published articles on their products. In addition, a number of companies may have available a database of unpublished articles. For a headquarters site, this may be an enormous worldwide database and require many staff to maintain. However, in all cases the key to a successful and useful database is the quality of the information entered. Therefore, staff will be involved in journal scanning, indexing, abstracting and highlighting key articles from the worldwide product literature for future use.

### Promotional Material Approval

It is essential that all promotional material complies with the ABPI Code of Practice, the UK Medicines Act and European legislation. The medical information department often have a key role in ensuring that the information used in such materials and the material itself is:

- up to date;
- accurate;
- represents current medical opinion;
- complies with the Code of Practice in all respects.

This will involve a lot of contact with the company's own marketing department, advertising agency and medical staff. It also requires highly developed interpersonal skills!

## QUALIFICATIONS AND PERSONAL ATTRIBUTES

### Qualifications

Essential entry qualifications are either a good life science degree (preferably pharmacology, physiology, biochemistry, microbiology etc.), or the candidate should be a registered pharmacist. The exact life science degree preferred will vary from company to company depending on their product range.

Although some companies may take new graduates straight from university in a training role, most would prefer somebody with at least one year's work experience in a relevant area, e.g. elsewhere in the industry or at a hospital. In some companies with over-the-counter (OTC) or nursing-orientated products, nurses or nutritionists may also be employed.

However, with the high cost of investment to train medical information staff, companies are looking more and more for experienced medical information officers *or* pharmacists with drug information experience. In addition, an MSc in information science may be considered useful, but is in no way essential, and individuals considering such a course as a way into medical information should talk to companies first to assess current views.

### Personal Attributes

As the role of medical information officer interacts and interfaces with so many different people—external customers, sales, marketing and clinical research staff—the skills required are many and it is often difficult to find all of these skills highly developed in one individual. Some of the skills are as follows:

- quick-thinking—able to evaluate a situation and act appropriately;
- good technical knowledge—able to *use* and remember knowledge gained during formal studies and from work experience;
- willing and able to learn quickly—ability to assimilate knowledge;
- flexible—able to handle different tasks and people and switch between them;
- high energy level—able to cope with high volumes of work-loads and associated pressures;
- able to meet deadlines;
- personable/friendly—face to face and on the phone;
- outgoing;
- assertive;
- good communicator;
- even tempered;
- able to work in a team;
- thorough and conscientious;
- able to act on own initiative;
- willing to ask for help;
- mature;
- confident;
- responsible;
- lateral thinking/creative;
- a good ambassador;
- evaluative;
- well-organised—able to prioritise a large work-load;
- able to keep calm under pressure.

## TRAINING AND EDUCATION

Training is primarily on the job and will include such areas as:

- product knowledge;
- therapeutic area knowledge;
- company contacts/procedures;
- information skills—use of resources, enquiry handling, customer care, literature evaluation, use of external databases, writing, industry appreciation, advertising material review, current awareness, legal aspects of information use.

Training is generally provided in-house by more experienced senior medical information staff. However, external courses may be used for therapeutic area knowledge and external databases, depending on available company resources.

In addition, staff will require training in personal skill areas such as presentations, communication skills, interpersonal skills, time management and problem solving. Initial training will be provided either by internal or external courses, depending on the resources available inside the company. Follow-up training and development will usually be by means of personal coaching and counselling by the manager.

In addition, where possible new medical information officers may attend a training course run by the Association of Information Officers in the Pharmaceutical Industry (AIOPI). This is a co-operative annual training course using 10 host company venues. Subject coverage includes:

- adverse reactions;
- biomedical literature searching;
- chemical information;
- computers and information technology;
- communication skills;
- current awareness;
- evaluation of literature and medical writing;
- external literature searching;
- in-house databases;
- intellectual property;
- legislation and ethics;
- marketing and business information;
- patient information;
- promotional material;
- records management.

The course provides not only an awareness of a wide range of information skills but also gives trainees an opportunity to visit other company sites, exchange ideas with colleagues, and make valuable contacts for the future.

Most medical information officers will join AIOPI and gain considerably from attendance at meetings and at the annual conference, and by receiving their regular news-letter, where significant issues are tabled for discussion. Some medical information officers also join the Institute of Information Scientists (IIS) or the Association for Information Management (AsLib), depending on their job functions.

As medical information officers are continually needing to learn new skills and keep up to date with developments, reading of journals and attending meetings and exhibitions plays a vital part in their development.

## CAREER COURSE

Depending on the level of entry of the individuals into an organisation, a number of grades of medical information officers tend to exist;

- trainees—new graduates;
- medical information officer;
- senior medical information officer—further responsibility;
- principal medical information officer—further responsibility;
- manager.

Progress and development will depend on the size of the department, the size of the company, the opportunities available and the aptitude of the individual.

It is important to bear in mind that the exact job title may not always be an appropriate reflection of the individual's role and status in the company. A single person providing a medical information service in a company may have all the responsibilities of a manager in a larger department, with the exception of staff responsibility.

In some companies, medical information managers may progress to be in charge of international teams and may be responsible for areas such as regulatory affairs, the library, drug safety, business information or public relations.

Although there is plenty of scope for an individual to expand his or her horizons within medical information, a number may wish to explore opportunities elsewhere, especially in the commercial areas of the business.

Medical information officers liaise with so many staff that they gain a good appreciation of most other roles in the company. Most medical information officers adapt well to their new roles, which may include:

- sales;
- market research;
- clinical research;
- drug surveillance;
- product management;
- regulatory affairs;
- training;
- public relations.

Similarly, a number of the above professionals may make an excellent medical information officer. In fact, some senior business managers in the industry have had valuable early experience in medical information.

Outside the industry, medical information officers have developed successful careers with:

- external database providers;
- public relations;
- publishing;
- training;
- freelance/consultancy, depending on the individual's aptitude.

### Expanding the Role

There is always plenty of opportunity for the proactive individual to expand their role for the benefit of company and him or herself.

The position of the medical information officer at the hub of so many vital activities offers plenty of opportunity routes for those motivated to become involved in a number of other areas, as can be seen from the section on 'Job content'.

## THE FUTURE

Information is becoming more and more important to all organisations, but particularly to the pharmaceutical industry.

The timely provision of appropriate information to the right individual at the right time is essential to help keep the company at the forefront of development in research and may help provide the competitive edge over its competitors.

The role of the medical information officer is likely to develop as more and more information becomes available. In particular there are moves towards increasing information provision directly to the end-user— whether the patient or senior business manager. As expectations increase, end-users are likely to place increased demands on information professionals. Each of these individuals is going to need help to select the appropriate sources to match their needs.

There will always be a promising future for the flexible medical information officer. In an industry where few individuals are as ideally placed to gain such an overview of the business and of the pharmaceutical industry as a whole, the opportunities are almost endless.

In addition, the individual who has a proactive approach to their work is likely to recognise such opportunities and where they can be of benefit to their companies.

*Remember: information is worthless unless it is communicated!*

# 22
# Medical Writing as a Career

## Brenda M. Mullinger

### Tonbridge, UK

Good communication skills are regarded as a prerequisite for many of the careers outlined in this book. Nowhere is this more relevant than in the capacity of medical writer, a broad title that encompasses many job descriptions. Common to all is the need to produce well-written documents that fulfil their function to inform the reader adequately, effectively and unambiguously.

This chapter focuses mainly on medical and technical writing, a relatively new but rapidly expanding field within pharmaceutical research and development (R&D). Medical copy-writing, a more creative communication mode which has been well established for many years, will also be mentioned briefly.

The need for specialist writers has emerged in recent years largely as a consequence of Good Clinical Practice. Many companies have groups of technical writers, while others frequently have recourse to independent communication agencies or freelance writers.

Medical writers provide a service to others, such as those responsible for international clinical research, product registration (regulatory affairs) or sales and marketing activities. The next few pages provide a review of career opportunities for all those who relish the challenge of communicating medical findings in an accurate and responsible manner.

*Discovering New Medicines: Careers in Pharmaceutical Research and Development.*
Edited by P.D. Stonier
© 1994 John Wiley & Sons Ltd

## JOB DESCRIPTION

A medical writer is someone whose primary function is to produce written communications about the use of pharmaceutical products in man, either through original writing or substantive editing. Job titles vary; the term 'medical writer' is often used by independent agencies and freelance writers. Within the British pharmaceutical industry titles such as 'clinical documentation scientist', 'reports production unit', 'medical affairs scientist' and 'editorial executive/assistant' may also be encountered.

Before discussing the qualifications and personal attributes that are needed for a career in medical writing, it is worth considering the type of documents that are required.

## DOCUMENTS PREPARED BY MEDICAL WRITERS

All pharmaceutical companies are faced with producing a variety of texts, often of considerable volume, in support of their clinical research and marketing activities. Although the types of documents required are fairly standard across the industry, responsibility for writing them can fall within several departments and to many and various personnel. Consequently the work of a medical writer will vary from one company to the next and from one agency to the next. In my experience company writers seem to concentrate on a limited range of documents in support of one main function or therapeutic area within their organisation. By contrast, freelance writers and agencies have to be 'jacks of all trades' in the medical communications field.

The major types of documents that might be prepared by medical writers, with a brief description of their purpose and contents, are as follows.

### End-of-study Reports (Clinical Trial Reports)

At the end of each clinical trial a full report must be prepared which details every aspect of the investigation, such as who did it, where, when, in what disease and patient population, using which medications and methods, what was found and what the results mean. These substantial reports are needed for internal record keeping, as part of quality assurance activities and Good Clinical Practice (GCP), to meet statutory requirements of the regulatory authorities and often as part of a submission for marketing authorisation.

Writing a study report is a demanding and time-consuming activity which, owing to the day-to-day demands of running clinical trials, is increasingly relinquished by clinical research personnel. Such reports are the *raison d'être* for the majority of medical writers within pharmaceutical R&D and for many freelances. They are generally written using a standardised and often highly circumscribed format, specified by a company's standard operating procedures (SOPs); some sections may be common to all study reports on the same medicine. In companies where the final study report is produced by those conducting the trials, the medical writer may initially create a report template to facilitate the process.

### Expert Reports and Integrated Summaries

These components of the dossiers needed for product licence applications may well be drafted by a medical writer for use by the national or international regulatory department. Expert reports are key documents which not only provide an unbiased distillation of the important clinical research findings detailed in the individual study reports but also a critique of the methodologies, studies and, indeed, the whole development plan. Their preparation requires skill and experience. The final copy must appear above the signature of an appropriately qualified expert.

### Investigator's Brochure

This comprehensive document is written at the beginning of a clinical research programme on a new medicine and it is updated as additional information becomes available. It informs the doctors and support staff at a centre where a clinical trial might be conducted about the new medicine, its pharmacological and toxicological profile in animals, its pharmacological and pharmacokinetic properties in healthy volunteers, together with any preliminary data from studies in patients. Investigators' brochures are often prepared by the pharmaceutical physicians or clinical research scientists in the project team. However, medical writers are increasingly becoming members of such teams and in some companies they make a significant contribution to writing or editing the investigator's brochure.

### Protocols

Every clinical trial requires a protocol detailing the objectives and methodology of the trial. When a new clinical research programme becomes established the medical writer may be involved in producing a core protocol, containing many standard sections, that can be amplified as needed for individual trials.

## Papers for Publication

The pressure to publish the results of clinical trials in one of the thousands of biomedical journals around the world generally stems from either the investigator's wish for recognition or a commercial desire to publicise the new medicine. Whereas once this was the treasured responsibility of the investigator or the company's clinical research personnel, now they turn frequently to the medical writer for assistance. There are several reasons for this. First, writing a good paper is neither a simple nor a straightforward task; it requires ordered thinking, succinct writing and a feel for the language—skills that are not always displayed by modern physicians or scientists. Second, as in many writing tasks, a quiet environment and protracted periods free from interruption are considered conducive to maximal productivity; such opportunities are rare in the corporate environment or the busy hospital. Last, the chances of having a paper reporting a good scientific study accepted by a prestigious journal are enhanced by paying attention to that journal's requirements on structure, length, style of references and so forth—activities which are second nature to an experienced medical writer.

There are three potential roles for the medical writer in the production of papers for publication. The first is to help the original authors prune and improve their draft manuscript. This capacity as an 'author's editor' has been in existence in the USA for several years, notably in academic medicine. Within Europe it is particularly valuable to authors wishing to publish in a language, generally English, which is not their mother tongue.

Freelance writers and communication agencies are increasingly being employed as ghost-writers for papers which are then embellished by the acknowledged authors before they are submitted for publication. This is a legitimate and valuable activity since it ensures an accurate and well-written paper which, if the science is good, should not be returned by the journal for lack of information, muddled presentation, ambiguity or inconsistent arguments. I find the motivation in writing such papers is the challenge of communicating important clinical information to the profession, the interest from working in diverse therapeutic fields, the opportunity for interacting with international specialists and the satisfaction of seeing a project completed. Finally, it is rewarding to see the paper in print—and pleasing when asked to write another!

In the third role the medical writer has a fair chance of being the acknowledged author of the publication. Review papers, in which all published and/or unpublished data on a particular medicine are summarised, are valuable publications, particularly to the marketing department. Whereas some companies employ their own marketing-based medical writer, such projects are often commissioned outside the company. Indeed, some independent communication agencies specialise in producing their own reviews of pharmaceutical products.

## International Conference Communications

The many conferences around the world provide an opportunity for the rapid publication of important clinical results, and a chance to access an audience interested in the speciality field of your company's product. These conferences generate a lot of work for the marketing-orientated medical writer both within and outside the industry.

Preparing the abstract of a talk, for publication in the conference proceedings, is an art in itself since a lot of data must be condensed into a small space. The actual presentation is a similar challenge, trying to convey in 10 or 15 minutes the results of, say, a two-year long study. In this case, when preparing the text the author must consider the different constructions and syntax used in the spoken language, to ensure a natural flow which captures the audience's attention. Consequently the medical writer may assist clinical research staff in writing either the abstract or a presentation outline.

Most conferences include sessions at which authors can present research findings on posters for viewing by the delegates. The production of such posters is becoming big business, as each vies with the next to catch the eye and communicate a message. It is a field where the medical writer with a flair for presentation can make a significant contribution.

## Medical Information

This is a speciality in itself which is the subject of another chapter. Suffice it to say, some medical information officers spend much of their time writing: answering queries on products from the public or professions and providing reviews or abstracts of current literature in specified fields.

## Product Monographs

Written to inform doctors and pharmacists, the product monograph provides a comprehensive picture of a new medicine, including the rationale for its prescription and an outline of prescribing information.

This is a key marketing support document that does not require the fine detail invariably found in research reports.

### Educational and Training Materials

Medical writers, particularly in communication agencies, help to provide the large variety of materials used in the education and training of company personnel, such as clinical research associates (CRAs) and sales representatives, as well as their customers, such as physicians, nurses and pharmacists. All may benefit from generalised training materials on, for instance, a specific disease or health problem and from product-orientated educational packages. Versatility and creativity are essential as all possible media are used in this highly competitive field.

### Advertising Materials

The scope of work handled by medical copy-writers varies. Certainly, they produce advertising copy and other promotional aids. As this is a specialised field calling more for a flair in advertising than a sound technical background, many pharmaceutical companies retain agencies to undertake this work for them. This approach also allows for flexibility in creative ideas, through access to a number of copy-writers.

### Other Tasks

None of the documents mentioned in the previous sections is the exclusive province of a medical writer. Some may form part of the wider job of other staff within a pharmaceutical company. Equally, writing may not be the sole task of a medical writer. For instance, editing the contributions of others, particularly those from overseas, is a common responsibility. This requires distinct skills that not all writers possess and for which training is limited. Also, many writers have to interact with agencies or freelances when in-house resources are limited, and in some companies the writer heads a team of people involved in the study completion/submission process. These roles provide further scope for the ambitious medical writer.

## PERSONAL ATTRIBUTES

Anyone wishing to be a medical writer requires, above all, an intuitive feel for the flow of language. Although such an intrinsic characteristic cannot be learned it can be developed; many people do not recognise their own writing skills at the beginning of their working lives. Being a grammarian may well be helpful but certainly it is not essential; many writers can tell instinctively whether a sentence is right or wrong. It follows therefore that the vast majority of writers are best able to communicate in their mother tongue.

When producing documents for the R&D function, technical writers also need to be logical thinkers with an eye for detail and a tidy mind. These are not uncommon characteristics in a well-trained scientist. An ability to appreciate the key points within the detail is, in addition, crucial for the writer of reviews and manuscripts destined for publication. For writers on the commercial side, there is a need for greater creativity while maintaining an understanding of the technical background.

Tact, diplomacy and negotiating skills are not the most obvious attributes of a writer, and yet all come in useful. The writer often interacts with others and may have to resolve differing views on interpretation of data or presentation of a report. Some become team leaders working towards a consensus and a goal, while others in their capacity as editors may assume the role of teacher to aspiring authors, or mentor to key researchers.

Self-motivation is an obvious necessity for the freelance writer; in an agency there is also a need for flexibility, stamina and good humour! Burnout is recognised by many as a real problem for writers, for some due to the volume and repetitive nature of the reports, for others due to constant pressure and tight deadlines. Successful writers develop resilience and their own ways of coping; I find plenty of variety is the best solution.

All potential writers should seek to set and maintain high standards and derive satisfaction from seeing a job completed within given time limits.

## QUALIFICATIONS

Despite what seems to be implied by the job title, medical writers in the UK, USA and Australia do not generally need a medical degree although such a qualification may be useful. In some other European countries a medical training is likely to be essential.

Medical writing rarely provides career opportunities for new graduates, as it is a job in which some understanding of the health care industry is essential. Consequently there are no obligatory requirements for qualifications and experience.

## Formal Qualifications

A degree in one of the biomedical sciences, such as pharmacy, pharmacology, physiology or biochemistry, is probably the most useful background, particularly for an R&D-related writing job, although any science degree may be acceptable. In some companies a higher degree is considered desirable whereas in others, with appropriate experience, non-graduate qualifications may suffice.

## Experience

Relevant experience is as important as formal qualifications. Previous industrial experience in laboratory or clinical research is particularly useful for technical writers although some come from academic or hospital medicine. Medical information can provide a valuable background particularly for more commercially orientated jobs.

The most important qualification is the hardest to define—an affinity with writing! Any prospective medical writer must provide evidence of their writing ability: research papers, a degree thesis, even an article for the local newspaper will help! In addition, all must expect some sort of writing test as part of the interview process. This may vary from preparing a précis of a technical report or editing a paper, to proof-reading an article or preparing a news-letter. Needless to say, the CV will be scrutinised too.

## Other Desirable Skills

Keyboard skills are now essential for all industry and agency writers; only freelances have the freedom of choice! An interest in data is necessary, coupled with the ability to evaluate and communicate numerical findings. Other desirable skills and qualifications will depend on the nature of the job. For instance, knowledge of foreign languages, statistics, kinetics or certain therapeutic areas may well be helpful.

## AVAILABLE TRAINING

At present in Europe there is very little training available either within or outside the pharmaceutical industry that is specifically targeted for the full-time medical writer. The majority of courses on technical writing are designed for personnel who write reports and papers as part of their wider job. Such courses can be valuable to the scientist who aspires to medical writing at a later stage in their career.

In North America the American Medical Writers Association (AMWA) has, for many years, been providing specialist training and recognised examinations. A European chapter (EMWA) of this association has been established which hopefully will extend and improve the training situation in Europe.

Companies vary enormously in the provision of in-house training; most seek candidates with established writing skills, then provide necessary training on specific products or therapeutic areas. The availability of training is definitely a worthwhile topic for discussion at interview. Probably the best kind of training is on the job, learning from an experienced writer. Also, much can be gained from observant reading and from the constructive criticism of others.

## OPPORTUNITIES

It is not possible to assess the number of job opportunities for medical writers, partly because of their varying titles and areas of responsibility but mainly because the situation has changed so rapidly in recent years. Several companies which five years ago had no medical writers, now employ a group of eight or more. Although established groups may not be expanding, other companies are following the trend towards employing specialist medical/technical writers within their R&D function.

Since medical writers provide a service, groups are generally located within the company's head office or regional centre. The differing priorities and occasional language barriers often mean that subsidiaries choose to use local freelance writers or communication agencies. They can be found almost anywhere!

Within the UK, advertisements generally appear in the national newspapers, journals such as *Nature* and *New Scientist* and pharmaceutical industry communications. Recruitment agencies may also be involved in finding candidates.

## CAREER COURSE

As yet there is no clearly defined career path for medical writers; this speciality is still evolving. Within the larger pharmaceutical companies and contract houses there are generally two or three levels of seniority for writers which involve increasing administrative and/or management responsibilities. Perceptions of opportunity after that vary enormously. Certainly, some in industry regard medical writing as a relatively quiet environment from which there is no obvious way forward. However, it is increasingly viewed as a good point from which to enter planning, regulatory affairs, quality assurance, international medical affairs or even clinical research, since the medical writer becomes well aware of what is going on elsewhere in the company.

A good medical writer, with broad experience, is generally welcomed by the communications agencies, as deadlines and budgets are often tight and opportunities for training are limited. Agencies can provide the opportunity to work on a wide variety of projects, both in terms of the product area and type of communication.

## Freelance Writers

Many people consider becoming a freelance medical writer, often for the wrong reasons. It is not an easy career solution for every redundant CRA or pharmaceutical physician! Not only is an enjoyment of writing essential but so, also, is the right personality. Self-motivation and self-discipline are obvious attributes; so too are an ability to work alone, generate business, negotiate realistic deadlines and establish a repu-tation. These are not easy tasks when starting from scratch; networking is essential and a contract from former colleagues is generally the way most freelances get started.

Confidentiality, integrity and reliability play an important part; clients must be able to rely on all three. Anyone who works independently is only as good as their next contract, so repeat business and good recom-mendations from a client are essential for survival. But however good, the freelance will always have to handle the irregular ebb and flow of the work-load and income, while being psychologically prepared to refuse work when time constraints are impractical.

The uncertainty of work, together with the isolation, lack of training opportunities and the limited sense of involvement and feedback mean that working on a freelance basis does not suit everyone. Additionally, there is the knowledge that only rarely does an outsider get projects on the latest pharmaceutical breakthrough. More often, communications concern lower-priority products for which the company medical writer may lack motivation.

All this should be of little concern to the freelance writer who wel-comes the opportunity to work in as diverse fields as possible. The var-iety, flexibility, opportunity to exercise choice and above all, the independence, make freelance writing an ideal outlet for those with the necessary experience.

## CONCLUSIONS

For anyone with an interest and ability in medical writing, there is a range of opportunities which is generally expanding. Career paths are as yet unclear and prospective candidates should be prepared to carve their own. Certainly, in this relatively new field, each individual has a chance to develop their own position.

Within Europe, medical writers seem to have an ill-defined image which lacks professional status and recognition. This situation is changing and no doubt in the not too distant future they will occupy a recognised role similar to that enjoyed by medical writers in the USA.

Since the ability to write is an eminently transferable skill, and the need for written communications is unlikely to diminish, the long-term future for medical writers is encouraging.

## ACKNOWLEDGEMENTS

I thank all those who gave freely of their time in answering my queries.

# 23
# Careers in Drug Regulatory Authorities

## Keith Fowler

*Formerly*: Medicines Control Agency, London.
*Present address*: Roche Products Ltd, Welwyn Garden City, UK

The control of medicines is now accepted throughout the developed world and most countries have followed the example of the US government, which in 1906 passed the Food and Drug Act and hence led to the establishment of the Food and Drug Administration (FDA)—the first governmental agency in modern times to be charged with regulating drugs intended for medicinal purposes. Where America led, the rest of the world has followed and most countries now have a governmental department or agency to control the marketing of new drugs according to strict criteria relating to their quality, safety and efficacy, to monitor their performance in clinical use and to ensure that they continue to be made to the highest possible standards. For example, the UK has its Medicines Control Agency (MCA), Ireland its National Drugs Advisory Board (NDAB), Germany its BGA, and the European Union is soon to have its European Medicines Evaluation Agency (EMEA). The common factor in all these regulatory authorities is that they are part of government, and those who work in them are first and foremost civil servants.

It is unlikely that anyone sets out with the stated ambition of working in a regulatory authority. Many, however, do so and find the work interesting and rewarding. Most come to it with experience from other areas. Until some five years ago, most of those working in the UK

*Discovering New Medicines: Careers in Pharmaceutical Research and Development.*
Edited by P.D. Stonier
© 1994 John Wiley & Sons Ltd

authority were full-time career civil servants working for the government Department of Health and Social Security. A similar arrangement
continues to apply in the USA at the FDA and in most European countries. Recruitment to such a system is thus primarily to the Civil Service
and only secondarily to the regulatory authority. This was how the then
Medicines Division of the Department of Health got (and lost) its
managers and administrators who saw a few years working in 'the
windswept wastes of Vauxhall' as a useful but essentially temporary
career move before 'moving on to higher things' such as running the
National Health Service (NHS)

For doctors and pharmacists things were a little different. Most were
recruited directly from the pharmaceutical industry, academia or the
NHS to work in the Medicines Division. They became civil servants and,
after a probationary period, became established and effectively had a
permanent job until their sixtieth birthday, when they could draw their
pension. Promotion was possible both in the division or elsewhere in
the Department of Health, with increasing emphasis on the management of people and budgets. Most European countries' agencies continue to do something similar, indeed in the USA the FDA continues to
employ full-time civil servants who, when established, have no fixed
retirement age and virtually have jobs for as long as they want, but in
the UK things have changed somewhat with the advent of 'next steps
agencies'. These are effectively separate governmental businesses
charged with a specific task for which they are given control of a budget
and a certain amount of freedom to run things their own way. The Medicines Control Agency (MCA) is one such and is now charged with the
control of medicines in the UK, while enjoying considerable autonomy
in organising its own affairs including the power to 'hire and fire' and
set terms and conditions of employment. Those who work there are still
civil servants and continue to enjoy the five or six weeks annual leave
and index-linked, non-contributory pension of others in the service,
while remaining free to apply for posts in other government departments if suitably qualified.

That part of the EC Commission which deals with medicines is
different again. There are some full-time civil servants employed by the
Commission in Brussels, but many more who work there have been
seconded for limited periods from member states, while others are on
short-term contracts, mainly to perform specific tasks. There is a feeling
of impermanence at present due to the advent of the new European
Medicines Evaluation Agency (EMEA). Apart from the fact that it is to
be sited in the UK, little is known yet about how this will run or even
where exactly it will be located, but it will certainly provide
interesting—exciting even—employment for a chosen few, perhaps no

more than a hundred or so managers and professional advisers in the first instance. After that, who knows?

So what happens in a regulatory agency? There is, of course, plenty of fairly humdrum office work such as happens in any large organisation. Paper has to be pushed and numbers have to be crunched just as they do the world over, but the overriding function is the protection of the public health by the control of medicines for human use. It should not be forgotten, however, that animals take medicines too, so there are agencies for controlling medicines for veterinary use just as for those used by doctors. Indeed, the principal medicines legislation in the UK, the Medicines Act 1968, applies equally to human and animal medicines.

All medicines need to be approved by the regulatory authority even to do the clinical trials which will support the applications for authority to market them. These applications have to be evaluated and again when successful result in the granting of a licence or marketing authorisation so that the drug can be manufactured, advertised, distributed and sold. Once on the market they have to be continually monitored for quality and safety in use. These, in broad terms, are the functions of the regulatory authorities.

Licences have to be applied for, and an application to license a new medicine will usually be supported by scientific evidence filling as many as 250 or more volumes, each containing two or three hundred pages of text and tables. This mass of paper has to be catalogued, stored, moved, checked for completeness and evaluated. It contains the information that the sponsor company hopes will persuade the medical, pharmaceutical and scientific assessors, and the independent advisory bodies such as the Committee on Safety of Medicines, that the medicine is safe, effective and of good quality, so that they can recommend the granting of a licence to market and promote the product. Assessment of this mass of data generally involves the production of an assessment report, which is essentially a summary and commentary on the application. Even this may run to one or two hundred pages, and considerable skill and experience is required to produce a report which identifies the key issues relating to the safety, quality and efficacy of the product for which a licence is being sought. This basic process is common to all regulatory authorities, although the actual details of the process may vary. Applications on computer disk are beginning to appear and probably represent the way ahead, but for the time being the professional assessors working in regulatory agencies have to do a very great deal of reading before writing their 'short' assessments.

Another important part of medicines control is drug safety or pharmacovigilance. All drugs cause some unwanted effects. These range from the trivial to the very severe, even fatal. It is thus essential for authorities to keep a close watch on the performance of drugs which are licensed and on the market. Most countries operate a system whereby reports of adverse reactions are sent to the national authority by pre-scribing doctors. The UK Committee on Safety of Medicines operates a successful system of adverse reaction reporting using the yellow reporting cards, after which the system is named. The Yellow Card system is, in fact, a very sophisticated, advanced, computer-based system which records, stores and analyses the data from many sources, including the reports from British doctors. Naturally, this work calls for considerable expertise from disciplines such as medicine, pharmacy, toxicology, statistics and informatics. The people who work in this area have frequent contact with the regulatory and drug safety departments of pharmaceutical companies and while, like all civil servants, they do not deal directly with the media their work can and often does attract considerable public interest. Processing tens of thousands of yellow card reports (many of them in traditional doctors' handwriting!) is a daunting task. However, this is the only method by which adverse drug reactions (ADRs), which occur too infrequently to have appeared in the clinical trials done in three or four thousand patients before the drug is licensed, can be identified. Remember, *all* drugs produce some unwanted effects and it is clearly of the greatest importance to balance these against the benefits of the particular drug. This is the remit of pharmacovigilance and its importance to the community cannot be over-emphasised, as may be deduced from the great attention the media pay to this vital aspect of medicines control.

The manufacture of modern medicines requires processes, people and machinery of the highest quality, and systems to ensure that the highest standards of purity and batch-to-batch reproducibility over time are maintained. The application of agreed standards of Good Manufac-turing Practice (GMP) are monitored by most authorities through medi-cines inspectors, whose job is to visit manufacturing sites and wholesale dealers' premises, sometimes unannounced, to examine in detail how companies' products are made, controlled, stored and distributed. The inspectors are usually chemists or pharmacists with years of experience in the manufacture and/or testing of pharmaceuticals. Unusually among those who work in regulatory authorities, they spend a considerable part of their time out of the office on site inspections. These are not only in the UK but can be almost anywhere in the world where drugs are made for the British market, although the evolution of reciprocal inspec-tion agreements with other countries is tending to reduce the need for foreign travel. These inspections are important to companies. A seri-ously adverse report from the inspectors can lead to withdrawal or suspension of a licence to manufacture drugs or classes of drugs at a particular site, or to operate as a wholesaler. This can have considerable financial implications for the company involved.

In the UK people not directly concerned with regulatory affairs have tended to think of the Medicines Division as if it were synonymous with the Committee on Safety of Medicines (CSM). This is much less the case now that the Medicines Control Agency (MCA) has established a separate corporate identity for itself, but some confusion still exists. The CSM is one of a number of advisory bodies, established by law and made up of part-time experts appointed for limited terms by government ministers. There are other similar bodies, such as the Committee on Dental and Surgical Materials (CDSM), and it must be emphasised that the members of all these committees are *not* full-time civil servants. They are invited to serve on a particular advisory committee because of their knowledge and experience in particular specialities relating to medicines. You do not *apply* to become a member of the CSM!

There are also various subcommittees of the main committees, again made up of experts, and all of these are serviced by the full-time civil servants of the secretariat. There is an enormous amount of paper involved in even a single monthly meeting of one of these committees or subcommittees. The documents are written by professional assessors—doctors, pharmacists, dentists, scientists, lawyers—and administrators, and then have to be printed, collated, packed and distributed in time for members to prepare for the next meeting. Deadlines are tight and dedicated work is required from the support team in order to meet them: there is, however, an awareness of taking part in something of real value to the common good. This may have something to do with why people choose to work in regulatory agencies. Those who do, enjoy the satisfaction of being 'on the side of the angels' as part of a system which, while often having to say 'no' to pharmaceutical companies trying to license new drugs, is also expected to advise and help companies to get good drugs licensed.

So how do you set out on a career in a regulatory authority? This will, of course, depend on your qualifications and experience, and, importantly, the country where you hope to work. If your aim is clerical or administrative, in most countries you will first need to become a civil servant, usually by examination. Your choice of job at the most junior level may be limited, and an expression of interest in working for the national regulatory authority may be insufficient to get such a posting, but as you gain experience you will become eligible to apply for specific, more senior appointments in your chosen field. After that, you are constrained only by your abilities, qualifications and the availability of suitable posts. Up to a certain level of seniority, posts tend only to be advertised internally, but after that, particularly where professionals with particular skills and experience are required, they may also be advertised outside the Civil Service in the relevant scientific journals.

The system of employing professional assessors, i.e. doctors, pharmacists, scientists etc., in the UK is probably not typical of practice in other countries at present. Appointments are now made for limited terms of three years' duration, with the possibility of the initial term being extended for further limited periods. The enforcement of compulsory retirement at age 60 for both sexes has been dropped, so contracts can now be extended more or less indefinitely, depending on fitness, performance and employee preference. The old Civil Service concept of a permanent job until your sixtieth birthday, after satisfactorily completing an initial probationary period, seems to have gone for good. Of course it has to be said that this no more than reflects what is happening in the Civil Service as a whole and in large parts of the private sector. If this sounds negative, it must be emphasised that those assessed to be doing a good job and continuing to meet the high standards set by the agency will probably be offered renewal of their contracts, while others who perform less well may not. Among the perceived advantages of the 'next steps' status of the MCA is its ability to reward superior performance by bonuses or salary increases and to promote to managerial posts, free from the constraints of the old Civil Service pay and conditions structure which among other things had separate promotion paths for administrators, doctors, pharmacists and scientists.

With regard to management, this is very much the key to advancement in regulatory authorities, just as it is any organisation, whether it be governmental or private sector. You do not become chief executive simply by being the best assessor in the business, and it is no longer necessary for doctors to be managed only by doctors and pharmacists by pharmacists. Management skills are a scarce and highly prized commodity and for those identified as having them, whatever their initial discipline, promotion to the highest levels is a real possibility.

The decision to site the new EMEA in the UK and the intention to have it up and running in 1995 may have some effect on the MCA and its staffing, but this is expected to be minimal. Redundancies are *not* anticipated. Curiously, the establishment of the EMEA could even *increase* the work of national authorities such as the MCA. In a word, there is unlikely to be any reduction in the need for regulators, especially experienced assessors, as a result of the EMEA.

So what sort of background is needed to become an assessor? A recent

MCA advertisement for physicians may help. This speaks of:

> UK-registered physicians with a proven record of achievement in clinical, academic or pharmaceutical medicine. A higher qualification in medicine, pharmacology or epidemiology would be an advantage. Knowledge of, or experience in drug development, whilst useful, is not essential. You will work to the highest professional standards, and be capable of assimilating complex information quickly, and making decisions that impact on how medicines will be developed and used.

The same advertisement confirms:

> Positions for a period of three years, in the first instance, and renewable on review.

Those contemplating a response to such an advertisement should grasp the opportunity, where available, of talking to someone in the authority who is actually doing the job for which they are thinking about applying. In this way it is possible to get a feel for the environment in which you will be working, see what sort of person is actually doing the job, how they do it and whether they seem to be enjoying it. My own view is that if you cannot identify with the aims of medicines control and take pleasure from so doing, you may well find the work more than usually tedious. As I have already said, the masses of paper involved can be daunting, but there are compensations. The satisfaction, excitement even, of teasing out the clinical implications of a mass of data can be very satisfying. Working with top experts in deciding whether to license a major new drug is educational and intellectually rewarding. Consideration of a new toxic event associated with an established drug, and deciding whether the drug should be withdrawn from the market, imposes a huge responsibility on those involved in balancing risk against benefit for patients. Above all there is the sense of taking part in something vital to the public health, which makes work in the regulatory authority a more than usually satisfying career.

# 24
# Pharmaceutical Law—A New Legal Speciality

## Ian Dodds-Smith

McKenna & Co., London, UK

It is perhaps surprising that, until recently, a student of law would have searched in vain for textbooks in the English language even remotely concerned with European pharmaceutical law as a special subject. The industry has naturally been a fertile field for the practice of intellectual property law for a long time but most lawyers in the patent and trademark field would have a practice where pharmaceutical matters were common rather than their exclusive diet. Legal texts on subjects such as medical negligence now often have a token chapter on specific issues relating to the supply of medicinal products but even this is a relatively recent development. However, there are no legal texts that deal with the relevant law in the type of detail so common in other areas of activity such as the aviation industry.

This is despite the fact that the pharmaceutical industry is one of the more discrete industrial sectors, European industry is at the top of the world league and has had specific European Community (EC) legislation, let alone national legislation, devoted to its activities since 1965. The picture is changing fast and it can confidently be stated that a new legal speciality has developed that springs largely from the unusual regulatory features of the industry, the special ethical and legal problems relating to clinical research and the complexities of personal injury litigation concerning its products.

*Discovering New Medicines: Careers in Pharmaceutical Research and Development.*
Edited by P.D. Stonier
© 1994 John Wiley & Sons Ltd

## REGULATION IN THE PHARMACEUTICAL INDUSTRY

The pharmaceutical industry is today undoubtedly the most regulated of all industrial sectors. At every stage in the marketing of products there is governmental intervention. The normal way in which such intervention is achieved is through detailed legislation backed by criminal sanctions. On some matters voluntary government schemes exist (e.g. pricing) but the control is no less formal for that.

In comparison to the USA, which has had extensive regulatory controls for more than 50 years, most controls within Europe have been imposed in the last 20 years, with the thalidomide tragedy adding a new urgency to the political pressure that already existed for control of dealings in medicinal products. In the UK, from the relatively small beginnings of product licensing under the Medicines Act of 1968 (in fact, not operational until 1971), virtually every aspect of supply has been controlled, partly in response to harmonising Directives within the EC. Within the EC regulatory control of the industry was an early candidate for attention, with Directive 65/65/EEC laying down the framework for licensing based upon safety, efficacy and quality, but the pace of adoption of Directives quickened in the last five years with attempts to complete the internal market by 1992. Twenty-five out of 29 of the Directives relating to human medicines were adopted in the period 1983–1993.

Legal specialities develop out of the demands of commerce for advice, which in turn tend to be dictated by the increase in the complexity of relevant laws and uncertainties in their application. Whilst lawyers working within industry naturally develop knowledge and skills specific to their employer's business, legal knowledge in private practice will only develop if companies find the need to seek legal advice in a particular field on a regular basis. Until recently, that simply did not happen in the regulatory field.

One of the reasons is that regulatory control was not treated as a natural arena for lawyers. Initially such control focused upon obtained marketing approvals and despite the fact that the controls ultimately had their origin in legislation—often some of the most detailed and opaque texts on the statute book—regulation was treated essentially as an issue of administrative rote in most companies. Regulatory personnel tended to operate as adjuncts to either the medical or marketing functions and legal input was minimal. Even in-house lawyers seldom became involved in the licensing process. The ethos of such groups was to get the product to market as soon as possible, and companies would operate the procedures imposed by the regulatory authorities, frequently without any real understanding of the statutory basis for such procedures. If a regulatory authority wanted something done, it was done and with little or no thought being given to whether there was a sound legal basis for the request or restriction imposed. This is not to be critical of such an approach because in most cases the interests of a company may be better served commercially by complying with a request rather than questioning the powers of the regulator.

One feature of the regulatory framework in the UK is that the full expression of the controls is not to be found in statutes in any event but rather in 'administrative directions' issued under the Act through notices published in the Medicines Act Information Letters (MAIL). Perhaps the best example is in the field of adverse drug reactions, where the statutory controls are, in fact, described very simply as a requirement to maintain a record and provide details as and when the licensing authority direct. However, based on this simple statement, periodic and changing directions (often of a very detailed nature) were issued in MAIL. In short, the practical controls on companies were to be found as much in interpretive and 'how to do' guidelines and notices of the Department of Health as in the statute book. For many years industry was very comfortable with this.

What changed to cause the demand for regulatory advice to increase? First, national regulation has increased not only the complexity of controls (and particularly the relationship between them) but also the potential for conflict with the regulatory authorities. Controls developed progressively in the UK through the late 1970s to cover commercially critical areas such as advertising. The prosecution in 1986 of one company and a responsible officer in relation to the advertising of a product undoubtedly increased the concern of companies to ensure compliance. Legal as well as medical sign-off of advertising copy became much commoner. More generally, with increasing controls companies became more concerned that one could not always be confident that different companies were being treated fairly and consistently in relation to the same issues. Undoubtedly, the authorities were sometimes grappling with similar problems of interpretation and positions changed from time to time, sometimes depending upon the attitude of individual assessors or officials. As a result companies became more concerned to establish that their 'rights' were not being infringed in an increasingly competitive market-place.

The second complicating factor has been the addition of a raft of European legislation, often with limited consultation and text that is frequently not a great advertisement for careful thought and precise drafting. In fact, of course, if Directives are to harmonise practices and decision-making within the European agencies, drafting that is imprecise merely facilitates (and frequently enshrines) lack of consistency in approach. English lawyers are sometimes criticised for applying a too rigid interpretation based upon what the words alone mean and are told that in the European context one must apply a 'purposive approach' to interpretation based upon the recitals to the Directive. If a purposive approach is adopted it is suggested that all will become clear and the need for lawyers will evaporate. This is, of course, fallacious because few Directives have a single, clearly defined purpose; most seek to balance somewhat conflicting principles, namely the need to ensure safety and promote public health, but to do so without hindering the free movement of goods and the innovation and development of the European pharmaceutical industry. It is therefore not difficult to reach different interpretations of a Directive's provisions according to the weight you attach on any given matter to one or other of these underlying principles. Moreover, sometimes provisions are so vague and conflicting that incorporation into national law is delayed. The difficulties experienced in the UK in implementing the Advertising Directive and Labelling Directive illustrate such problems very clearly.

Explanatory documents such as the Notice to Applicants and Guidelines from the Committee for Proprietary Medicinal Products (CPMP) seek to assist in interpreting Directives, and these documents frequently go into considerable and useful detail not found in the Directives themselves. Companies are guided in their planning by such documents but in fact the documents carefully eschew any claim to be legally authoritative and at the end of the day they reflect an opinion that the courts can, and do, frequently disregard when asked to adjudicate on the law. It is small wonder that companies, perplexed by the uncertainty that European legislation injects for a business that must take long-term decisions, and for which uncertainty is therefore particularly unwelcome, turn increasingly to their lawyers for assistance and hopefully a degree of certainty.

The problems are compounded by the need to translate Directives into the domestic legal framework. Frequently, member states persuade themselves that their existing legal provisions will already comply but often, while the main thrust is consistent, the wording of key provisions is, in fact, different. Thus when Organon sought the assistance of the English courts in determining their rights in relation to the product Bolvidon (mianserin), the judges identified a significant number of ways in which even relatively basic provisions of European law were not accurately reflected in the Medicines Act legislation. This was of great significance because as a matter of European law a company is entitled to rely either upon the provisions of the domestic law (in which case the licensing authority cannot seek to apply a European provision that it has failed properly to implement) or, if they are more favourable to the company, the provisions of European law (and the licensing authority cannot rely upon domestic provisions that are at odds with the European law that the state was obliged to implement). Companies consider it novel to have an option in the law they may follow and the demand for legal advice will obviously rise in such circumstances!

An additional factor predisposing to uncertainty and, therefore, the need for legal advice is that Directives may be implemented not by legislation but merely by administrative action. The latter converts into statements of practice which the Medicines Control Agency in the UK usually issue in MAIL. It is normally considered optimal that when the law changes on a given matter those affected by it should receive a clear statement of the new position at the time the change becomes effective. In the UK there have been several instances where statements of administrative practice have been issued many months after the operative date. Such was the case with the far-reaching changes in relation to abridged applications generated by Directive 87/21/EEC. It was not until the SmithKline French litigation concerning generic copies of Tagamet had raised one of the issues arising out of that Directive that the Department of Health issued a statement in MAIL in August 1988 describing the administrative action that implemented the new law which had become effective long before in July 1987. Total absence of information creates the most uncertainty of all!

Finally, whilst the EC has not yet fully implemented the Future Systems, the European regulatory authorities are in certain cases (e.g. pharmacovigilance) already acting as though they were in place. Often this makes extremely good sense, particularly with a view to getting consistent and speedy decisions on safety issues. However, the existing legal function of the CPMP, outside the concertation procedures for multi-state and biotech/hi-tech applications for marketing authorisation, is to advise member state authorities rather than to issue directions to the holders of national marketing authorisations. Such *de facto* developments towards centralised decision-making add a new dimension to the problems of those in regulatory affairs, who in the pharmacovigilance field, for instance, increasingly have to understand the legal requirements in all member states because adverse drug reaction (ADR) reporting remains unharmonised as to both type and timing of reports and the controls remain firmly rooted in national law.

Not only are companies keener to establish their legal position, but also as the relationship between the regulatory authorities and industry has become more open it has perhaps also become more professional. There has developed a greater willingness on the part of companies to defend their interests, if necessary by resort to law. The traditional concern that to argue with the authorities over the licensing of one product would only provoke difficulties for the company with other product applications, is giving way to an appreciation on both sides that where uncertainty exists or companies are aggrieved by an issue it may be necessary to seek clarification of the law by judicial review. This naturally increases the demand for lawyers with expertise in regulatory affairs.

There are, of course, dangers in assuming that the courts are equipped to resolve all regulatory disputes, particularly those that genuinely arise from scientific assessment. However, as successfully prosecuted cases of judicial review show, there are cases where a company has little choice but to seek judicial review and it would be strange if, against the complexities of law described above, there is not an increase in cases of judicial review. Recent case law has clarified that European law gives standing to any person aggrieved by the wrongful application of European law by a regulatory authority to seek the assistance of the courts. In contrast, in the Medicines Act itself (S. 107) an attempt is made to restrict any challenge to the regulatory decision to the licence holder or prospective licence holder rather than a third party directly affected. This, together with the development of European law suggesting that in appropriate circumstances damages may be obtained from the regulatory authority for breach of European law obligations and the possibilities of obtaining interim relief pending the substantive hearing such as the suspension of the licence in issue, will increase the willingness of companies to litigate to protect their interests. On one view, regulatory law alone will provide sufficient material for specialisation, without necessarily encompassing expertise in the matters that are discussed below.

## CLINICAL RESEARCH AND ETHICAL ISSUES

Regulation of commercial activities—in the broadest sense of the word—takes many forms ranging from legislation to application of the general law principle requiring the exercise of reasonable care at all times. Despite the growth of European regulation described above, at the present time no Directive has been adopted directly controlling clinical research. This reflects in part the difficulties of harmonising activities that touch upon different medical traditions and practices. A few countries such as France and Ireland have legislated in advance of European harmonisation. Phase I research in healthy volunteers is not directly regulated at all in some countries, including the UK. Nevertheless, the last 10 years have witnessed markedly increased interest in issues relating to the ethics of research and its organisation. Of particular concern have been issues of 'informed consent', the increased commercialisation of research notably with healthy volunteers at phase I, and compensation for injury suffered during the course of research. Lacunae or uncertainties in the law have been partially filled by a plethora of guidelines from various organisations, some European (e.g. the Guidelines for Good Clinical Practice (GCP) of the CPMP), some national/governmental (e.g. the Department of Health Ethics Committee Guidelines), some trade association (e.g. the GCP Guidelines and Compensation Guidelines of the Association of the British Pharmaceutical Industry) and some professional (e.g. the Royal College of Physicians of London Guidelines on Research).

To a large extent Ethics Committees, operating by reference to these guidelines, have filled the regulatory gap and during recent years both their constitution and procedures have been formalised. Ethics Committee approval is now of considerable importance and more problematical. Delay in obtaining it can have significant commercial implications. The application of ethical guidelines (which by their nature tend to be flexible) to different factual situations creates significant problems of interpretation which are accentuated when, as is often the case, pharmaceutical companies conduct multi-centre (including foreign centre) trials. Legal training is seen as an advantage in considering the interrelationship between such guidelines and general law principles, and very many ethics committees now include a lawyer. Expertise in the law and ethical guidelines relevant to research is now very much a requirement for lawyers advising pharmaceutical companies and the contract research organisations that serve such companies.

## PRODUCT LIABILITY

The trend towards legal specialisation arising from regulatory developments has been given added impetus by the significant increase in litigation concerning the products of the pharmaceutical industry. The thalidomide tragedy led to the first major case, but in the event the litigation was fairly limited as media pressure brought about a settlement of claims that had become bogged down in legal and technical uncertainties. Many of the uncertainties remain and it is still the case that no litigation in England involving a pharmaceutical product has yet proceeded to trial and judgement on both negligence and causation—the two key components that traditionally a plaintiff has had to prove to establish a right to compensation. In the mid-1970s claims concerning the marketing of Eraldin (practolol) by ICI were settled by a compensation scheme established very quickly after withdrawal of the drug. The Primodos litigation (concerning a hormone pregnancy test) which began in the late 1970s was the first case to proceed any distance and involved several hundred claimants and allegations of teratogenicity. However, the proceedings were discontinued after four years by the plaintiffs (a matter of weeks from trial) on the basis that the expert evidence exchanged showed that there was no real possibility of the plaintiffs establishing that the product was capable of causing the alleged injuries at all.

However, the 1980s witnessed an explosion of major cases with claims in respect of particular drugs being numbered in the hundreds and sometimes in the thousands. Claims involving pertussis vaccine, steroids, oral contraceptives, blood products, non-steroidal anti-inflammatory agents, intrauterine devices, contrast media and benzodiazepines have been raised. One of the most significant was that involving pertussis vaccine, where the court ordered a preliminary issue on causation and the Wellcome Foundation was able to demonstrate that on balance of probabilities the vaccine was not capable of causing brain damage. This result was achieved in large measure by dissecting the principal epidemiological studies upon which the association was based and showing that the epidemiology was severely flawed, mirroring to a considerable degree a key factor in the discontinuation of the Primodos litigation where base data underlying central epidemiological studies had also been obtained and assessed for the first time with a critical eye. The relationship between legal principles of probability (each component of a cause of action including causation must be established on the balance of probability) and tests of statistical significance in epidemiology raises interesting issues.

Other cases were either discontinued, settled or, in a few instances, are still pending. The largest pending litigation concerns benzodiazepines and has involved directly or indirectly all of the manufacturers of benzodiazepines from the 1960s onwards. It is unusual in that physicians prescribing the drugs have been made defendants in a number of cases. It is also noteworthy that the Legal Aid Boards in Northern Ireland and Scotland have in this litigation contributed to the funding of the more advanced litigation in England on the basis that there should not be parallel proceedings in all jurisdictions within the UK based on public funds. The benzodiazepine litigation developed into the largest personal injury litigation that has ever been seen in the UK where the nature of the claims (the essential allegations concern dependence), the long period of usage of products and the similarity between the symptoms of the underlying conditions for which benzodiazepines were prescribed and the symptoms alleged as injuries, obviously contribute to its complexity.

The 1990s have seen new additions to the lists of products where material litigation is or has been threatened including human insulin and, for the first time, veterinary products in the shape of products used to dip sheep. Indeed, if today one opens the 'Help Please' column of the *Law Society Gazette* (where solicitors advertise to other solicitors their interest in particular types of claims and their desire for coordination) in some weeks well over half the entries relate to possible claims in respect of medicinal products. Of course, many of these claims do not develop and others develop very slowly. Frequently claimants are encouraged to 'forum-shop', and if the UK licence holder has an American parent one will often find that an attempt is made to have the claims heard against the parent in the USA, arguing that testing took place there or the product information was 'controlled' by the parent company. In recent years the American courts have become firmer in their resolve to dismiss such claims on the grounds that the American forum is not convenient, but lawyers advising pharmaceutical companies need to have a working knowledge of the jurisdictional and choice of law rules applicable in other countries.

Most major pharmaceutical companies are multinational and the possible international dimensions of litigation are increasingly important. Publicity surrounding claims in the UK are picked up by the foreign press and there is then a considerable potential for claims developing in other countries, particularly in Australia or New Zealand where the legal system and legal remedies are similar. Finally, an added difficulty for companies is that one can no longer assume that claimants in Scotland or Northern Ireland will join in, or await the outcome of, English litigation relating to the same product. The same factors at work in England are present in those jurisdictions and a company can quickly find itself fighting on a number of fronts. Careful coordination is at a premium both to safeguard the client's interests and control costs, with the result that the English lawyer advising the pharmaceutical industry today needs to have a good knowledge of the relevant procedural rules in those jurisdictions too and have developed contacts with lawyers there in whom he has confidence.

What are the factors that have led to the pharmaceutical sector being at the forefront of product liability litigation? Clearly we have a more litigious environment, where the public are quicker to sue if they believe (or more accurately have been led to believe) that use of a product might be to blame. The explosion in claims certainly does not reflect reduced standards in the industry (controls are greater than ever before) and increased litigation has affected the practice of medicine too. The fees for membership of the medical defence organisations in the UK continue to soar, reflecting the legal costs of defending and sometimes settling claims. The trend is not restricted to the UK; in the Republic of Ireland premiums have risen by 139% for surgeons and 143% for physicians over the past two years, reflecting both the increase in litigation and the higher personal injury awards (40% higher on average than in the UK). Procedural changes have in some respects made litigation easier in the UK and the Republic of Ireland than in many other European countries, but primarily it is the very nature of medical treatment and the use of medical products that makes it easy to commence (though usually difficult to prove) claims. Relevant factors are the inevitability of an association (though very often not causal) between the symptoms of illness and use of a drug or other medical intervention, the relative ease with which negligence can be alleged in fields with few absolute standards and the difficulties in proving the negative in relation to medical causation.

Media interest and changes in the approach of the legal profession to advertising have also contributed. The media (and public) love health issues and this, combined with the 'David and Goliath' scenario to which claims against multinational corporations automatically give rise, is an irresistible combination. Invariably unbalanced publicity about one claimant's 'battle' with a 'drug giant' can quickly create a snowball effect, with anyone who has taken the drug in question and contemporaneously experienced ill-effects quickly discounting the possible relevance of the underlying condition for which the drug was taken in the first place and believing that he or she may have a valid claim for compensation. Moreover, media interest is now fuelled by solicitors seeking to develop their own reputation in this specialist field who, since changes in the rules of professional conduct in 1990, may now more freely advertise their involvement in particular cases. This is accepted as a legitimate way of promoting the client's case and bringing further pressure to bear on the manufacturer to settle claims. Media comment often invites other patients who believe they may have a claim to contact particular lawyers already involved on behalf of claimants. While all of this is perfectly legitimate, in the pharmaceutical field there are certain risks attached because many patients are naturally suggestible; if such patients are eligible for legal aid they can participate in litigation at no cost to themselves, and the question arises: what have they got to lose by putting forward their case for consideration? In recent years some firms of solicitors have advertised in the press by reference to named drugs that have been withdrawn or had their licences suspended. Such advertisements note that patients might be entitled to compensation if they have used the particular drug and offer free first consultations. Whilst defendant corporations are much less comfortable about their own lawyers participating in the media debate, lawyers advising pharmaceutical companies need to have experience in dealing in the media with what are frequently highly emotive issues.

A further factor in the growth of litigation is ironically the development of court procedures for 'controlling' multi-claimant (and sometimes defendant) cases in the management sense. The concept of a 'group action' is not unknown in other fields but most experience has been gained in the pharmaceutical field. Part of the aim of these procedures is to ensure that claims are coordinated and proceed roughly in parallel, usually under the supervision of a single judge. Such procedures can only operate efficiently according to a strict timetable with the imposition of 'cut-off' dates by which all claims must be notified. In fairness, however, such dates have to be given some publicity and the courts have encouraged plaintiff lawyers to advertise the dates freely. The effect, of course, may be to encourage the submission of claims of varying merits and viability solely to ensure that the opportunity to proceed is not lost. In the benzodiazepine litigation, the increase in claims following advertisement of the names of the various benzodiazepine drugs marketed over the years was phenomenal, with almost 20 000 claims notified by the cut-off date. Whilst some of these factors ought also to encourage litigation in other sectors (and environmental claims are certainly increasing), the fact remains that the pharmaceutical sector is particularly vulnerable to product liability litigation and this is reflected in the fact that nearly all the group actions raised have been in the pharmaceutical field.

As regards the future, there is little reason to imagine that pressure from claims will abate. First, substantive law has moved in favour of claimants. Strict liability was introduced in 1988 under the Consumer Protection Act 1987 and adds an additional cause of action that is meant to facilitate the pursuit of compensation for injury due to defective products. If a product fails to offer the safety persons are entitled to expect, it is deemed 'defective', and if causation is demonstrated the manufacturer is left with the burden of proving one of the statutory defences, the most important of which is the 'development risks defence'. This bars liability if the manufacturer can show that at the date he put the product into circulation it was not possible, in the state of scientific and technical knowledge, to discover the defect in the product. Strict liability only applies to a product that was put into circulation after 1 March 1988 and so virtually all the litigation to date has required proof of negligence. Although there is little experience with strict liability (in either the pharmaceutical or any other commercial sector) the effect is not likely to be to reduce litigation, and the general principle of 'a consumer's expectation of safety' and the 'development risk defence' raise special problems of interpretation in pharmaceutical cases.

Secondly, plaintiffs are increasingly better advised than they used to be. Lawyers in private practice instructed by companies have developed expertise in the field, although in practice defendants tend to go to a few firms with a 'track record'—a sure sign that the need for specialist advice is recognised. In parallel and perhaps to an even greater extent, as instructions have been more widely spread, considerable expertise and knowledge of the sector have been developed within firms traditionally acting for plaintiffs in the personal injury field. The English Law Society's proposals for panels of specialists in personal injury and medical negligence work and the Legal Aid Board's move towards franchising of firms to conduct major litigation for claimants based on proof of expertise are expected to lead to greater specialisation. Whilst the number of firms handling the work for plaintiffs will diminish, identifying where specialist legal advice can be obtained should become easier. The Law Society's plans for a specialist panel for personal injury is well advanced and curiously pharmaceutical product liability has been assigned to the personal injury panel rather than to the medical negligence panel, despite the overlap with the latter. As an adjunct to these developments, specialist support services have blossomed in recent years. The Association for Victims of Medical Accidents (AVMA) has become increasingly important in advising people who may have claims. The recently formed Association of Personal Injury Lawyers (APIL) and even more recent formation of the Forum of Insurance Lawyers (FOIL) is further evidence of increasing specialisation. There is also an international dimension, with lawyers acting for plaintiffs in different countries getting together and exchanging know-how and thoughts on strategy, and information and documents relating to particular products and the way they have been marketed in different countries. With the help of such technical advisers and with greater coordination of effort, lawyers are in general more willing to take on, and more adept at conducting, claims against pharmaceutical companies.

Finally, there is the issue of contingency fees. The financial limits for eligibility of legal aid have not kept pace with inflation and very recently, amidst much criticism, the government has restricted eligibility still further in the UK. In response, the government has bowed to pressure to revoke the prohibition on contingency fees and allow them, albeit not in the form of the American model. The new rules will allow conditional fee arrangements to be made between solicitors and their clients, thereby facilitating litigation and shifting some of the risk and financial burden onto the legal profession and away from the individual litigant and the public purse. In the USA the lawyer is able to agree with his client that a charge will be made only if the litigation is successful. In those circumstances the lawyer becomes entitled to a percentage of the damages, normally about 40%. The UK proposal is not to give the solicitor a direct interest in the damages but rather to allow him to increase his fees above the norm in the event of success. It was, at first, proposed that a limit of 20% uplift would apply but this was clearly too low to make the option attractive and the government very recently agreed that the uplift may be 100%. Whilst conditional fee arrangements are unlikely to cause an increase in personal injury claims generally which is outweighed by the reduction in eligibility for full legal aid, there is real concern that the identity of the defendant rather than the merits of the claim will more frequently be a factor in determining the decision of the lawyer to take on the case or avoid it. The 'deep pocket' principle of which American lawyers speak not only reflects the natural consideration that litigation should not be commenced against someone without resources to meet a judgement, but also tends to encompass the principle that some litigation may be 'viable' because the defendant is likely to be more willing to settle a case for (quite high) nuisance value to avoid cost, management disruption and adverse publicity. It is too early to say how precisely these new arrangements will affect litigation in the pharmaceutical sector but there are reasonable grounds for suggesting that they will increase litigation, and as they incorporate a performance incentive they will, in their own way, encourage specialisation still further by plaintiffs' lawyers.

Litigation in the pharmaceutical field is characterised by wide allegations, normally including failure to research and failure to warn. This translates into the need to collate and disclose massive quantities of documentations, invariably covering the whole life of the product. Such litigation combines the special nature of personal injury law and practice with the law relating to product liability, as applied in an industry with distinct characteristics. The procedural problems are accentuated by its propensity to be multi-plaintiff. For its optimal conduct it requires a thorough appreciation of the nature of the pharmaceutical industry and the regulatory system within which the industry operates (the regulatory authorities may also be co-defendants), together with an appreciation of the legal issues to which the interposition of the prescribing physician between the supplier of the product and the patient gives rise. The concept of the learned intermediary (as US lawyers call such physicians) in its purest form is peculiar to the pharmaceutical field and creates special problems related to the application of general law principles, particularly in 'failure to warn' cases.

Also required is an understanding of the scientific disciplines raised by the issues in the action, which invariably include pharmacology, toxicology, epidemiology and pathology. Dependent upon the nature of the claims and disease the drug was marketed to treat, lawyers must also become conversant in other disciplines as diverse as teratology and psychiatry. The instruction of experts and the assessment of the cogency of their opinions depend upon an understanding of the scientific fields within which they are practising. In the author's own firm this has led to the recruitment of a number of physicians, some but not all of whom have gained a further professional qualification in law. This reflects the fact that as many cases turn on science as upon a substantive or procedural law issue. The major multi-plaintiff pharmaceutical cases are administratively onerous and extremely costly to conduct. Optimal conduct requires the legal advisers to both plaintiffs and defendants to possess special skills and knowledge. Neither the Legal Aid Board nor the industry is prepared any longer to pay to take the lawyers they appoint 'up the learning curve'.

## CONCLUSION

Although as yet aviation law finds a special place in legal directories but pharmaceutical law does not, this reflects only a lack of appreciation by the authors of these texts of the complexities of the regulatory environment and the fact that most pharmaceutical cases have been settled or discontinued with limited publicity. Behind the scenes a specialisation has recently developed in response to an explosion of regulation and litigation, and while it is not as widely developed as in the USA it is likely to become so in the next decade and be European in focus.

# 25
# Pharmacoeconomics—New Careers in Pharmaceutical Medicine

## Nick Bosanquet and Anna Zajdler

St Mary's Hospital Medical School/Imperial College,
University of London, UK

The first generation of economists working in the industry have been mainly involved in adding economic information to clinical trials and in generating information for regulators, but market pressures seem likely to give economists a more central role in contributing to company strategy and decisions on product development. Economists were mainly involved in contributing information on specific products, but their role will widen to issues about the longer term future. From a mainly defensive and fact-finding role economists are now likely to be involved in developing more active strategies for the industry's future.

The original role of economists was in contributing an additional dimension to clinical trials. In a pioneering contribution in 1984 two economists, Drummond and Stoddart, argued for a phasing policy for the collection of economics data so as to minimise unnecessary work (Drummond *et al.*, 1988). The aim was to collect as much data with as little cost as possible. Data would be collected during use of services, then towards the end of the trial additional economic analysis could

*Discovering New Medicines: Careers in Pharmaceutical Research and Development.*
Edited by P.D. Stonier
© 1994 John Wiley & Sons Ltd

be carried out. This could cover:

- detailed costing of alternative therapies;
- estimates of resource savings from more effective therapies;
- estimates of costs to patients from treatment.

This model of involvement in clinical trials was adopted by many leading firms. Thus Schering-Plough's annual report for 1992 stated that 'The Company's new pharmaco-economic and QOL [quality of life] research unit is integrating economic and QOL evaluations into world-wide clinical trials and new product development, providing support to therapeutic and marketing teams' (Schering-Plough Corporation, 1992).

## GENERAL CONCEPTS OF PHARMACOECONOMICS

Economists have already started to develop pharmacoeconomics in distinctive ways. Classic economic studies used to rely heavily on cost–benefit analysis (CBA). In CBA all costs and benefits are translated into monetary terms. The approach was most viable where health care was an investment programme; it worked less well when health care was basically aiming at improving consumption of health or quality of life. There has been much more development in recent years of cost effectiveness analysis (CEA). Benefits can be measured in terms of changed life expectancy or reduced morbidity. Increasingly research methods have been able to cover psychological dimensions such as reductions in depression or anxiety and improvements in social functioning.

CEA studies still form most of those carried out in the pharmaceutical industry, but there has been a rapid growth in another type of study which seeks to measure quality of life in a much more explicit and con-sistent way. This is cost-utility analysis (CUA). Here life years gained in treatment are adjusted by utility weights reflecting the relative values which individuals place on different states of health. The output measure most commonly used is the quality-adjusted life year (QALY). There is particular interest in this measure because of its potential in allowing for comparison between different health programmes.

Pharmacoeconomics is an important part of a new wider culture of health economics. It is important to assess how pharmacoeconomics has made a distinctive contribution to this culture. Economists distinguish between the demand for health and the demand for health services.

Individuals seek to improve their stock of health by various kinds of investment. They make decisions about lifestyles and they may allocate varying amounts of time and energy to improving health. Health is affected by individual decisions about smoking, alcohol, exercise and road safety. Social programmes and incentives can also affect these decisions. Thus, the UK has low speed limits on the road and a much lower level of deaths and injuries from accidents than Germany. On the other hand, UK citizens have persisted with high-fat diets. The productivity of health services has to be assessed against other alternative ways of bringing about improvements in health outcomes.

Economists have a range of different possible measures of effectiveness. Some of them are economic, involving measurement of lost output from early mortality. This kind of calculation was used to support nineteenth-century public health programmes for clean water and sanitation and is still used to support the case for public health programmes in developing countries.

There is increased emphasis on more personal utility based on different measures of output. The QALY, for example, is an index that health economists have developed which weights survival and freedom from pain together into one composite measure. Economists are unusual in their interest in 'psychometrics', which has been a way of dealing with the difficulty of measuring output and the return on investment.

An effective treatment is one which increases health benefit. An efficient programme is one which delivers effective treatment at the lowest cost. This could be a matter of early detection of disease, or of changing location of treatment. Treatment in a day hospital might be more efficient than treatment as an in-patient.

Economists have been critical of health care agencies on the grounds that they have concentrated on administrative routines and blank cheque financing rather than seeking to promote more effective and efficient treatment. Economists were most active to start with in designing incentives to greater efficiency in terms of cost containment. They are now also urging adoption of incentives to greater effectiveness such as the setting of health targets and the measurement of health needs.

In summary, there are four basic techniques of economic evaluation which can be used by pharmacoeconomists.

## Cost Analysis

This can cover direct budgetary costs to health agencies. It would also be possible to measure monetary costs and psychological costs to patients. The treatment costs are calculated without any consideration of benefit.

## Cost Benefit Analysis (CBA)

This measures both costs and benefits in money terms. The earliest forms of the analysis concentrated on benefits in reduced costs of medical treatment and production gains from an earlier return to work. This is the ideal form of economic evaluation which in practice is very rarely used, because of the difficulties in allocating monetary values to intangible health gains.

## Cost Effectiveness Analysis (CEA)

This method allows the assessment of output in terms of health gain with measures such as 'cases successfully treated', reductions in mortality and years of life gained. This is the most common form used by medical scientists and researchers and is being used increasingly by health policy-makers. Thus the World Health Organization (WHO) has set targets for reductions in mortality by the year 2000.

## Cost Utility Analysis (CUA)

This is the newest form of evaluation and can be applied to a wider range of programmes through measuring changes in quality of life. It can be used to assess benefits from programmes that are in part palliative, such as chemotherapy for advanced cancer or for treatment of chronic illness which cause loss of quality of life but which do not reduce mortality. It can also allow the patient's own views and preference to be taken into account, so that patients can define what is quality of life for them.

## DECISION MAKING TECHNIQUES

These concepts have also been translated into decision-making techniques, incentives and guidelines to managers. Again there is a common culture not least because of individual carriers such as Professor Alain Enthoven of Stanford University, who has made a fundamental impact on thinking in the UK, Sweden and the Netherlands, and the work of the OECD in a series of reports. Among the most influential of these concepts are the following.

## The Diagnosis Related Group (DRG)

This divides all hospital treatment into 467 different diagnoses and standard costs are attached to each. Hospitals are then reimbursed according to these standard costs. The aim is to increase efficiency and to lower cost. For example, the reference pricing system in Germany has adapted this principle to pharmaceutical markets. A buyer sets a price that he is willing to pay based on ideas about what is reasonable.

## The Cash Limit

This sets an annual budget which the health services provider cannot exceed. The aim is to ensure budgetary control. This has been a key element in UK policies and has also been used in the French hospital system.

## Increased Co-payment

This shifts more of the burden of payment directly on to the consumer. This system has been used to reduce costs of Medicare by increasing amounts paid by elderly Americans for hospital treatment. It has also been applied to prescribing in Denmark, Germany and the UK, where patients have been asked to pay more in prescription charges.

## General Management

The UK has pioneered the use of business management approaches in health services through defining aims and targets with rewards for performance. This has implied a stronger role for managers relative to professionals. The old role of the manager or administrator in many health systems has been similar to that of a caddy on a golf course.

## Provider Competition

This is designed to increase both effectiveness and efficiency. Providers are expected to offer more attractive programmes with higher health benefits. They are also expected to offer lower costs. Provider competition has been a strong theme in the US health system since 1980 and the concept is now being used in the UK and in the Netherlands. The UK internal market system is trying to harness provider competition to local health needs. Purchasers will have freedom to buy services to meet local health needs from a range of providers, public and private.

## THE WORK OF PHARMACOECONOMISTS

Pharmacoeconomists have been mainly involved with the middle stage of CBA, CEA and CUA. Much of their work has been product specific and carried out as part of the development process within companies. They have not yet been involved in much assessment of the impact of new management systems but there is likely to be greater activity here in the future. Already new pharmacoeconomics departments are concerned much more with demands from external regulations. Ontario produced guidelines on presentation of economic data which became mandatory both for initial registration and for inclusion of new drugs in formularies (Ontario, *Draft Guidelines*, 1991). Australia also introduced requirements for cost effectiveness studies as a condition for registration. Pharmacoeconomists are coming to be concerned with the preparation of cases for these outside agencies.

Pharmacoeconomics had begun as a service function within corporations. Each company had a small unit or department contributing to the development process. Companies had to face very real constraints on outside recruitment. The shortage of experienced health economists was greater in the UK; as a result many companies filled posts in the new units with staff transferred from other development functions who had an interest but no formal training. In the USA it was more common to recruit from the larger pool of economists with some experience in health or related sectors.

Although the number of pharmacoeconomists is small, many departments within companies have had an interest in using their time. Brian Lovatt, Manager of International Outcomes Research at Zeneca Pharmaceuticals, has set out 'the principal aims' of any pharmacoeconomic programme as those of 'providing competitive advantage by describing and demonstrating the economic and quality of life benefits of suitable products' (Lovatt, 1993). This endeavour could involve the marketing department, the medical department and those concerned with regulation. All these have an interest in the timing and organisation of the development process.

Health systems are moving from short-term cost containment to longer-term measures designed to increase effectiveness. The first-generation systems involving the use of DRGs and cash-limited budgets have generally succeeded in containing costs in Germany and in the UK. The most rapid movement to second-generation systems involving provider competition has come in the UK, Sweden and the Netherlands. In the past countries may have been content to contain spending; now they may even be prepared to reduce it unless it can be related clearly to health aims, as is particularly clear in Sweden.

These changes are now leading to new options and choices for pharmaceutical companies. They have to take decisions in a very different environment with much greater uncertainty. The content of pharmacoeconomics is likely to change and move towards these issues of strategic choice. In the second generation pharmacoeconomics is likely to make a more varied contribution. The involvement with clinical trials will continue but there will also be more involvement in head office roles concerned with strategic development. Pharmacoeconomics is likely to be able to offer a greater variety of roles and career progression.

New issues affecting business development are likely to include the following.

### The Greater Impact of Cost Containment

The implied target in the 1980s was that of holding down the growth rate of health spending to 3–4% a year in real terms: for the 1990s the target is likely to be that of holding real spending constant, and some countries may even be seeking reductions in real spending. The budgets for pharmaceutical spending will be rising much more slowly than in previous decades.

### New Threats to Health

For decades since 1945 health indicators in Western Europe have been reassuring in registering steady progress. The 1990s may well see a reversal in which the lines change directly. The full effects of increased smoking have yet to come through in terms of premature mortality and smoking-related disease. Overall WHO forecasts for Europe, which includes Central Europe and Russia, show a likely rise in deaths from smoking-related disease from 800 000 in 1990 to 2 million in 2025, with additional effects in terms of morbidity and chronic illness (Trigg and Bosanquet, 1992). Many European countries are likely to see increases in poverty and unemployment, with the return of some of the diseases of poverty such as tuberculosis. Increased migration is also likely to bring higher morbidity. In the more mobile society of the USA more than one in five Americans are infected with sexually transmitted disease. Numbers can be expected to rise in Europe, but this is only the most obvious problem. Contact is likely to lead to greater resistance problems in treating infection.

Europe faces a challenge of greater health needs and greater pressure on services at a time when funding in real terms is likely to be static or falling.

## Pressure for Change in Secondary Care

Most hospitals in developed countries were built near traditional city centres. In a number of countries these locations are not well suited to the enlarged suburbs. At the same time new techniques such as minimally invasive therapy are making it much more possible to treat patients on a day basis. Consumer pressure to introduce such techniques is now growing.

## The Gains to Extended Primary Care

Within the UK the 20-year investment in primary care through the Family Doctor Charter has created a potential for much greater service in the primary care setting. Extended primary care can involve a more effective and accountable service in consultation and a wider range of services from the primary care base.

## CONCLUSIONS

The industry is entering into a period of much more intensive change, which is likely to bring an upturn in career prospects and career interest for pharmacoeconomists. All these wider changes will have major impacts on the markets for pharmaceuticals.

One pioneer, Nicholas Wells, Chief Economist from Glaxo, has concluded that 'Pharmacoeconomic analysis is perhaps most appropriately viewed as a research activity still undergoing development and refinement as work continues on its theoretical and technical underpinning and practical experience is gained through its application to contemporary therapeutic issues' (Wells, 1993b). There are an increasing number of good quality studies. As the field expands there might well be ethical issues over possible publication of results which are unpleasant to sponsors. Companies might also face more competition from buyers of pharmaceuticals trying to make the most effective use of fixed budgets (Barrett *et al.*, 1992).

In the new climate, activity in pharmacoeconomics is likely to expand on the 'demand' side among large buyers and regulatory agencies as well as on the 'supply' side among companies. Pharmacoeconomists are likely in the future to have a more varied choice of employer as well as a greater variety of roles within pharmaceutical companies, but they are likely to experience new market pressures and ethical stresses in carrying out these roles. In the late 1980s an increasing number of new products together with more active health promotion has put more pressure on budgets. Now pharmacoeconomists have to relate to a health world in which QALY measures are increasingly being used for rationing services rather than for planning expansion. Pharmacoeconomists seem in fact about to end their age of innocence.

# 26
## Careers in Industry Associations

### Frank Wells

Association of the British Pharmaceutical Industry, London, UK

Let me be quite realistic. The chances of making a total working life career in a pharmaceutical industry trade association are remote. Only a handful of people work in them—currently just 54, including the secretaries, in the UK trade association (the Association of the British Pharmaceutical Industry, known best as the ABPI), acknowledged as being one of the best in the world—and the graduates tend to come from elsewhere or to be going elsewhere. Turnover at the ABPI, however, is low, indicating a higher than average degree of job satisfaction.

Nevertheless, now is not the best time worldwide, to consider a career in this particular field. At the time of writing, the trade association in Germany has collapsed, that in the USA is generally regarded as being in thrall to the regulatory authority, and officials of the trade association in Italy are in prison. Fortunately, no two trade associations are the same, and as this book largely deals with the British scene, for the purposes of this chapter I will base my comments on the situation as it applies to the ABPI, and I will concentrate on graduate careers.

*Discovering New Medicines: Careers in Pharmaceutical Research and Development.*
Edited by P.D. Stonier
© 1994 John Wiley & Sons Ltd

# ASSOCIATION OF THE BRITISH PHARMACEUTICAL INDUSTRY

The ABPI was founded in 1930, and its responsibilities are to work on behalf of its member companies, particularly in relation to government departments. It is governed by the board of management, which is advised by a wide range of expert committees. The association is funded wholly by the subscriptions of its member companies, based on a formula which is applied to turnover. When the industry is under financial pressure, then so is its trade association. However, the overwhelming majority of pharmaceutical companies in the UK choose, voluntarily, to belong to the ABPI, which is encouraging for those who work there. Approximately 92% of the research-based pharmaceutical companies in the UK, and approximately 85% of the generic manufacturers, are currently in membership.

The offices of the ABPI are located in central London, which is an essential prerequisite; previously in Regent Street, near to Piccadilly Circus, it has occupied offices at the Trafalgar Square end of Whitehall since 1984. Partly because the majority of member companies are situated within 80 km of London, committee members and other visitors find this venue as convenient as anywhere, and members of staff are able, relatively easily, to reach a central location, or sally forth from it, whithersoever they have come, and wheresoever they are going.

## CHARACTERISTICS OF JOBS AND HOLDERS

Since the skills that are seen to be necessary at the ABPI tend to reflect many of those required in the industry, it is not surprising that graduate recruitment is largely from pharmaceutical companies. The role descriptions and salary structures are based on comparisons with equivalent conditions within such companies. There are currently five directors or associate directors of various departments in addition to the 'führer', plus six other graduate managers. The departments are of medical, scientific and technological affairs, public and parliamentary affairs, commercial and international affairs, and legal affairs and intellectual property. The Centre for Medicines Research, the Office of Health Economics, and the Prescription Medicine Code of Practice Authority are all associated with the ABPI, but they are staffed independently.

The qualifications of the present senior staff of the ABPI demonstrate appropriate training: for example, I am obviously medically qualified, my associate director is a biologist, the director of international affairs is a legally qualified pharmacist, the secretary of the association is a legally qualified vet, and the manager of commercial affairs is a pharmacist, as is the person responsible for pharmaceutical technical affairs, who also happens to have a degree in business administration. Higher degrees and qualifications might be an advantage but in practice these appear to be less important than having a considerable amount of relevant past experience and the right attitude to the job in general.

Past experience is important, though obviously different people will have had different backgrounds, and nobody can have done everything which might be considered relevant for a particular job. In my case, for example, I did not have any previous experience within the industry at all, but I had been a GP for nearly 20 years, and an under secretary at the British Medical Association (BMA) for seven, and what I had to offer was felt appropriate. As a GP I had pursued a number of different 'extramural' interests, including phase III and phase IV research as an investigator, the training of potential GP principals, the teaching of medical students, chairmanship of the Local Medical Committee, membership of the Suffolk Area Health Authority, involvement with the BMA Board of Science, and so on: and during my time with the BMA I sequentially had responsibility for science and ethics, GPs and hospital doctors, and throughout had responsibility for the Joint Formulary Committee, devising and producing the new-style British National Formulary. The BMA years brought me into contact with a large number of government officials and others, and I am sure that my first career component, followed by the second, led to my appointment with the ABPI having some credibility.

## STAFF SELECTION

Head-hunters are used to fill posts at director level, but not at manager level. Once a decision has been taken to create or fill a vacancy, the sequence of events is in accordance with standard practice, i.e. job analysis, advertisement, pre-selection, interview (usually two) and then appointment. Because the association reflects confidence or otherwise throughout the industry as a whole, every now and again there is a freeze on recruitment, and it would be unrealistic to anticipate the association being in an expansionist mode for the foreseeable future.

Two people are usually involved in assessing a job when it falls vacant—the personnel manager and the relevant director—using Hay MSL criteria and their own assessment of the role. The situation is then either discussed with a head-hunter, or an advertisement is placed in the relevant journals that are widely read by the target population.

My own post would probably be handled by a head-hunter, but other posts might appropriately be advertised in *SCRIP*, *New Scientist* or the *Pharmaceutical Journal*. Such an advertisement would give details of the position, organisation, location and salary range, with key information on the dimensions of the job and on reporting relationships. My own job requires me to head a department which includes an associate director, a manager, an executive officer and three secretaries; the associate director and my own secretary report to me, the other members of the department report to the associate director, and I report to the 'führer'.

Responses to advertisements vary, but there are usually many respondents. The personnel manager sifts out any applications which are manifestly unsuitable, and the remainder go to the relevant manager. We do not use application forms, but prefer to rely on the presentation of the response, including the contents of the candidate's curriculum vitae. A finite number of candidates are called for a first interview, which will usually be with the personnel manager and the relevant director, together. If the candidate is successful, he or she will be called for a second interview, this time involving the 'führer' as well. If the face fits and the chemistry works well, the most applicable person will be appointed.

Despite having said that jobs within the association tend to reflect those within its member companies, the working environment is quite unlike that within a pharmaceutical company. The whole organisation is numerically small, and is situated in the heart of a big city. The premises are, frankly, not as luxuriously appointed as the equivalent offices of member companies—a feature which raises some comment when we are visited. No one can accuse the UK trade association of wasting its members' money in this—or indeed any other—regard.

The broad purpose of my own job—and it is unique, at least within the UK—is to give medical support, and with the associate director scientific and technological support, to the aims of the association in the following ways:

- managing the service which the department of medical, scientific and technological affairs gives to member companies;
- representing the industry's views on medical, scientific or technological matters through personal dealings with outside bodies, including the Department of Health, BMA, medical Royal Colleges, Medical Research Council, and many others;
- acting as medical adviser to the association, the 'führer', and ABPI committees and working parties;
- supervising and supporting the work of the departmental team;

- ensuring that the efforts of the department of medical, scientific and technological affairs are coordinated with those of other departments within the association.

All that sounds rather prosaic; essentially what I do is service the Medical, and Medical and Scientific Information, Committees, and the Statistics Working Group, and all their various working parties and liaison meetings. 'Servicing' in this context includes producing agendas and minutes and taking all necessary actions arising from these meetings. There are about 60 meetings a year which require this spectrum of involvement. Additionally, approximately three one-to-one meetings, are held per week with relevant persons from outside the association. Liaison meetings with relevant outside bodies such as the medical Royal Colleges also occur regularly.

With regard to paper-work, the processing of a large number of incoming documents takes up a significant amount of time; some of these—together with internally generated reports, queries or comments—are sent on a consultation process, and this is referred to below. Literally hundreds of queries have to be handled during the year, and either (usually) answered direct or (infrequently) passed on to others. A great deal of public speaking is involved, including television and radio work, much of it at unsocial hours. The repertoire of topics which have to be known in outline, and some of them in depth, is extensive. I personally have any one of 14 different basic subjects on which I may be excepted to lecture, literally sometimes, at the drop of a hat. Writing definitive documents, articles, chapters, and indeed editing whole books may follow as a natural sequence, once one becomes familiar with a particular topic or series of topics.

The job is therefore essentially complex; most of the tasks involved are demand-driven, but there is considerable freedom to be proactive or to use initiative, within the overall interests of the association. Directors and managers at the ABPI have to be self-confident, and need to know how to listen as well as how to communicate. They have to be able to assess what they hear so as to retain what is important, and to reject what is unimportant, and they have to command the confidence of those with whom and for whom they are working that they are capable of this critical assessment, as well as being able to communicate in a way which gains and holds respect inside and outside the industry.

Personal attributes are relevant; graduate staff working in a trade association have to know when and how to take low or high profiles, be good humoured at all times (including when feeling extremely bad humoured), and they need to be able to generate and hold the respect of senior management and technical staff in both member companies and in outside organisations such as contract houses, sister associations and above all government departments. There is now also bound to be a European element to the job, and liaison with the appropriate persons in the European Federation of Pharmaceutical Industry Associations (EFPIA) is essential. To a lesser extent, liaison with the International Federation of Pharmaceutical Manufacturing Associations (IFPMA) is important, because of its relationship with the World Health Organization (WHO).

Anyone working in a trade association soon realises that project management and prioritisation are important skills, as there are very many different demands on one's time. Another important skill is how to handle a committee: my own job involves looking after the ABPI Medical Committee, which is made up of senior and distinguished pharmaceutical physicians from 18 member companies. They are all extremely busy in their own right, and give up valuable time to serve on the committee, and must therefore quite justifiably be handled with great respect. On the other hand, they all know that they are on the committee to do a different job of work, and must be treated firmly if they do not appear committed. Their opinions are invaluable, but there may be 18 different opinions, and the act of defining a compromise or a consensus is one of the skills needed for this particular type of job. The paper-work generated for and by a committee can be formidable, and decisions have to made regarding the extent to which the members of a committee are involved in consultation processes; they cannot be expected to comment on everything, but a representative industry view on important issues can only be formulated as a result of consultation, and so committee members expect to, and do, receive a number of discussion papers on which they are expected to comment within a finite time-frame.

At the same time, the job involves achieving a balanced appreciation of the needs of member companies collectively, whilst looking at the impressions which this might create with the professions, the government and the public at large, and deciding how to cope with these impressions, and any reactions to them. This sounds like having the proverbial wisdom of Solomon combined with the patience of Job, but most of the time things fit into the general scheme of things intended to create the best possible environment for the industry in which to operate.

# Part V
# Getting Started

# 27
# Recruiting Professional Staff

## John Hawkings

Eames Jones Judge Hawkings, Welwyn, UK

The 1990s will be the 'era of the recruiter'. This quote from a former president of the Institute of Personnel Management was made at the end of the 1980s when the UK was experiencing significant skills shortages during an economic upturn. At the time of writing this chapter a seemingly endless recession has changed the predicted vision of the 1990s. Recruitment problems are still there, but they are different and present equally difficult challenges for recruiters to overcome. Perhaps, therefore, every decade could be called the era of the recruiter because recruitment will always be with us, with a range of ever-present but varying problems. The recruitment process is costly, time-consuming and yet, in essence, is still very hit or miss. The consequences of mistakes in loss of time, money, disruption and even psychological damage can be significant. Recruitment may appear easy to those with little or no direct experience of the process, but it is not.

In this chapter I have looked at the processes and methods of recruiting professional staff. The view is from a recruiter's perspective because it has been my part in the process over many years. However, I think an appreciation of the objectives of the recruiter could help those on the other side of the process—the candidates being recruited—to understand the exercise in which they are taking a part.

Recruitment has always been with us since masters started selecting their servants. In essence this master/servant association is still at the

*Discovering New Medicines: Careers in Pharmaceutical Research and Development.*
Edited by P.D. Stonier
© 1994 John Wiley & Sons Ltd

core of the employment relationship. Probably the two world wars of this century and the need to select vast numbers of people have had the greatest influence on recruitment styles as they have developed today. The 1930s saw developments in the behavioural sciences which could be tested in the large-scale recruitment drives of the Second World War.

For most people involvement in a recruitment process is probably a sporadic activity. However, it is a widespread activity. About 7.4 million vacancies were filled by employers in the UK in a single year at the end of the 1980s according to Department of Employment research.

## PHARMACEUTICAL RECRUITMENT

Narrowing down the perspective to the pharmaceutical sector, the statistics of recruitment activity are still impressive. In 1991 the Institute of Manpower Studies reported on a survey they conducted into recruitment activity in the pharmaceutical sector, examining specifically the extent of manpower and skills shortages amongst managerial and professional staff. Surveys rarely receive a full response, but the results of this one suggested that about 7500 professional staff were employed in research and development (R&D) and the medical/clinical departments of pharmaceutical companies in the UK. In 1990 almost 2900 experienced professional and managerial staff (from all functions) were recruited. One of the groups with significant levels of recruitment activity was in the medical/clinical area. It was noted that vacancies for clinical research associates (CRAs) had increased in recent years, causing recruitment problems. The demand for medically qualified staff had been greater than supply over a considerable period. The fact that such staff were at a premium was reflected in the relatively high turnover of this group.

However, although this may sound gloomy for the recruiter and hopeful for the potential CRA or pharmaceutical physician, the overall conclusion of this detailed analysis was that apart from severe shortages in certain groups, e.g. PhD chemists, pharmacists and statisticians, overall the industry was not suffering from real shortages as had been suspected before the survey. Predictions for the future were also optimistic, with three-fifths of companies expecting growth and another three-fifths of companies expecting growth in professional and managerial staff members.

This background presents a promising picture for those proposing to join the industry or move within it, especially if they are at the early stage of their careers. However, as I indicated at the start of this chapter, predictions made one day which can seem both sure and clear to the predictor can be completely turned around in the future by change of circumstances.

## CANDIDATE EXPECTATIONS

So, what can a potential new entrant to a professional-level appointment in the pharmaceutical industry expect from the recruiters? Even in an industry as developed and well organised as the pharmaceutical industry, sadly what you experience in a recruitment process can vary enormously. At one end is the textbook recruitment exercise carried out with concern for the candidate and with conscientious attention to reach the right decision by the recruiter, and at the other a muddled process with no clear objectives where the candidate comes away with so many unanswered questions and concerns that they probably have decided that they do not want the job anyway.

Candidates should feel that they are going through a well-ordered and planned process in which every aspect of their background, experience, personal approach, style, motivations and beliefs is examined thoroughly. The recruiter should ideally have examined areas of skills and expertise that the applicant may not even know they possess. The aim should be to find the perfect fit of candidate to job, which might be the job as it exists now or as it might develop and change in the future.

Also the choice is not one-sided. The potential employee needs to be given enough information about the vacancy, its current and future status, the department and company to be able to make a decision as to whether they actually want the job. Portraying this essential information accurately might be difficult for the recruiter. For the manager in a panic to fill a vacancy there must often be a temptation to sell the job; to emphasise the advantages and play down the drawbacks; to try and attract the favoured candidate whether it is the right job for them or not. The responsible manager will present the job with all its faults and advantages so the candidate can make their own assessment based on the most accurate and true facts. If candidates suspect they are getting a one-sided picture they should question deeply to unearth potential drawbacks.

Another aspect of recruiting professional staff which, if it goes wrong, can have disastrous consequences for both candidate and company is the speed and pace of recruitment. Rushed recruitment could be as disastrous as a slow, inactive recruitment exercise. Rushed recruitment, often the result of panic and pressure from the manager who is living with a vacancy, can only produce a poorer result. For example, some of the best candidates may apply at a late stage of the recruitment exercise and may be omitted, stages of the recruitment process could be left out, or the candidate may not be given enough time to consider whether they really want the job. Similarly a too slow selection process, with long gaps of inactivity and too many interviews, could result in lack of interest developing in a candidate who was originally excited by the vacancy and, more importantly, the candidate accepting another job offer or being persuaded to stay with their existing company. Recruiting at the right speed is, therefore, not easy but can be an instrumental aspect of the success or failure of a recruitment exercise.

Timing is an aspect that candidates need to consider as well. If a candidate is not sure how long to allow to attend an interview, or any other part of a selection process, it is far better to find out beforehand the amount of time to allow than half an hour into an interview announce that they have to leave in a quarter of an hour.

## RECRUITER TECHNIQUES

So how can the recruiter find the right professional staff effectively? They must follow a systematic approach that starts with analysis of the job and the ideal person to do it. A selection process is then designed to find as close as possible a match to the ideal person they have identified. Everybody concerned in the process must have a clear and common understanding of what the recruitment process is expected to achieve. It seems self-evident that you cannot find what you need until you determine what it looks like. Yet it is not uncommon for a recruiting manager to rush out to look for 'one the same as the last job holder' or 'a standard CRA'. This approach has little chance of success.

Firstly a detailed job description must be prepared. This may be an appropriate time to consider whether the vacant job should be eliminated, split up between other people, or redesigned. It is an opportunity to make changes that may improve the jobs and responsibilities of other staff. Various processes may contribute to the preparation of job descriptions, such as watching somebody do the job, interviewing people doing the same or similar jobs, analysing termination interviews or previous appraisal reviews or simply the manager writing the description on their own. A candidate being recruited should ask for a job description. Absence of this document could perhaps be a warning sign.

The next stage is to predict the essential and desirable characteristics of the ideal person for the job. This analysis is usually carried out to a pre-designed plan, of which there are some long-established and well-known ones in existence. One example of such is Roger's Seven-point Plan whereby an employee specification is written down under the headings physical make-up, attainments, general intelligence, special aptitudes, interests, disposition and circumstances. As well as determining the essential and desirable characteristics under each heading it can also be useful to identify the contraindications, i.e. the attributes that would preclude someone from the appointment. Before recruitment starts it is also useful to work out the induction programme and training programme for a new employee. If this is left until later when the recruitment exercise becomes more active it may not be completed and once the new employee is joining the company it is too late.

All the activities mentioned so far should take place whatever the type of vacancy or level of recruitment. What happens next in the procedure will vary in relation to the type of job and type of people to be attracted and assessed. Having decided recruitment is necessary the next stage is to look into the people market-place.

For recruiters there is a vast pool of advice available, usually free, about the most appropriate methods of attracting candidates, where to advertise and how to prepare an advertisement. Advertising agencies will write advertisements at no cost to advertisers, and a well-written advertisement will not only be more effective in targeting the right people, but should also deter applications from those who are totally inappropriate. With so much advice available there should be no excuse for getting recruitment advertising disastrously wrong, especially where the choice of media is obvious, and yet it is still possible to see advertisements in totally inappropriate media which must result in no applicants and be a complete waste of substantial sums of money.

The job seeker's role in this part of the process is easy. They only need to watch advertisements in the professional journals they normally read. They can also contact appropriate recruitment consultants dealing with their specialism and, of course, they can write speculatively to companies to see if they are recruiting.

## SELECTION

### Interviews

Candidates have applied for the job and the next step for the recruiter is to apply methods for selecting the most appropriate. The range of techniques available is vast, but according to an Institute of Manpower Studies survey of over 300 organisations most employers' selection procedures are 'unscientific, subject to bias and unreliable'. The three most common selection techniques were interviews, references and application forms, which are the least valid and reliable measures of future job performance. Another survey indicated that most employers use no more than two or three selection methods although over 12 were in use in the UK.

The interview requires most comment. It is almost universally used by employers in the selection process and most employers believe they are a reliable selection method, although research evidence suggests the opposite. Generally candidates can expect two or more interviews, usually with two or three interviewers together or singly. The interview can be improved significantly if the interviewer has been trained. The trained interviewer should have worked out what information they want to collect from candidates. They should have an interview plan which provides an outline and prompt to ensure the main areas of interest are covered and none are omitted. They should be skilled questioners, following up the facts given in an answer with more questions until a full picture emerges and there are no uncertainties or inconsistencies. They should not ask questions that will just elicit yes and no responses or suggest the answer expected from the candidate in the question. They should submerge all personal prejudices and biases. An American study of selection interviews found interviewers reached decisions to accept or reject in the first four minutes. They should show respect and they should take full notes. How many people can accurately recall the contents of a $1\frac{1}{2}$ to 2-hour discussion if they make no notes at all? They can only come away with a general impression and research shows that the general impression is likely to be more favourable than warranted. Pressure tactics, stress interviews and trick questions are all bad practice, although difficult questions are certainly allowed. Above all the interviewer should listen hard, talking for only up to 10% of the interview time.

Apart from being a method of collecting information about people, research has found that applicants decided whether or not to accept job offers partly on the basis of how the interviewer behaved towards them. Interviewers who listened well were regarded more favourably by interviewees who seemed to form a more favourable impression of the organisation as well.

Most interviewees do not find it difficult to recognise a bad interview, but unfortunately there is little that they can do to correct such a situation. However, at least in an interview where the interviewer has done all the talking it may be appropriate to mention at the end that certain aspects of experience did not emerge in the questioning and tell the interviewer what they are. This may then prompt the interviewer to find out more by additional questioning.

## Psychometrics

But interviews are not the only selection method. There are many other assessment techniques that may be used in the recruitment of professional staff. This selection of techniques ranges from the useful and fairly common such as psychometric testing to the unusual and possibly dubious, like astrology.

Psychometric testing, if properly administered and interpreted, is amongst the most consistently reliable of all the assessment methods. However, in a 1990 survey tests were found to be used by only 16% of employers, although from experience it seems that in the pharmaceutical sector that percentage is higher. The most widely used tests measure aptitudes (verbal, numerical and abstract reasoning), general intelligence, personality and typical performance. They can either be given individually or in batteries. However, although in general they are regarded as more valid and reliable predictors of performance, not all tests are good tests. Some of the widely marketed quick tests which require no training to administer and interpret should be viewed with caution.

Although there is a large volume of data to support the predictive value of tests it is apparent that testers and those being tested frequently have firm views on the subject and sometimes the question of testing needs to be put into perspective. In essence tests are a further tool in the recruitment process. They can be used as a source of information to be further discussed, checked and examined at an interview. It is also essential that test results are reported back to those who have been tested. There is no excuse for allowing the impression to persist that testing is a secret and underhand method of finding out facts that candidates may want to hide.

Some of the processes on the borders of psychological testing should, however, be looked at with caution. Into this category comes graphology: the analysis of handwriting. Although more popular in mainland Europe, especially France where it is widely used, it is still rarely used in the UK. The predictive validity of handwriting analysis is not great, and there remain many questions surrounding its usefulness.

## References

Very straightforward methods of assessment are reference and qualification checks. Most employers check references. They are very cheap to obtain for the cost of a stamp or a phone call, but the subjective aspects are not considered particularly reliable. References rarely say anything critical and many personnel staff learn to read between the lines.

However, they can confirm dates and facts and from time to time they can bring to light problems that remain hidden in interviews and for this alone are worth doing. From my own experience I recall a particular candidate with a behavioural problem that remained undetected through several detailed interviews, emerged as a possible problem through personality testing and was confirmed as a definite problem from a reference with a former employer.

Another reference check that is rarely carried out but is simple to do, and dangerous if not done, is a check on qualifications. It may seem unbelievable, but I have met cases of invented qualifications from applicants for pharmaceutical industry jobs.

Biodata is worth mentioning because, although it is only used by a small number of companies, it is claimed to be both reliable and valid and it does seem to produce consistently good predictions of future performance. Specific types of biographical data are chosen generally because on a statistical basis they are good predictors of future performance. The data are collected from applicants, either from application forms or biographical questionnaires. Although it has faults, as have all other methods, its high predictive value may mean that in future it could come into wider use.

## Assessment Centres

Assessment centres are a widely used form of group assessment, more especially for graduate and junior professional-level appointments. With their origins in the UK in the selection of army officers by the War Office Selection Boards during the Second World War, they have become increasingly popular. They typically consist of one to two days spent with other candidates undergoing tests and group exercises which are objectively analysed and scored. Leaderless group discussions and group problem-solving exercises are typical of the processes used. They will more generally be used where the field of candidates is wide and so are most common for the junior professional appointments. Where the number of candidates is small or the experience of candidates is great they are probably less appropriate and there is always the issue that the identity of each candidate is known to the others, which might not be appropriate at higher levels.

## Other

Other assessment methods used are presentations, written projects on job-related topics, work sample tests and many more, but those described above represent either the most widely used (interviews) or interesting (biodata) or unusual (graphology). For the professional employee about to be recruited it at least may give some pre-warning of what could be expected.

## RECRUITMENT DECISIONS

By this stage the recruiters should have collected enough information about candidates to be able to make some decisions. A common way of describing the main decision-making techniques is through either actuarial or clinical predictions. Actuarial decision-making involves the objective statistical analysis of data about candidates. The clinical method involves the review of information that is available and on the basis of this and the decision-taker's own experience a choice is made. There has been much debate over time about which is the best method, but at the end of the day it is still the case that most decisions on whom to appoint rely on 'gut feeling' and intuition.

## LEGAL ASPECTS

Finally, I am going to mention briefly the legal constraints on recruiters. I am sure that many potential recruits do not immediately associate recruitment with legal requirements. They will be wrong. As with most areas of employment, Acts of Parliament also dictate what the recruiters can and cannot do. I hope nobody recruited to a professional-level appointment in the pharmaceutical industry experiences discrimination that breaks the law. However, an overview of the laws that govern recruiters may add a further perspective to the complexity of their role.

The Sex Discrimination Act 1975 and the Race Relations Act 1976 make it unlawful to discriminate on grounds of sex, married status (but not single status), race, colour, nationality or ethnic or national origins. The Act lays down rules covering selection arrangements, the decision on whom to appoint and the terms on which employment is offered. An employer cannot refuse to offer someone a job if they are, or are not, a member of a trade union because of legal requirements in the Employment Act 1990.

Those who recruit on behalf of companies or employment agencies or consultancies have to comply with all the laws mentioned. This can be difficult if a recruiting company asks the consultancy to select for recruitment in a way that would break the law and the recruitment consultancy should refuse to comply with such a request. In addition these bodies are bound by their own regulations, the Employment Agencies Act 1973, which regulates their activities.

Any agency or employer who keeps information about applicants on computers must comply with the registration provisions of the Data Protection Act 1984. Another activity tightly controlled is the writing of advertisements to attract applicants for a job. The contents of job advertisements must follow the requirements of the Sex Discrimination Act and Race Relations Act. Finally the disabled are also protected in theory. The Disabled Persons (Employment) Act 1944 provides for recruitment quotas which require employers with 20 or more employees to employ at least 30% registered disabled employees unless they apply for a permit excusing compliance.

But what happens in reality? For some time a view has existed that although the legislation has worthy intentions and has been in existence long enough for an effect to have been experienced, in fact the wide-reaching changes in employment practices that were expected have been slow in coming. Perhaps it is difficult to legislate for universal change in beliefs and attitudes and perhaps the examples set by the tolerant employer will in the long run have the greater influence.

## CONCLUSIONS

Every aspect of the process of recruiting professional staff into the pharmaceutical industry can be characterised by a range between extremes. Speed can be very quick or slow. In my experience this has ranged from under a week to over a year. It can be simple: one interview with one person, or complex: interviews with many different people in different countries using a variety of selection techniques. It can be an enjoyable, informative experience for the candidate or it can be a nightmare. In the main it is likely to be on a range somewhere between the extremes.

Throughout the process both sides are taking decisions, with either side free to withdraw from the proceedings. Usually a developing relationship between the two sides with the increase of mutual trust is occurring. At the point of writing this even after several years of severe recession, cut-backs, mergers and redundancies, in the area of recruiting professional staff into the pharmaceutical industry there still seems to be a shortfall of skilled, high-quality staff as there has been, in my experience, over all varieties of economic climates. It seems unlikely, therefore, that this situation will change and I find it difficult to envisage that the type of professional staff recruited into the pharmaceutical industry will ever become a glut commodity.

Against this background recruiters need to realise that although they retain the right and duty to assess and select carefully, they should not regard recruitment as purely putting candidates through a range of tests and exercises. Both sides need to clarify their views of each other and reach agreement through negotiation. Negotiation, openness and compromise are more likely to characterise recruitment in the future than the straightforward selection of the servant by the master, and, hopefully, if this occurs the process will be the better for it.

# 28
# Preparing a Curriculum Vitae

4Cs Communications, Borough Green, UK

Lest familiarity breed contempt: the time and skills needed to prepare the *right* curriculum vitae (CV) for the *right* job are far too often and with ill effect, sadly underestimated.

Preparing and presenting a CV entails much more than jotting down a few chronologically ordered facts about you and your career and sending it off to 'whoever's' advertisement offers 'excellent prospects', or even better, matches your skills, experience and aspirations—on paper! Preparation of a successful document (and satisfying future career) begins long before the first draft.

## DEFINING THE CURRICULUM VITAE

A cogent CV reflects personal and professional awareness (by the author of him or herself); clear, realistic ambitions built on that appraisal; and structure and content matched to relevant job opportunities and demands (Figure 1).

The CV should be considered, not as an isolated item, but as Volume II of an essential trilogy:

- Volume I:   *Targeting the future* (setting career priorities);
- Volume II:  *Targeting the goal* (preparing the right CV for the right job);
- Volume III: *Opening the door* (the interview and beyond).

*Discovering New Medicines: Careers in Pharmaceutical Research and Development.*
Edited by P.D. Stonier
© 1994 John Wiley & Sons Ltd

---

A cogent CV:

1. addresses no more and no less than is asked for—*pertinent and current*
2. presents a favourable but realistic impression of the applicant—*constructive*
3. presents the information with clarity and economy of expression—*clear and concise*
4. displays neat typography and logical layout—*legible, pleasing to the eye*
5. stands on its own—*self-contained*

but

6. is accompanied by a covering letter—*introduction*

---

**Figure 1.** The CV profile.

*Emergency procedures,* a brief appendix to Volumes II and III, reassures unsuccessful applicants that all is not lost and refers them back to basic principles of preparation. They should evaluate their efforts before repeating the process. 'Losing' erodes confidence and performance. 'Losing' might not mean that the best candidate won: but, in a very competitive situation, the winner will be he or she who understands and answers the employer's requirements precisely; who is confident about personal talents and motives for change. He or she will probably present the best CV.

## An Introduction: 'Tailored' or 'Standard'

The CV is an introduction—would-be employee to employer: primarily, a summary of skills and experience, requested by or judged to be of value to the employer. The employer usually has the advantage. A successful CV quickly attracts interest against stiff competition; proves its pertinence for a specific purpose; or suggests valuable new possibilities to the employer. The writer should therefore be clear about why he or she is applying for:

1. a specific position (solicited response); or
2. possible employment (unsolicited inquiry).

The submissions will be 'tailored' accordingly. That will be easier and more effective if the writer has first worked through *targeting the future* (Figure 2 and below).

A 'standard' (basic details only) CV is generally *not* appropriate for specific job applications. It may however, serve well for:

1. *initial inquiry,* addressed, with a covering letter, to an appropriate source—e.g. to the *named* manager of the recruitment service offered

1. Analysis—*personal and professional profiles*
2. Exploration—*information gathering/perspective*
3. Organisation—*classification/review*
4. Reflection—*career options/priorities*
5. Targeting the goal—*the right CV for the right job*

**Figure 2.** Targeting the future: selecting career priorities.

by a company. The correct name and title changes the perceived approach from 'fishing' to one more soundly based on 'interest and research'—principles pleasing to a scientific, market-orientated industry. It should be planned—not luck!

2. *informal reference* which clarifies the author's areas of interest and expertise for colleagues and associates (not necessarily new!)—e.g. in team or multi-centre projects; committees; international meetings and correspondence. If seeking change, don't forget potential head-hunters!

3. *emergency 'stop gap'*. CVs prepared in haste or while under stress rarely impress. Emergencies and 'opportunity', however, defy prediction. A current 'standard' CV at hand is a wise investment.

Deficiencies in a hurried response (e.g. to a casual meeting or advertisement noticed just before an application deadline) may be addressed in a covering letter or conversation. The writer will still be at a disadvantage against a carefully targeted CV prepared for open competition. That disadvantage can be reduced by a recently revised standard CV; by the candidate giving priority to background research, of both job and employer, before interview is offered. Such initiative is rarely wasted, even if the application is unsuccessful.

This chapter focuses on *Targeting the future* (Volume I) and *Targeting the goal* (Volume II). Volume I sets the scene for success; Volume II uses that information to prepare the CV most appropriate for the chosen goal. Volume III consolidates their combined wisdom and *opens the door*: here, to careers in pharmaceutical medicine; to challenges and opportunities discussed in the preceding chapters. The emphasis, the key to success, is *preparation*: keeping in touch and up with professional perspectives; keeping 'yourself and yours' in the career planning picture.

## CAREER PRIORITIES: TARGETING THE FUTURE

### The CV and Pharmaceutical Medicine into the Twenty-first Century

The degree and pace of change in pharmaceutical medicine have been dramatic over the past 40 years and show no signs of slowing down, stressing the need for frequent career review and revision.

*Options* is a 'buzz-word' of the technological age. However, several such others limit the kaleidoscope of opportunities implied: *competition, qualifications, skills* and, increasingly, *mobility*. Next, struggling for precedence in career development, come *potential* (under 30–35?) and *experience* (never 'too much too soon'; but over 40–45?). These factors strongly influence employers. Prospective employees must allow for them when planning career moves and selecting jobs; when preparing CVs.

Despite the rhetoric, and undoubted effects of first impressions at interview (*opening the door*), personality, and personal interests and responsibilities are not always high-profile priorities. Companies which pay them due attention are worth noting; those with a doubtful record, worth avoiding—especially in this age of constant change and rising expectation. Applicants cannot *afford* to ignore them when *targeting the future*. The CV should reflect research and understanding of general and professional management attitudes to personnel and arrange personal details accordingly. *Analysis* (see below) will help with this process.

CVs which imply uncertainty about the writer's commitment rarely succeed—e.g. perhaps seeking 'anything better on offer' after publication of 'Medical and Dental Staffing Prospects in the NHS' dashes hopes for quick advancement in a preferred field. The work of the faculty, the first professorial chair and MSc in pharmaceutical medicine (Surrey University), and George Poste's insights into the twenty-first century, indicate the speciality's dynamism and growing prestige. Candidates must show excellent ability and potential, appropriate training and experience, and valid reasons for making theirs a 'first option' decision. The CV must address these messages clearly; succinctly; persuasively.

### Before the First Draft—Steps in Clarification

Analysis, exploration, organisation and reflection are the foundations for setting career priorities.

*Analysis* asks basic questions about professional and personal life and relates the answers to career development (see Figures 3 and 4). The process helps clarify issues at work and at home: perceived versus actual problems and assets; professional performance/prospects/satisfaction;

---

Current interests and commitments 'outside office hours'

(examples only)

Main responsibilities: *family, including elderly parents, asthmatic son; my own health*

Main commitments: *school governor, 'Age Concern' committee; tennis club secretary*

Main interests: *sports activities; play clarinet; photography; theatre; travel*

Main aspirations: *enjoy work and personal life; raise a happy family; retain rural home base*

Main areas of conflict (work v. home demands): *is the balance reasonable? Necessary? Why?*

---

**Figure 3.** Changing jobs? Personal inventory.

---

Current career: prospects for progress and change

What job am I doing?                     Where am I headed (natural progression v. change)?

What are the prospects/problems?         Is this what I want? (use a debit/credit balance sheet)

What are the options?                    Do I know enough to make such major decisions?

What do I need to know?                  Where are/who have the answers?

What to do with the information?

---

**Figure 4.** Changing jobs? Professional inventory.

possible alternatives; and current or potential conflicts between career and personal interests.

*Exploration*—broad-based information-gathering focused by *analysis*—is an essential precursor to progress: to the right CV. It penetrates façades, develops balanced perspectives. Advertisements (and employers) do not highlight pitfalls or problems! All jobs have them, but the quality of management and the working milieu influence their frequency and their impact. An 'informed' CV can handle contentious issues; subtly address difficulties in ways which suggest the candidate would manage well. A key question to ask is: 'Why change the setting but not the problems?'

The first matter to reconsider, keep open perhaps, during *exploration* is evaluation of the current appointment. Was the first *analysis* sufficiently objective and broad? Was 'wise counsel' sought ('outsider'/'the boss'/college)? This latter may be impractical. Discretion in the exploratory stages is prudent, but reasoned inquiry should not offend or prejudice prospects. A professional parting on good terms has definite benefits: positive presentation of the 'last' appointment and references for the CV; confirmation when *opening the door*. A clear picture of the 'here and now' helps detect problems and opportunities, often in different guise, when considering future options.

Sources of information featured throughout this book reveal the exciting variety of openings and the pace of change in pharmaceutical medicine. Exploration is not an option. In summary:

- *Professional and public libraries* provide ready access to current thought and opinion worldwide. Librarians are invaluable allies. Relevant trade and professional journals give a sense of the main issues affecting both industry and the profession and where they might be heading. Local and international meetings are listed. Company annual reports provide insight into their main structure, interests, finances and operational networks. Comparisons may spark new interests.
- *Direct inquiry* to professional and commercial organisations—e.g. the Faculty of Pharmaceutical Medicine (FPM), the British Association of Pharmaceutical Physicians (BRAPP), company personnel departments—even legal specialists—yields up-to-date job profiles and career prospects (vital for tailored CVs!).
- *Conferences and local meetings* attract pitface professionals with different backgrounds and opinions. 'Just listening' can replace illusions with challenging perspectives—for people changing course within the field, as well as newcomers. Organisers, if asked, may arrange introductions to colleagues with common interests. Personal contacts are a rich source of ideas—and opportunity. CVs, benefiting by them, must honour their tacit confidentiality.

*Organisation* of information as it is gathered improves the speed and quality of the review. Categories should cover both the profession as a whole and special interests and options. Those outlined in this book provide an excellent quide. Practical options will emerge, identifying potential positions, employers and plans for action. The CV will be forming among the ideas. First impressions benefit from informal discussion with objective colleagues; with family—partner or spouse; with children old enough to understand—especially the implications, for school and friends, of relocation; of a parent's increased absence, working for(?), but not very often with, the family. More formal contact with official sources should refine impressions; confirm or banish doubts.

*Reflections* on this background research and discussion clarifies priorities; selects realistic goal(s) for action. Volume II—the CV—can now be prepared with confidence. Figure 5 summarises the clarification process.

**Analysis**

Develops *professional and personal profiles*; clarifies job/home conflict and compatibility; indicates what, if any, changes may be an advantage

Matches job descriptions with professional and personal profiles; determines what skills are needed; identifies options for *exploration*

**Exploration and organisation**

Gathers and classifies information about career opportunities in spheres of interest suggested by *analysis*; prepares them for review

**Reflection**

Translates messages gained from the data and opinion review and clarifies how best to pursue in the chosen field, keeping a healthy balance between professional and personal interests

These priorities form the basis for an *action plan*; introduce:

**Targeting the goal!** preparing the right curriculum vitae for the right job

**Figure 5.** Preparing the right CV: before the first draft.

## THE RIGHT CURRICULUM VITAE FOR THE RIGHT OCCASION: TARGETING THE GOAL

Clearly, neither the CVs' contents nor format will be static. Each should offer variations of the standard, able to show an applicant's talents to best advantage, in different but appropriate circumstances.

Definite advantages can be realised in *opening the door*. The CV becomes a resource: provides a safe focus for discussion. Candidates so equipped perform better at interview; respond better to unexpected or trick questions. They have a realistic view of the position, the profession and the organisation. They can more accurately assess whether the interviewers and the job match general expectations; whether further questions should be answered before accepting final offers—especially if those differ from the original and a quick response is required.

## STRUCTURE

No one template gives the 'ideal format'. A CV is a personal document which must, however, fulfil a defined purpose. That purpose is a key guideline in preparation. A covering letter addressed to a named recipient (see below) should introduce it. This section therefore deals more with principles and guidelines than 'role models'.

**Warning!**

Technology compensates for poor handwriting and artistic inadequacy. Not for poor content.

**Potted Reminders**

1. *Targeting the future* is not an option.
2. Guidelines for a cogent CV (Figure 1) matter.
3. Ensure the CV delivers positive perspectives, not unsustainable illusions.
4. Read advertisements and job descriptions carefully. Remove doubts before preparing the CV.
5. Prestigious positions attract high-standard submissions. Your CV will be only one of many.

*Presentation*, unless otherwise stated, is best set on one side only of A4 paper (preferably white or pastel). Typed or printed text (simple fonts and clean paper!) ensures legibility. Elaborate or 'bound' versions offer no advantage. CVs are often photocopied for selection committee members who quickly recognise 'commercial' productions. The document is therefore best sent unfolded.

*Language* and style must be clear: short sentences; no unexplained jargon or abbreviations—even if very common. Foreign graduates tempted to use commercial editors must recognise that, if qualifications are otherwise appropriate, language difficulties will be apparent at interview. Special courses in medical terms and writing, as held in London, may boost language proficiency.

*Format* follows a fairly standard order:

- personal identification and contact information;
- education/career details;
- personal background;
- miscellaneous (relevant skills, publications, referees ...);
- synopsis (may precede main CV).

**Content**

*Personal identification* opens the document, preceded by a heading which identifies the CV's nature and purpose and the person responsible for its receipt. 'In confidence' may be added at the author's discretion. Identification details present the applicant's full name and contact (usually home) address and phone/fax numbers. The name may be added (in small print) to each numbered page in case they become separated. Office contacts should be offered with caution if a new job is being pursued without the knowledge of current employers. An obvious note (e.g. in bold type) should direct correspondence to the preferred address. Overseas applications need care with address details (e.g. area codes, unfamiliar abbreviations), titles of address and the date. Many countries reverse the month and year in figures. If in doubt, write the month in full, the day and year in figures. This is important to check when noting deadlines published in 'foreign' advertisements. Details such as age, sex (if the gender is not clear from the name), nationality and marital status may be added here or under personal background.

*Career and educational background* form the heart of the CV. The author must address the employer's priorities. A call to 'further inquiries' to clarify ambiguity before applying is worth the effort. A senior professional CV rarely needs information before the course which conferred the basic professional degrees. Postgraduate qualifications (with source and explanation if uncommon) are listed chronologically with the career history or in a separate block. Foreign candidates should ensure that their qualifications are appropriate and language ability adequate.

Appointments traditionally appear in reverse chronological order (most practical for long histories). The current/last appointment of importance and its relevance to the advertised post is described in most detail. (The relevance of *each* post to the latter should be highlighted!) Reasons for application may be included here, in the covering letter—or, especially the details, left until interview. The career history should, even if unusual, show logical progression and use of opportunity (or misfortune) to enhance knowledge and skills pertinent to mainstream interests. For example, the ability to anticipate and cope with change; to budget and use resources imaginatively and effectively; to be trustworthy. The clue to acceptance of the 'unusual' is insight (preparation) and presentation. The tone of the text should be positive, but suggest ability to compromise: where possible, indicative, rather than definitive or prescriptive. Interview will fill in required details. Remember, the CV *stimulates* interest; *suggests* potential!

*Personal history* is not a pseudonym for autobiography! The CV is an invitation—to interview. This section should present the candidate as a person whose 'private' interests and activities are compatible with the job, in both personality and commitment (*analysis* will have determined this much earlier!). Life experiences may be used constructively: e.g. foreign residence or travel to suggest global perspectives and languages; energy and curiosity; adaptability; good people and organisational skills; mobility. If in doubt, leave it out! Gaps in the CV may be explained, at least in part—e.g. maternity leave, overseas family postings, illness. Personal health is a confidential matter which may be pursued at interview. It is usually wise to omit details at CV stage, but a condition likely to interfere with performance is also likely to deteriorate under the resultant pressure. *Targeting the future* will help select suitable openings.

*Miscellaneous* items include anything of interest to the proposed post. Each is kept brief and placed in order of relevance. For example:

- *Publications.* List the most recent and/or meritorious 5–10. Indicate that a full list is available on request. Be prepared to discuss their relevance to the post advertised.
- *Computer skills.* Indicate levels of competence with which systems and packages.
- *Languages.* List in order of proficiency and indicate oral fluency compared to ability to read and write. Remember, you might be asked to show your skills at interview!
- *Professional affiliations.* These may highlight complementary interests and useful connections.
- *References.* These are often optional at the CV stage. If so, their availability 'on request' could be mentioned here or in the covering letter. Referees must be asked beforehand for their cooperation. They also need a clear idea of the kind of reference needed. References from the two most recent appointments are advisable, unless particular requests or features from other positions supplant them. If either post ended on unfavourable terms, explanations are best left until interview. 'Preparation' will direct how this might be best handled. A general principle is—be as positive as possible, if asked.

*Synopses* are just that—insight, at a glance, to details of the full CV. Each should ideally cover only one page (maximum two); present basic personal identification, career outline and miscellaneous items most relevant to the application. It usually lies behind the letter of introduction as the first page, or at the back, the last page, of the CV.

*Standard and tailored CVs* tell the same basic story. The latter vary their emphasis in response to specific requests. 'Standards' probe potentials carefully selected by analysis. Both rely for success on meticulous preparation; on rigorous review and currency. Both benefit during preparation from informal comment by a 'disinterested' reader.

*Letters of introduction* addressed to the person identified in the advertisement, or as otherwise directed, should also keep to one page. A handwritten submission may be requested. If not, the choice is yours. Take the opportunity to introduce the application 'with pleasure'. If appropriate, explain briefly your interest; draw attention to, and explain, possible disadvantages such as absences or unconventional qualifications. Make them a focus of interest, for exploration at interview. And be prepared for a grilling if you are invited! The principle here is to identify possible stumbling blocks; interpret less conventional experience likely to be undervalued; subtly make the most of your assets. Avoid saying too much. The written word is easily misinterpreted—particularly when it is one among very many and time is limited.

## CONCLUSION

The CV is ready for inspection. Volumes I and II of the trilogy are complete. Volume III will open the door to new horizons in a world whose possibilities already range 'beyond imagination'. May the best-prepared man or woman win!

# 29
# Training and Education in Pharmaceutical Medicine

## David K. Luscombe

Welsh School of Pharmacy, University of Wales, Cardiff, UK

Rapid expansion of the pharmaceutical industry during the early 1950s resulted in a significant increase in the number of medical doctors employed in the development and assessment of new medicines. To provide for the specialist needs of these doctors in the UK, the Association of Medical Advisers in the Pharmaceutical Industry (AMAPI) was launched in 1957. In keeping with the aims of other professional societies, AMAPI organised regular symposia to keep members up to date with advances in their chosen speciality. Such continuing education programmes were designed specifically for AMAPI members with several years experience. No provision was made for doctors newly appointed to the pharmaceutical industry who had to learn their skills 'on the job' under the supervision of a more experienced doctor (Snell, 1985). This situation might have continued to this day, as indeed it has in many other countries, but for a number of events which took place in the UK and brought about an urgent need to establish a structured training programme for medical doctors newly recruited to the industry.

*Discovering New Medicines: Careers in Pharmaceutical Research and Development.*
Edited by P.D. Stonier
© 1994 John Wiley & Sons Ltd

## THE NEED FOR TRAINING PROGRAMMES

During the 1950s the role of the pharmaceutical doctor was primarily that of a medical adviser. However, the job gradually became more varied and the responsibilities increased significantly with the advent of the Medicines Act 1968 which necessitated a substantial increase in the quality and quantity of clinical information required in obtaining new product licences. As a result, the knowledge and skill requirements of the medical adviser increased greatly. Indeed, this newly acquired expanded role was recognised by Snell (1970), who introduced the term 'pharmaceutical medicine' to describe the specialist work carried out by medical doctors employed in assessing the efficacy and safety of new medicines. The widespread acceptance of this new term and that of 'pharmaceutical physician' led AMAPI to change its name in the mid-1980s to the British Association of Pharmaceutical Physicians (BrAPP), which more closely reflected the work being carried out by its members.

With the ever-increasing knowledge base and skills required by the pharmaceutical physician in carrying out their daily duties, there became a real need for AMAPI to establish some form of structured training programme for new entrants to the industry. This need was reinforced on publication of the report of the Royal Commission on Medical Training (1968) and that of the Joint Committee on Higher Medical Training, which emphasised the need for medical doctors in the pharmaceutical industry to undergo an appropriate form of training and, furthermore, to seek recognition for their particular expertise.

It was initially assumed that industry doctors would be eligible for accreditation in clinical pharmacology and therapeutics by the Joint Committee on Higher Medical Training. However, it was soon realised that for the great majority of doctors employed in the industry this was an incorrect assumption. Thus, it became essential to seek some other form of recognition for pharmaceutical physicians. The possibility of the Royal College of Physicians providing this recognition was investigated and resulted in a formal proposal being submitted to the Joint Committee of the three Royal Colleges of Physicians of the UK, inquiring whether a postgraduate diploma might be established to meet this need. In 1975 the Joint Committee acted positively to initiate such a diploma and after a brief gestation period the new Diploma in Pharmaceutical Medicine was launched, with the inaugural examination taking place in November 1976.

This was a historic landmark in the development and recognition of pharmaceutical medicine in the UK, despite the fact that the General Medical Council (GMC) at that time would not recognise the Diploma in Pharmaceutical Medicine as a registrable qualification. This was in keeping with the GMC policy of restricting the registrability of post-graduate qualifications. However, it was stated by the then secretary of the GMC that the new diploma would be 'useful in identifying doctors who would be entitled to a certificate of completion of specialist training in clinical pharmacology and therapeutics for the purpose of EC directives'. The fact that the regulations for eligibility to sit the Diploma in Pharmaceutical Medicine stated until 1992 that candidates should normally have undergone a two-year period of part-time postgradute education in pharmaceutical medicine (in addition to at least two years of post-registration medical training) meant that such a programme had to be available for those candidates wishing to be eligible to sit the new diploma examination.

## ESTABLISHING A STRUCTURED TRAINING PROGRAMME

The first structured postgraduate training programme designed to meet the specific needs of the pharmaceutical physician was organised by AMAPI in 1974. The prime purpose was to convert the newly recruited hospital doctor or general practitioner into a specialist in pharmaceutical medicine. The course was part-time and consisted of eight one-day meetings per year covering the following subject areas: toxicology and the extrapolation of data to man; animal pharmacology and its relevance to man; biopharmaceutics, pharmacokinetics and chemistry; practical aspects of pre-clinical studies, regulatory affairs; business management, marketing functions, personnel and training methods; medical information, literature retrieval; therapeutics, adverse reactions and drug efficacy. In addition, a one-week residential course was held dealing with the clinical evaluation of medicines in man. This included a clinical trials workshop and provided some coverage of medical statistics.

Whilst the one-year training programme was well received by AMAPI members, it was not considered comprehensive enough by the Royal Colleges of Physicians to be recognised as a course suitable for preparing candidates for the Diploma in Pharmaceutical Medicine examination. In consequence, it was necessary to expand the initial AMAPI training programme to a two-year course in order to provide the equivalent of eight weeks of full-time study, which was the minimum requirement for eligibility to sit for the Royal Colleges of Physicians diploma. Interestingly, in a survey of pharmaceutical physicians carried out some 15 years later, the majority of respondents confirmed that the basic knowledge and skills relating to pharmaceutical medicine requires a two-year period of part-time training (Stonier and Gabbay, 1992).

The revised two-year AMAPI programme commenced in the autumn of 1976, the course contents being based on the same syllabus as that used for the diploma examination. Furthermore, the regulations governing eligibility to sit the examination were used as the criteria for entry to the course. Thus, participants had to hold qualifications in medicine, surgery and midwifery recognised by the Board of Management of the Royal College of Physicians and be either fully registrable in the British Medical Register or fully registrable in the country in which the qualification was granted. This latter clause was particularly important since it actively encouraged industry doctors working in mainland European countries to attend the training programme and sit the diploma examination. In fact, in the first four examinations which were held, some 18% of those who attended the course and sat the examination were resident in continental Europe. One doctor was working in the pharmaceutical industry in the USA, whilst another was resident in Nigeria (Macleod and Goldberg, 1981). By November 1990, some 297 candidates had sat the diploma examination, with 234 being awarded the Diploma in Pharmaceutical Medicine (Shelley, 1991).

## THE BrAPP/UNIVERSITY OF WALES POSTGRADUATE COURSE IN PHARMACEUTICAL MEDICINE

In 1978, AMAPI (now BrAPP) invited the University of Wales (UW) to collaborate in organising its two-year part-time training programme. This scheme became known as the BrAPP/UW Postgraduate Course in Pharmaceutical Medicine and was the originator of all later part-time postgraduate courses in pharmaceutical medicine. This course continues to be the leading one of its type in the world. Consisting of five modules per year, each of three days' duration, the course is fully residential, being held at a variety of hotel conference venues in the UK. To be eligible to enrol on the course, participants must be medically qualified and employed either by a pharmaceutical company, a clinical research organisation or a regulatory authority. Approximately two-thirds of course participants reside in the UK, with the remainder working in countries as far afield as the USA, Denmark, Germany and Italy.

The aims of the BrAPP/UW Postgraduate Course in Pharmaceutical Medicine are two-fold: (a) to provide medically qualified personnel with the specific knowledge and skills needed by a doctor to carry out the daily duties of a pharmaceutical physician, and (b) to prepare doctors for the Royal Colleges of Physicians Diploma in Pharmaceutical Medicine. The objectives of the course are to provide the new entrant to a pharmaceutical company, clinical research organisation or regulatory authority with the specialist knowledge and skills to practise pharmaceutical medicine and to provide the core knowledge necessary to be successful in the diploma examination.

The course contents are based on the recently revised syllabus for the Diploma in Pharmaceutical Medicine issued by the Faculty of Pharmaceutical Medicine of the Royal Colleges of Physicians of the UK (Shelley, 1991). For organisational purposes, the syllabus is grouped into 10 free-standing modules considered the key areas to the discipline of pharmaceutical medicine. These 10 modules which comprise the BrAPP/UW course are listed below. Formal didactic teaching has been reduced to a minimum, most teaching being based on interactive sessions in which case studies provide course participants, working in small groups, with the opportunity to apply their knowledge to the types of problem-solving situations which regularly confront the pharmaceutical physician in the work-place. In general, the course contents are biased towards providing new knowledge rather than developing personnel skills such as management skills, creative thinking and media skills. Admission to the course takes place each summer, with module 1 (discovery of new medicines) commencing yearly in October. The remaining four modules in year one of the course are scheduled in November (pharmaceutical development), February (clinical trials), April (toxicity) and June (regulatory affairs, legal and ethical issues). The second year of the course commences in October with module 6 (development of medicines and economics of health care) and is followed by module 7 in November (medical statistics), module 8 in February (principles of clinical pharmacology), module 9 in April (information, promotion and education) and, finally, module 10 in June (safety of medicines).

The role of such a structured training programme should not be underestimated. It is vitally important to the development of the discipline of pharmaceutical medicine and is greatly appreciated by new entrants to the industry. For example, in a survey of pharmaceutical physicians who had previously attended the BrAPP/UW Postgraduate Course in Pharmaceutical Medicine, some 87% recommended others to enrol on this course on joining the pharmaceutical industry (Bax *et al.*, 1982). Clearly, structured training programmes should be freely available to all pharmaceutical physicians in whichever country they are employed. Hopefully, the steps currently being taken to internationalise the UK course, its contents and syllabus, will help to bring this about. In contrast to the limited availability of structured training programmes, the experienced pharmaceutical physician has a wide variety of continuing education courses to choose from in order to keep abreast of advances in pharmaceutical medicine. Unquestionably, the availability of both structured training programmes and continuing education programmes provides the means by which pharmaceutical medicine will gain universal acceptance as a medical speciality, resulting in substantial benefits to the doctors who practise this discipline.


## THE ROYAL COLLEGES OF PHYSICIANS DIPLOMA IN PHARMACEUTICAL MEDICINE


On completion of the two-year BrAPP/UW Postgraduate Course in Pharmaceutical Medicine, participants normally present themselves for the diploma examination. To be eligible, candidates must hold qualifications in medicine, surgery and midwifery recognised by the Royal Colleges of Physicians and be either (a) fully registrable in the British Medical Register or (b) fully registrable in the country in which the qualification was granted. Although originally mandatory that candidates should have attended a two-year postgraduate course in pharmaceutical medicine such as the BrAPP/UW course (Macleod and Goldberg, 1981; Goldberg and Smith, 1985), since 1992 this is no longer the case. Thus, candidates may now sit the examination without having attended a training programme although they are strongly recommended to do so (Shelley, 1991). To date, the examination has been held annually (in November). To be awarded the Diploma in Pharmaceutical Medicine, candidates must satisfy the examiners in a written paper (including a multiple choice component) and an oral examination. From 1994 the Faculty of Pharmaceutical Medicine will take over responsibility for the examination within the Royal Colleges of Physicians. To date (October 1993), some 383 candidates have sat the examination, with 299 of these being awarded the Diploma in Pharmaceutical Medicine. This represents an overall pass rate of 78%.


## MEMBERSHIP OF THE FACULTY OF PHARMACEUTICAL MEDICINE


A major advance in gaining recognition for the discipline of pharmaceutical medicine was attained in 1989 with the inauguration of the Faculty of Pharmaceutical Medicine of the three Royal Colleges of Physicians of the UK. The primary objective of the new faculty is to raise standards in pharmaceutical medicine for the benefit of both the general public and the membership. Following the model of other colleges and faculties in the UK, membership is gained by a two-step process. The first stage of membership (Associateship) requires a candidate to obtain the Diploma in Pharmaceutical Medicine (Gabbay and Goldberg, 1991). Candidates who obtain the diploma may apply for Associateship of the Faculty of Pharmaceutical Medicine (AFPM). In addition to the diploma an applicant should be a fully registered practitioner with at least two years' general medical training and two years in an appropriate post in pharmaceutical medicine. The second stage of membership (Membership) is open only to those who have satisfied the requirements for Associateship and is based on the practical side of a speciality. It requires submission of a dissertation (20 000–25 000 words) relevant to pharmaceutical medicine (Gabbay and Goldberg, 1991). On acceptance of the dissertation and after a satisfactory oral examination, Membership of the Faculty of Pharmaceutical Medicine (MFPM) is awarded, provided that the applicant has completed six years post registration training, of which four would normally be in pharmaceutical medicine.

## OTHER STRUCTURED COURSES IN PHARMACEUTICAL MEDICINE

Postgraduate training programmes have recently been established in a number of other countries. Following the UK lead, these are collaborative ventures between various national associations of pharmaceutical physicians and universities. For example, in Spain the diploma is managed by the universities of Barcelona and Madrid working in conjunction with AMIFE, the Spanish equivalent of BrAPP. In Belgium, a structured postgraduate course has recently commenced at the Free University of Brussels in collaboration with the Belgium Association of Pharmaceutical Physicians. In the Far East, a course leading to a diploma has been established by the Philippine College of Pharmaceutical Medicine. Not surprisingly, other associations are actively considering the setting up of formal training programmes in pharmaceutical medicine. These include associations in Portugal, Italy, Germany, France and perhaps the USA once the proposed American Academy of Pharmaceutical Physicians has become established.

In Switzerland, the Center for Research and Teaching of the University Policlinic of Basle organises a course in pharmaceutical medicine attended by both medically and non-medically qualified personnel. Under the auspices of the European Confederation of the Upper Rhine

Universities of Basle, Freiburg i. Br. and Strasbourg, the European Course in Pharmaceutical Medicine is designed for people employed in clinical and pharmaceutical research in industry, in regulatory authorities or universities. Started in 1991, the course is organised over a two-year period and consists of six modules each of three days' duration. The topics covered include: drug development—meeting the needs of the future; toxicology and clinical pharmacology; clinical trial methodology; biometrics in drug development; regulatory affairs; project management. A certificate is awarded following attendance and successful accomplishment of the course. A multiple-choice questionnaire is used as a means of self-assessment on completion of each session, with a written examination (multiple-choice) being held at the end of the two-year programme.

## DIPLOMA COURSE IN CLINICAL SCIENCE

In addition to physicians, the evaluation and monitoring of medicines today involve a large team of people of varied educational training and qualifications, including scientists, pharmacists, nurses and many others. Whilst most of the tasks involved in setting up and monitoring clinical research projects make similar demands on these different team members, their varied undergraduate backgrounds bring a different emphasis and need for postgraduate training. As a result, the University of Wales in Cardiff established the postgraduate Diploma Course in Clinical Science in 1987 to provide basic scientists entering the medical department of a pharmaceutical company with the clinical and scientific knowledge and skills relevant to the clinical evaluation and safety assessments of new medicines. This unique two-year part-time training programme is organised in collaboration with the Association for Clinical Research in the Pharmaceutical Industry (ACRPI) and is designed specifically to meet the educational and vocational needs of clinical research associates with backgrounds as varied as pharmacology, geology and nursing. Unlike its sister course, the Postgraduate Course in Pharmaceutical Medicine, therapeutics is a major component of the diploma course in clinical science. Other subjects include: the principles of pharmacology, toxicology, clinical pharmacology and pharmacy; clinical trial methodology; medical statistics; adverse drug reactions; regulatory affairs; communications; ethics and legal aspects of drug research. Formal written examinations are conducted at the end of the first and second years. Candidates also have to complete formal course work and a dissertation of approximately 20 000 words and may be required by the University Board of Examiners to present themselves for an oral examination on completion of the course. Candidates who satisfy the examiners in all parts of the examination are awarded the Diploma in Clinical Science by the University of Wales.

## DIPLOMA COURSE IN REGULATORY AFFAIRS

Although some medically qualified doctors specialise in regulatory affairs, most regulatory affairs departments within the pharmaceutical industry are staffed by non-physicians. In Europe, these staff are represented by organisations such as the British Institute of Regulatory Affairs and the European Society of Regulatory Affairs (ESRA). In attempting to fulfil the training requirements of its members, BIRA and ESRA formed a partnership with the University of Wales in Cardiff to develop a postgraduate diploma programme similar to those already organised for pharmaceutical physicians and clinical research associates. This resulted in the establishment in 1989 of a two-year part-time course of modular design leading to the Diploma in Regulatory Affairs. At present 12 modules are offered, each consisting of approximately 25 hours of lectures, interactive workshops and seminars. To receive the diploma, a candidate must have attended a total of eight modules in a minimum of two years and a maximum of five years, and passed the written examination associated with each module. Course work must also be satisfactorily completed, together with the successful submission of a dissertation of 12 000–15 000 words, which has to be completed within five years of initial registration for the diploma course. Candidates may also be required to undergo an oral examination on completion of the written examinations (one per module) and/or the submission of the dissertation. Currently, the following 12 modules are being offered: strategic management of regulatory affairs; regulatory strategy for a new active substance—pre-clinical development; regulatory requirements for a new active substance—chemistry and pharmacy; core clinical studies—the regulatory input; clinical regulatory compliance; regulatory strategy—the market-place; regulatory strategy for submissions for established active substances; data requirements for registration of established active substances; registration of biological and biotechnology products; registration of veterinary products; USA—the regulatory environment; regulation of devices. The modules are organised as a rolling programme with six being taught each academic year. Whilst the majority of modules are held in hotel conference facilities in the UK, the module on regulation of devices will be held outside the UK at the end of 1994. This movement towards modules being held in countries other than the UK reflects the increasing number of

Europeans registering for the BIRA/UW Diploma Course in Regulatory Affairs.

## MASTER OF SCIENCE IN PHARMACEUTICAL MEDICINE

Recently, as part of its modular postgraduate degree programme, the University of Surrey has commenced a taught Master of Science course in pharmaceutical medicine, the first of its kind. This is aimed at those graduates who wish to specialise in this newly recognised multi-disciplinary medical scientific speciality. The course involves 12 three-day teaching modules (eight compulsory plus four selected options) over a two- to five-year period, each module being accompanied by 76 hours of distance learning materials and exercises, together with a 20 000–25 000-word dissertation. The syllabus on which the curriculum is based is similar to those for the Diploma in Pharmaceutical Medicine and the Diploma in Clinical Science.

## CONTINUING EDUCATION PROGRAMMES

Unlike structured training programmes which aim to provide the new entrant to the pharmaceutical industry with the basic knowledge and skills necessary to carry out the duties of a pharmaceutical physician, continuing education provides the experienced individual with a means of keeping up to date with developments in a particular area of work. Such continuing education courses tend to be of only one or two days' duration, cover a plethora of subjects, and are organised by a variety of professional and commercial bodies. In the UK, for example, regular update meetings are held by BrAPP, the Royal Colleges of Physicians and the Faculty of Pharmaceutical Medicine. Whilst these are primarily for medical doctors, the Society of Pharmaceutical Medicine organises meetings attended by both physicians and scientists.

Inaugurated in the late 1980s (Burley, 1987; Salter and Gabbay, 1990), this society provides a forum through which all personnel involved in the discovery, development, evaluation and monitoring of medicines and the medical aspects of their marketing are able to exchange views and develop their skills in an interdisciplinary fashion. Many university departments throughout Europe and the USA also organise continuing education programmes, particularly in clinical pharmacology, pharmacoepidemiology, medical statistics and Good Clinical Practice.

## CONCLUSION

Despite the progress that has already been made towards establishing pharmaceutical medicine as a medical speciality, few medical schools include it in their undergraduate teaching programmes. At a result, doctors newly recruited to the industry have to rapidly acquire the specialist knowledge and skills relating to this new discipline. Fortunately, structured training programmes are available to convert the generalist medical doctor into the specialist pharmaceutical physician. The first and most widely known training course is the BrAPP/UW Postgraduate Course in Pharmaceutical Medicine, which has run successfully for 18 years. This particular course not only provides a training programme for newly recruited physicians to the industry but, equally important, prepares candidates for an academic postgraduate qualification, the Diploma in Pharmaceutical Medicine, and entry to Associateship and Membership of the recently established Faculty of Pharmaceutical Medicine.

For other non-medical personnel involved in the clinical research and medicines development and monitoring process there are a variety of specialist postgraduate training courses available as well as postgraduate diplomas and degrees. These training and educational developments in the newly recognised medical scientific speciality of pharmaceutical medicine are increasingly being adopted abroad.

It is considered that the increasing availability of both structured training courses and continuing education programmes provides the means for a broader understanding of pharmaceutical medicine, resulting in lasting benefit to those doctors, scientists and others who practise within the speciality.

# Part VI

# Changing Course

# 30
# Career Development in Pharmaceutical Medicine

Roger D. Stephens

Roger Stephens & Associates, Hatfield, UK

If a typical executive joins the pharmaceutical industry at age 27 and retires at age 62 having enjoyed an average annual 'package' worth, say, £35 000, then his or her career earnings in pharmaceutical medicine will be £1.2 million. You can adjust these figures how you like for personal career progression and local market conditions, but you will not change the fact that your career decisions will have multi-million pound implications. It never ceases to surprise me that people will cheerfully write pages of justification for a new photocopier or a new car, yet take back-of-the-envelope decisions about their careers. The career development literature does not help much: mostly it has been written for a management perspective by academics or human resources professionals and is designed to help personnel people and line managers plan organisational change. Very little has been written from the perspective of the individuals who actually own their careers, let alone that of pharmaceutical physicians, many of whom, by definition, have already made at least one radical change of direction. Few companies seem to have career development programmes which really work, for example, for physicians and clinical scientists. Understandably, none manages its programmes in ways which recognise the primacy of individuals as stakeholders in their own personal development: all very properly give primacy to the needs of their organisations.

*Discovering New Medicines: Careers in Pharmaceutical Research and Development.*
Edited by P.D. Stonier
© 1994 John Wiley & Sons Ltd

So the philosophical bases of this chapter are that you as an individual—not your employer—have the primary responsibility for the management of your own career, and that because the decisions involved are 'megabuck' decisions they deserve at least the attention which you would give to the placing of a clinical trials programme or a product launch for your employer.

The structure of the chapter is based largely on a contribution I gave to an industry symposium on career development in London in 1992. There I acknowledged the debt I owed to Dave Francis, author of *Managing Your Own Career*, the book which defined a practical, person-centred approach which I commend to people who are interested in taking charge of their lives. I am glad to have the opportunity to acknowledge it once more. Subsequently, I have learned much from Golzen and Garner, whose 'wise and subtle' book *Smart Moves* (1992) is well worth reading if you are serious about developing your own career.

## A WORKING PROCESS FOR DEVELOPING YOUR CAREER

### The General Approach

The approach is marketing-driven and quality/customer-orientated. It starts by asking individuals to regard themselves as products which exist to maximise the opportunities, or to solve the business, technical or regulatory problems of organisations. It is analogous to the process by which pharmaceutical companies develop drugs and market them. Thus, given that a compound is emerging from some programme of discovery, the first questions, designed to define its potential, might include:

- What is its structure?
- How does it work?
- What benefits will it offer to its users?
- Are there contraindications?
- Who needs one of these?
- Does the customer know they need one?
- What differential advantages is he or she looking for?
- Does my product offer such advantages?
- If not, can I develop it in useful ways?
- In short, how can I fit my product to meet the needs of the real world?

## Defining Yourself as a Product

This first part of the process is totally introverted. Analyse yourself as a 'product'. You may already have done some of the background work for this by writing a curriculum vitae (CV) or a career résumé. This is a valuable exercise but it does not provide the basis for a strategic pro- gramme of career development. Indeed, there is a school of thought which regards CVs as 'fictions about the past to help us feel better about the future'. If your CV is like that, throw it away.

To understand and define where your career is going, it is first essen- tial to understand where you are and how you really got there. So collect factual information about your past and your present, and assemble it in a big lever arch file. Make a kind of 'Book of Your Life'. Include:

- family memorabilia, notes of the addresses where you have lived and periods you were there;
- brief descriptions of the characters of parents, grandparents, uncles, aunts, cousins, teachers, bosses and very close friends you have had over the years;
- copies of your school reports, matriculation, degree and other certifi- cates of competence or qualifications;
- letters of appointment, psychometric or other test results, perfor- mance appraisal forms, congratulatory letters which came with, for example, bonus awards;
- if you have a family of your own, copies of your marriage certificate and the children's birth certificates; brief descriptions of the characters of your spouse and children;
- any other documentation or image which tells other people who you are and anchors you in your own personal reality;
- a page about why you chose your medical or scientific speciality in the first place—what influenced you; who influenced you; what per- sonal values were involved;
- another page or two about the rationale behind each separate step of your career to date.

Write each chapter and file it in the relevant place in the Book of Your Life. Leave each piece of writing for a few days and then review it. Try to make it 100% accurate and honest. Be especially rigorous in thinking and writing about your decision to go into pharmaceutical medicine. When you have finished, ask your closest friend to read and review it. He or she should be able to confirm whether you have developed the clearest, most reliable characterisation possible of the history and struc- ture of the product which is you: if so, proceed to the next step.

## Defining Your Aims and Objectives

To help you in defining your strategy for the future, you will need to give a lot of thought to your personal aims and objectives. You probably started out on your career with some wonderful dreams—to win a Nobel Prize, to be a master surgeon, to be as rich as Croesus. Now your ideas are probably more realistic and your situation more constrained by the need to fit yourself in with the opportunities which the real world offers. So prepare statements of the short-, medium- and long-term objectives which you have set for yourself and each member of your family. If you haven't set any, then get some down on paper. You cannot begin to plan without them. Try defining them under headings like wealth, power over people, expertise, creativity, working with like-minded colleagues, independence, security and personal status.

If you really want to be rich, then you are probably wasting your time being an employee: taxes will see to that. Try plastic surgery on Harley Street, or psychosexual counselling in Beverly Hills. If you seek power and influence, the obvious thing is to go into major-league politics—or if you are talented, to make your way to the top of a big company, academic institution, trade association or regulatory body. If exercising expertise excites you, then perhaps you should return to academia or to the clinical setting, or work in the more intellectually demanding areas of industry. Patients and companies seem to prefer steadiness to creativity in their advisers, so if you want to be creative perhaps you should have second thoughts about the entire direction of your career: consider following Jonathan Miller or Miriam Stoppard into the media. For the committed researcher in industry, a need for affiliation with like-minded people is often fulfilled by working in an active clinical research role offering frequent contact with clinicians, academics and colleagues who are life scientists. Autonomy and independence are generally contraindicated in industrial organisations: even at the very top you will be constrained by governments, stock exchanges and banks. There may be some autonomy left in the upper echelons of clinical medicine and academia—but even there, the managerial tendencies of modern governments and the inconvenient attentions of lawyers and the media will restrict your freedom. Security (in the sense of lifetime jobs with guaranteed pensions at the end of them) is going right out of fashion— even in the government service. But the consolation is that it seems to be getting more straightforward for people with marketable competencies (of which leadership ability is by far the most bankable and past qualifications the least) to build themselves secure lives, either as independents or as employees. Lastly, your perceived status in much of the professional and general community was certainly reduced by your move into pharmaceutical medicine: every head-hunter has his favourite story of the professorial recommendation of a candidate on the grounds that 'the poor chap has started drinking/has upset his colleagues/has submitted a really rather dreadful thesis ... so isn't going to make it here, but might well fit into the industry ...'.

When you have completed your analysis of the things which drive you, you should be ready to work out two or three alternative programmes of career steps which will help you to achieve a sustained sense of fulfilment in your career. Having done this, you can consider and assess the likelihood or otherwise of being able to take these steps with your present company.

## Development Moves Inside the Company

Matching people to the current and future needs of companies is a key responsibility of every manager at every level—perhaps assisted by the human resources function. It is absolutely in accordance with your own self-interest that you should help your management fulfil this responsibility by alerting them to your own career interests and objectives. Do not wait until the annual performance appraisal interview to do this. Initiate discussions—especially if you have changed your plans in ways which might offer advantages to the company in the achievement of its objectives.

Remember that advancement often requires the development and use of competences that are not needed in your present job. Accordingly, cooperate with your management to design your personal development activities to meet new challenges and improve your ability to remove obstacles which currently worry or frighten you. Get the widest possible experience of the work in pharmaceutical medicine. You can either 'sit still for long enough, and the whole lot will come to you' (Dr John Domenet, the symposium chairman) or move from unit to unit, or country to country. Get the widest possible exposure to executives who you perceive to be successful in your company: observe and emulate what they do; make sure they and other influencers are aware of your career plans. Become a volunteer in your company and in the relevant specialist societies and clubs. Approach opinion formers and senior figures when you see them in conferences, symposia and meetings; seek their advice and counsel: you'll be getting somewhere when they know your name and seek your advice in return. Make sure your company knows that they do this. Note that people who are doing well in their careers almost always manage to look good. They may not be especially handsome or expensively dressed, but there is usually a certain harmony between their grooming, clothing, coloration, body language and presence: study how they have achieved this and learn to emulate. Be strong and energetic. In situations of uncertainty, give management the benefit of the doubt. Don't whinge or cringe. Help identify and remove the obstacles which worry or frighten your seniors. Be known as the propounder of solutions, not the bringer of problems. In short, make yourself the logical choice for right next job when it comes along. But do not become too dependent on your company as the only source of training or career opportunities. It may not always be able to provide these at the right time or in the right sequence. Accordingly, your strategic plan should also include provision for self-motivated training and development, and for career moves which take you away from the company.

## Development Moves Outside the Company

The structure of your company is almost certainly pyramidal. As such, it sets natural geometric limits to the career opportunities lying on an upward path. However, upward opportunities are not the only kind of career development. You can move further into a function, or move sideways via a lateral job change or move out altogether. The important thing is that your career should continue to develop significantly at reasonable (say three- to five-year) intervals. It is not always appropriate to focus on the external trappings and higher salary of a more senior assignment. However, it is natural that from time to time you will feel that your company is taking too long to produce the right kind of development opportunities for you. You are especially likely to feel this if you have recently moved into pharmaceutical medicine from short-term research or clinical postings, perhaps involving many relocations, which will have habituated you to an expectation of instability and frequent change. Be careful about this. In my work as a recruiter, I meet too many highly qualified and ambitious candidates who have come to regret hasty decisions to change jobs. They have little or nothing to tell a prospective employer about their achievements. Conversely, those who have passively waited for years in the hope of promotion have often let golden opportunities pass them by—and then found themselves stuck in roles which have ceased to offer interest or challenge. They appear at interview as bored, frustrated, negative and narrow, and seldom get short-listed. So even if you are perfectly content, it makes sense to keep a routine eye on the outside world. Read the business press to keep in touch with major developments in the economy and the market; read the scientific and medical journals to monitor advances in the therapeutic fields which interest you; read the industry press to learn about developments in the pharmaceutical business. Monitor the job advertisements—not so much to find a new job, more so that you understand trends in the employment market and the kinds of things which are on offer. Bear in mind that a significant proportion of vacancies is filled by networking—shrewd recruiters often start by asking industry, clinical and academic opinion-formers for advice about potential candidates. This reinforces the need for you to be active in the relevant professional societies and clubs, at symposia and meetings. Just as industry, clinical and academic leaders may seek your advice, so they may also alert you to external opportunities which are perhaps still only at the planning stage. Include the reputable recruitment consultancies in your network, but avoid the cowboys. If the serious recruiters are not kept up to date with changes in your career situation and plans (or your new address and phone number!) they will be less likely to remember you (or be able to contact you) when they are briefed to propose a shortlist for a vacant job. And if you are actively seeking a new job, install an answering machine at home.

Above all, have a '*shopping list*' based on a clear vision of the features which will need to be present in any new job if it is to justify a decision to leave your present one. When this mirrors—or closely approximates to—the brief to which recruiters are working, you can justify the investment of a little time to explore the prospects. If the initial exploration generates too many doubts, back off. If not, continue with the exploration.

Go carefully: remember you are approaching a multi-million pound decision which could have a profound transforming influence not only on your own life and fortunes, but also on those people—colleagues and friends as well as family—who depend on you. But do not hold back if everything is clearly developing in the right way for you. If a new position matches most or all the key criteria in your plan—go for it!

# 31
# Physicians in Sales and Marketing

## John Hall

Allen & Hanburys Ltd, Stockley Park, Middlesex, UK

Doctors have a very low understanding of commercial affairs and are not particularly numerate. On the contrary, because of the broad span of their medical education, doctors are capable of fulfilling any one of a number of roles in the commercial arena.

These are two widely varying positions, both of which I have heard stated during my years in the pharmaceutical industry. As with all things, of course, there is an element of truth in both statements and the facts of the matter lie somewhere in the middle. In the course of this chapter we will explore some of the possibilities for physicians within the pharmaceutical industry who decide that they may wish to pursue a role outside of the mainstream medical department activities.

## BACKGROUND

Doctors are uniquely qualified to work in the pharmaceutical industry since they are the only group who have ever sat on the other side of the desk as a customer. You start therefore from a base of knowledge which is built upon several years of prescribing the very medicines that you will in future be promoting. In spite of this important background, it

*Discovering New Medicines: Careers in Pharmaceutical Research and Development.*
Edited by P.D. Stonier
© 1994 John Wiley & Sons Ltd

comes down to the personal attributes of the physicians themselves as to whether or not they will make a success in a commercial environment. Before 'burning your boats' it would be very useful if you can persuade your employer to allow you to undertake a secondment into either sales or marketing or possibly both. This will be possible only if you establish your role in the medical team first. Medical advisers are a very expensive commodity and you will have to work hard to persuade your medical director that he is prepared to carry on the functions of the medical department in your absence. If this can be arranged it will certainly give you a good feel for whether or not you want to make a permanent move.

There are several examples of doctors who have made a successful switch to sales and marketing and ultimately perhaps into general management. Remember, however, that when you move out of the purely medical arena you will be stepping into an area which although related to the practice of medicine is still nevertheless a very well-defined speciality in its own right, and having been a success in the medical department is no guarantee of becoming an overnight star elsewhere.

If you start the process early enough in your career, then beginning at the 'bottom' is a good idea. We have all sat on the other side of the desk from sales representatives on many occasions, but being out in the field as a representative yourself gives you a very different aspect upon what life is like from their point of view. Even if you only spend a very short time in the field, then I would still recommend that it is a good place to start since you will benefit from the kind of knowledge that this salutary experience will bring!

## SALES

Sales representatives really need to have a certain something which sets them apart as individuals. It is important to be both memorable and to be able to empathise and to get closer to doctors, which will then mean that they in turn are happy to share their experiences with you. Representatives need to have high energy levels and must always be willing to go that extra five miles out of their way in order to make a 'cold call', just in case there is a doctor who is prepared to see them. They need planning and organisational skills to a high degree; they need to be effective time managers and they need to be good at targeting their customers. They need to know what is the right number of times to call on a particular doctor and to be able to deliver the right message to the right person. Importantly, they must understand the needs of physicians in hospital and general practice. In understanding those needs they are then able to share in the whole support of the medical situation. They are effectively moving themselves around the table to sit on the same side as the doctor and are able to help him or her with the difficulty that they face in trying to set up a new clinic, look for a new practice nurse, find a new partner etc. Increasingly they also need to be the linchpin between hospital and general practice. A good sales representative can and should encourage this interface and develop this relationship and put the purchasers and providers together in this ever-changing National Health Service (NHS) situation. Doctors are of course well qualified to perform this role since they understand all of these issues as well as anyone does.

Doctors would probably not wish to remain as representatives for long, however, and will be looking for career advancement into sales management and then to progress ultimately to sales director, if that is the route they have chosen. Sales training can often be an intermediate step on this ladder, and doctors have all of the basic knowledge and ability to perform well in sales training. They cannot help only representatives with the sort of knowledge that they will need but they also have the ultimate ability to be able to role-play medical situations to help representatives to focus their minds on the key messages which they wish to deliver.

The sales manager will probably have all of the attributes of a representative but will also need to develop other skills and abilities in addition. They will need to have highly developed 'people' skills; they will need to have empathy with the needs of their representatives, and this is one of the main reasons why it is important to have progressed through that route; they will need to have insight into the problems that others are facing but they will need a lot of leadership skills as well; there will be a need to set objectives, to apply those objectives differentially between people in their team, and to have the ability to turn thoughts into action plans. They will need to have all of the influencing skills of a representative and also be able to resolve any conflicts between members of their team.

They have to use data and develop concrete examples to clarify situations so that others can understand and ultimately achieve. One of the most important issues these days facing representatives and managers is the ability to 'network'. This means that even if you do not have the answer to an issue yourself, then you 'know a man who does'. Collaborative working is the only way in which to function in the increasingly complex and varied environment in which we find ourselves. Not only are two heads better than one but sometimes many heads may be better than two.

A good sales manager will need to be task as well as people orientated.

He or she will need highly developed business knowledge and also knowledge of company procedures and administrative systems, which although apparently tedious are vital for the role. One of the difficulties that doctors may face in a pure sales environment is the need to marry ethics with business. This is not to suggest that sales people are unethical—far from it—but there is a need to work within procedures and policies and yet to apply innovative thinking and always to be looking for ways of doing things differently. The representatives that you manage will be seeing many of the same doctors several times a year and would be decidedly unwelcome if their approach to selling was the same on every occasion.

In order to put together a successful team around you, the right mix of experience and maturity is important. Good sales managers will be trying to improve business in each territory, whilst at the same time taking in the broader picture of a region of the country. Involving representatives in business projects encourages their understanding of issues. The prerequisite of any good sales manager is the ability to brief promotional campaigns to their team. Promotional messages must lose nothing in their translation from marketing into actions at the sharp end. You must identify what can be added to a promotional campaign in order to keep representatives motivated. Motivation is obviously a huge topic in itself and many books have been written on the subject. I do not intend to make any attempt to suggest what makes a good motivator of sales teams, because everyone has their own way of doing it. However, representatives must respect you for your business knowledge and they will be looking to you to manage geographically disparate parts in different ways, in order to fulfil targets across the whole region.

Communication is vital at all levels but extremely important in the area of sales management. Field visits should be carried out on a regular basis and the higher up the ladder you get the more you need to be aware of what is going on locally. With new technologies and the use of computers, faxes and various types of voice-messaging systems, there is absolutely no excuse for not being in constant touch with all parts of the network.

As sales director you will be managing a number of promotional campaigns and a number of people from quite different backgrounds. Your role as a coordinator of all these parts is vital. You should be aware of other resources within the company which can be brought to bear to handle local situations. As a doctor yourself it may be important that you visit a particular customer in order to discuss the issues of therapeutic management, so that they can understand that you have empathy with their situation and you are willing to listen to their problems as well. A sales director has a vast amount of country to cover and must look across the totality of the business. He or she will be a key member of the company management team and will need an understanding of the wider aspects of the business and an understanding of the five-year focus rather than just their main role, which is essentially to bring in the sales for the current financial year. He must see himself as part of a team and not just an individual focusing on several of the company's products, and must be constantly liaising with colleagues in senior management.

The sales director must be able to understand the feelings of the people in the audience when he addresses the entire sales force from the platform at the annual conference and on other occasions where he stands in front of a large group of representatives. The representatives are the ones who will generate the business on a daily basis and they will either go away charged with enthusiasm to sell their product, or not, largely on the basis of your words. Being a manager of so many disparate parts and being based in head office a long way away from all of those parts is a skill in itself. As sales director you will be managing through several layers of middle management, no longer able to relate to representatives on a one-to-one basis. On the three or four public occasions per year that representatives will see you, those are your only chances to establish leadership and credibility and to make this vital field force a cohesive group.

You will be scrutinised constantly by the sales force, many of whom will be wondering how they might one day acquire your job. It becomes more important than ever at this level to give positive as well as negative feedback. Sales people are never happier than when they are achieving what they saw at the beginning of the year as a stretching but realistic target for sales. They will quickly become demoralised by the setting of unrealistic sales objectives which they recognise as unattainable from day one of the new year. Incentives and bonuses are very important in the sales arena but they do not necessarily have to be financially related. Sales people may find incentive enough in being recognised publicly in front of their peers as a high performer. I am not suggesting that they would not relish the thought of an extra bonus as a result of being a high performer but the recognition in itself is worth almost as much as the financial incentive.

In summary, therefore, in the sales area there is no doubt that physicians by the nature of their general background and training will be perfectly capable of fulfilling any of the roles that I have described. One thing is certain, however: they will not be successful in those roles simply by believing that being a physician is enough. They will be clever enough and will have all of the background knowledge but it is as much about their character, their temperament and their personality as it is about any kind of knowledge or skill that they may possess. There is nothing new in this since the same is true of any senior management appointment within this industry or any other, but the sales manager or director par excellence needs to have a blend of people skills, task orientation and planning or analytical abilities. He will be in one of the high-profile jobs in the company and will be under constant scrutiny by all of his troops. He must be able to project himself and to give a clear lead on the few occasions when he will see all of the representatives together, and he must have a good understanding of the feelings of the troops on the ground.

## MARKETING

Let us now turn to the marketing area. A career in marketing will undoubtedly be enhanced by having spent some time in sales. It is important to understand the feelings of representatives who are presented with a promotional campaign which has been dreamt up by a product manager and creatively interpreted by an advertising agency. Let there be no doubt that the campaign as visualised in marketing may be quite different when it has been translated through sales management or sales training down to individual representatives, who will then reinterpret it in order to present it in the most plausible way to their customers, who after all know better than anyone. Time spent as a representative or in first-line management of representatives would be time well spent for anyone who wishes to make a career in marketing.

An integral part of many marketing departments is the marketing research group. Should physicians spend some time in market research if they plan to make a career in the commercial side of the company? I think the answer is 'not necessarily', but it would be another useful stepping stone to understand the overall process of marketing. The role of the market researcher is to enable the product managers and the marketing managers to make better-informed business decisions. It is possible these days to obtain audits of prescriptions, written or dispensed, of chemists or hospital purchases, of prescription changes in chronic disease areas, of sales force and advertising activity, even down to the level of what representatives said when they called on individual doctors. These data are mainly bought in from two or three large market-research data-collection agencies and need to be carefully interpreted.

Market researchers function best when they are members of the overall product-marketing team. They need to be highly analytical and numerate but are essentially in the business of adding value and contributing knowledge and understanding to a series of otherwise sometimes unintelligible numbers. They must be orientated to the needs of their customers because at the end of the day they are providing a service role. A good market researcher will never simply supply the numbers but will always supply an intelligent interpretation of the information. They must be open to whatever result comes out of the piece of research that has been commissioned. Research must never be ignored just because it does not fit with preconceived ideas. Equally, market research must not be used as a way of avoiding decisions since it can be all too easy to continue to commission further pieces of research until you reach the situation of 'paralysis by analysis'. Market researchers usually gain their job satisfaction from the fact that the work that they have done is accepted as a plausible answer to the question which was originally posed.

There is a different blend of skills and knowledge required for product marketing. The higher you progress up the marketing tree then the greater the understanding of medical knowledge that is required. Being a medic is useful in the sense that the strategic views of a senior marketeer have to be close to the views of the customers. Furthermore, the higher you climb up the marketing ladder, then the broader knowledge of concepts that you require, since you will be no longer simply selling your own product to doctors but you will need to understand all of the issues in the changing NHS environment. Marketeers need to be customer focused and it is vital to involve those customers, but you also need to have the ability to 'drive' the market. You need to have a vision of how the current market could be changed, but obviously that vision needs to be realistic and based upon good sense and medical logic. You need to visualise that things in your market-place could be totally different from what they are now and you need the ability to drive those changes through. The involvement of customers in this process is vital because in trying to change a market then you need to have a logical reason for doing so. In other words it is not so important to create the wave of change but it is more important to recognise that a wave exists and then to encourage it and 'ride it' to your advantage. I do not believe that creativity *per se* is vital in a marketing person: I believe that it is more important just to be able to think that things could be done differently. Innovation is important, along with an understanding that ideas which may appear to be 'off the wall' when they are initially floated might have a germ within them which could lead to considerable changes in the future.

Verbal communication skills are just as important in marketing as they are in sales. You need the ability to summarise in-depth data in order to give relatively simple concepts to an advertising agency. You must remember that you will not be personally selling any of your own products but all of the selling will be done on your behalf by sales representatives. The ability that is needed therefore is to be able to sell your ideas to others. The 'packaging' of yourself is very important. Your profile is important. There is an old but true saying that people buy people, not products. You will be responsible for the overall sales of your product even though individual representatives are of course responsible on their own territories. At the end of the day the sales force have to find you credible and they have to find your campaign plausible, otherwise it is doomed to failure right from the beginning.

As with any other area there is a high level of pressure. You will often be presenting to senior managers, sometimes to the board of management, and you cannot miss deadlines. Materials that are required for a sales conference are required for a particular date—the conference cannot be moved in order to encompass your difficulties with production of materials. Needless to say therefore it is vital that good planning is in place in order to be able to meet the many challenges that you will face.

As in medicine, you will need the ability to make decisions when all of the information is not available. The greater the breadth of experience that you have the better position you will be in to achieve this. You will certainly need high energy levels and you will need an element of the sort of traits that marketing people are sometimes accused of, i.e. being pushy, arrogant and highly persuasive. Needless to say these attributes must not be so far as to be negative traits, but an element of them is required to meet all of the aspects of the job. There is no doubt that you need to enjoy working with numbers because numeracy skills are vital in producing sales forecasts, five-year plans, analysing market research information, and looking at sales trends—all of which will be presented to you. You will need the ability to grasp quite complex concepts of managing budgets and sales, and one of the key ways in which your performance will be measured is on the overall contribution of your product to the company's profits.

Reward and recognition are very important in the sales area. In marketing, however, you are expected to get on with the job. The kind of people who are likely to be successful in marketing, however, will equally enjoy feedback and positive recognition. Ultimately, however, you will stand or fall by the commitment of the sales force to you and to your product.

If you do wish to progress ultimately to general management and aim to be managing director of the entire company, then some time spent in marketing will be a necessity because general managers need to have a breadth of marketing knowledge. Most of the questions or discussions at board meetings will revolve around marketing issues and sales performance, so all of the skills that are required in marketing, particularly as they relate to numeracy and understanding of the development of promotional campaigns, will be vital.

## CONCLUSION

In conclusion, therefore, there is no doubt that medics have all the basic intelligence and knowledge to be able to pursue careers outside of their chosen profession. At the end of the day, as with most things, it is the abilities of the person themselves to be flexible and to adapt to new environments and to have the right blend of interpersonal skills and technical knowledge which will be the final decider as to whether they make a successful career in a new area.

# 32
# Scientists in Sales and Marketing

## Elizabeth Langley

Langley Associates, Reading, UK

Graduate scientists most commonly encounter the pharmaceutical industry during the latter part of their degree course when they make their pilgrimage to the careers office. Those who have studied biosciences, particularly biochemistry, human biology, toxicology or microbiology at universities who have industrial links will be more aware of the research and development (R&D) activities of the industry. Some may even have spent time working within companies during industrial placement periods, which are commonplace in certain degree courses, or during vacation employment.

Those lucky enough to have worked in industry prior to graduation will have worn white coats, undertaken lots of menial tasks, attended meetings, but seldom have been party to the 'big' picture, namely, the long term goal of R&D to generate profit for the individual company. They will have worked amongst state-of-the-art equipment and with many dedicated and committed scientists. The commercial aspects of the organisation are likely to remain unexplained and indeed at this stage of anyone's career as a scientist perhaps that is appropriate. The day soon arrives, however, when those scientists aspiring to a career in the pharmaceutical industry find that there are not enough jobs in directly related topics to satisfy their demands. Hence the careers visit and the revelation that there is more to pharmaceuticals than R&D.

*Discovering New Medicines: Careers in Pharmaceutical Research and Development.*
Edited by P.D. Stonier
© 1994 John Wiley & Sons Ltd

## BACKGROUND

Without the efforts of the sales and marketing departments of the pharmaceutical industry many drug developments would have failed to reach their maximum potential in terms of financial return. Without this promised return many drug discoveries would have failed to make their way to the market. R&D have to be funded and, in basic terms, they have to be funded by profit from existing products. Skilful, knowledgeable sales and marketing can make a good product great and thus companies have found considerable benefits in recruiting scientists into the commercial end of the organisation as well as at the laboratory bench in order to help achieve high market share for any one company or product.

Whilst the disciplines of sales and marketing are linked, for the purposes of this chapter, each will be discussed separately. A generalised organogram of the main job roles in sales and marketing is shown in Figure 1.

The medical director will usually report to the managing director/Chief Executive Officer (CEO) at the same management level as the sales director.

## SALES

Most pharmaceutical companies in the European Union and the USA operate with teams of representatives who call on the 'end-providers' of their products, i.e. doctors, paramedics, nurses and therapists. These representatives differ from those in other industries because they seldom 'sell' their products to the 'end-user' (i.e. the patient). For

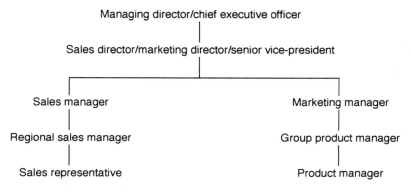

**Figure 1.** Generalised sales/marketing organogram.

ethical pharmaceutical products this is ruled to be unprofessional and unacceptable. These activities are governed by many codes of practice that operate throughout the world.

The salesperson in the UK, and other countries where socialised medicine is prevalent, seldom receives direct orders based on individual calls and thus has to use complex and often historic data to assess performance. Orders from retail chemists or distributors are more a measure of the anticipated success or current penetration of the product than a direct measure of the salesperson's impact. Thus the job can be frustrating because measures of success take time to establish and validate.

A doctor who says 'I will prescribe drug X' may forget to do so, not keep his promise, be sold 'better' by the next representative, or simply not see patients who are suitable.

The knack of the salesperson is to remain optimistic and persuasive in the face of a depressing call rate. The determination to succeed is paramount.

In a leading pharmaceutical company in the UK, with a sales force of 150 representatives, the proportion of science graduates has increased over the past 15 years to average approximately 65–75% graduates in 1993. The remaining percentage is made up of nurses, paramedics and career representatives, some of whom will have trained in pharmacy. The average age of an average sales force (not, of course, that one exists!) will be around 30 years. There remains a dominance of males but the balance is changing. It is probably a truism that the pharmaceutical industry offers fewer barriers to the career woman than other major manufacturing and export industries.

## SALESPERSON

An initial entrant into the sales arena of the pharmaceutical industry will receive in-depth product training and, of course, sales techniques training before visiting any customers alone. The technical product training is usually easy for a science graduate to grasp, especially if he or she has just left university. Indeed during certain sessions of the training course the trainer may use the expertise of those present to illustrate a point or offer current knowledge. This should not 'lull' the graduate into a false sense of security; knowing a subject or at least its technical details does not mean that you can relate it to others and it certainly does not mean that you sell it to others. The sales technique sessions are by far the most gruelling and frustrating for trainer and trainee when there is an 'expert' in the audience. Experience shows, however, that good selling skills learnt well at this stage and developed, adapted and 'naturalised' through practice will yield results much more quickly than a deep awareness of the relative importance of various cytochrome P450 isoenzymes in the hepatic metabolism of a particular drug.

## ABPI EXAMINATION

All representatives are required to sit and pass the ABPI Representative's Examination within two year's of joining the industry. Exemption is only available to those who became representatives before 1978 or who are medically qualified. A degree in biological or related sciences or a nursing qualification is not grounds for exemption. The examination requires candidates to have a basic knowledge of physiology, anatomy and drug-related effects, and an understanding of the functioning of the pharmaceutical industry. Whilst the prospect of this will not daunt any graduate scientist, the examination should not be regarded lightly. A highly qualified individual will be expected to do well by his or her peers and trainers.

## OTHER SKILLS

Learning listening skills, being able to adapt your drug's benefits to the customer's needs and responding to the customer's questions in a practical and helpful way are most likely to gain sales. Getting to see the customer on a repeated basis and developing a relationship where he or she is pleased and interested to see you are difficult lessons for many graduates to learn but are some of the most rewarding new skills in the end. Most doctors will not agree to see you simply because of your product knowledge They could obtain that data elsewhere. An effective representative will have to offer extra value, e.g. perhaps you present information in an easy-to-assimilate way or because you are particularly effective in providing information about one unit's practice to another and from one colleague to another. You are trustworthy and, although always on the periphery, will begin to be seen as part of the 'team'.

Humility, tenacity and a tough skin are all part of the character of a pharmaceutical salesperson. Most GP and some hospital doctor appointments are made so far in advance that you must maintain a sense of humour whilst accepting dates years in the future. Your objective must then be to meet with key doctors at an earlier opportunity. Numeracy and an ability to self-analyse also go with the job. You will be taught to analyse your own territory sales data but you must continually measure your own performance against goals set both by your manager and by yourself. Whilst gregarious people often thrive at this job it is not one for those who must have people they know about them all day. It is a lonely existence and, whilst lack of immediate supervision can be a welcome novelty, some people find the 'freedom' difficult to handle.

## REWARDS

The rewards of successful sales performance are gratifying and if they come after a period of personal training and development they can be doubly rewarding. Recognition by one's peers and indeed superiors is as important in the sales profession as in any other.

Being 'Number One' representative is not, however, the key to immediate promotion and often a new graduate or highly qualified individual will anticipate upward movement into an office-based or managerial role more rapidly than company procedure can accomodate. Patience at this stage of career development can pay dividends in the future and a strong experience base at what is often regarded as the 'grass-roots' job in the industry can help to build a broad career n the future.

## REGIONAL SALES MANAGER

The sales teams are usually managed by a field-based regional sales manager who will be responsible for up to 10 representatives. Most individuals who have experienced this important role will consistently remark that it is one of the most enjoyable jobs in the industry. There are, of course, a number of provisos attached to this remark.

To be a successful regional sales manager you must understand the selling role, usually having had sales experience yourself; you must understand people and you must be able to communicate up and down a management line. Essentially the team that reports to you will regard you as their main contact point when in the field. This can mean that you receive not just work-related problems but also domestic and social problems that are often created by the insular nature of a representative's job. Specialised interpersonal skills training is vital for most regional sales managers.

Acting as an intermediary between the strategy-setters based in the main office and those who work in the field can be difficult. Broad-based industry knowledge, perhaps experience in other internal roles within the company or other companies, helps to improve the sales/marketing communication and strengthens the individual.

Regional sales management is often used as a development tool for individuals who require rapid and concentrated man-management experience. There are many benefits in learning these skills out in the field away from the constant direct scrutiny of a line manager and with the ability to stand back from any one representative's problems simply because you do not meet them every day.

Analytical skills are very important in the role. The ability to interpret individual's sales data, develop strategies to improve weaknesses and enhance performance are the essential ingredients of the job. You will often be used by your representatives as a 'troubleshooter' for problems with customers. You will be seen as the first field contact for many departments in the company's office, and careful development of a broad spectrum of contacts throughout the company and active networking can be useful when problems arise or when promotion or job change looms.

Competitive spirit is critical to the salesperson and the manager, and the challenge of 'being the best' is often a major, and only, motivation on a wet Friday afternoon in winter!

## SALES MANAGER

Most organisations run with sales managers based in the office. In the past decade a number of companies have piloted entirely field-based sales management teams but in general it seems that the sales team prefers to have some central representation. Motivational skills are critical to the role of sales manager. Most good sales managers are charismatic and able to lead their team to ever greater success. Their selling skills are usually kept sharp by a constant battery of presentations to senior management regarding current and future sales.

## MARKETING

### Additional Qualifications

In the UK, those wishing to enter marketing either immediately following graduation or after undertaking other jobs within the industry would do well to consider the Institute of Marketing Diploma of Marketing. With a good science degree the diploma is most frequently studied for two years through attendance at evening classes held throughout the country. Internationally, and for those setting their sights on a high-flying commercial career, the Master of Business

Administration (MBA) is a recognised next step. This is somewhat more intense and may need considerable support from one's line manager regarding attendance at summer schools, etc. No qualification should be seen as the prerequisite to success in the industry and prospective candidates would be well advised to take specific career guidance before embarking on an MBA. Some companies may be willing to consider a one-year sabbatical for an individual and others may prefer to plan a development course that is better tailored to the company and industry needs.

### Product Management

'I want to get into marketing' is a familiar answer from many graduate interviewees aspiring to join the commercial environment. The aura of glamour that traditionally surrounds 'marketing' should be dispelled immediately. Product management is about knowing the market in which your product is positioned, strict attention to detail, forecasting your product's sales, and forward planning to ensure all sales force requirements for literature and samples are met.

The preparation of promotional material, including packaging, advertising, sales force literature and exhibition material, will be your responsibility and you will be badgered from all sides regarding content, colour, design concepts, quality of paper, cost, quantity, size and so on. You will be expected to be the product champion, to have a breadth of knowledge second to none about the therapeutic area in which your drug or range of products sells, remain up to date with journals and take the flak if it all goes wrong! And in this role do not expect to gain many accolades because success will usually be attributed elsewhere.

The satisfaction is gained from having a central role, liaising with many different departments both in and out of the company and from seeing the effects of successful and often novel campaigns.

You do not have to be 'creative' to be in marketing. You will discover that the world is full of creative people, some of who are employed to be creative, and truly are, and others who undertake the role as a sideline. The product manager's job is to develop a strategy for a product and utilise the resources available to increase the sales of that product. It is not the product manager's job to decide whether the packaging should be blue or red, but it *is* his or her job to know what the customer will respond to best.

Knowledge of the market is vital and market research both formal and informal, e.g. via regular visits to customers, feedback from the field or background reading, will help to give the product manager a clearer view of the direction the marketing campaign should take. Here the scientific skills of the individual can be very useful, especially when interpreting clinical papers or reports, liaising with medical department colleagues and talking to opinion leaders.

Presentation skills are important in this role and must be continually developed and refined. A poor presentation by a product manager to the sales force can mar the take-off of a new campaign. Equally, a good presentation to the board of management can increase a product's promotional budget and the confidence bestowed in the individual. As a product champion it is important to uphold one's product against others within a company's portfolio, and well-reasoned arguments can often gain your product more selling time than another. Direct representative selling is of course only one of the many different promotional routes available to help maintain a product's momentum. The product manager must constantly review and assess all avenues of promotion.

## Marketing Manager

Whilst the product manager's horizon must, by definition, remain limited to one or a group of products, the marketing manager, with responsibility for a range of products, must take a wider, more strategic, view. Skills learned as a product manager are important in this role but the easy refuge of 'doing' rather than delegating should be avoided. The marketing manager's role is one of liaison to facilitate the forward movement of all products within his or her remit. Close liaison with the sales management team is important, as is an intimate knowledge of the individual financial performance of each product. There is little point in promoting non-profitable product lines whilst other more cost-efficient ones wait in the wings. The marketing manager is a resource manager. The job holder must maximise the return from the finite budget and personnel resources. Creative thinking rather than creativity is an attribute for the marketing manager.

## NEW PRODUCT DEVELOPMENT

Depending upon the structure and relative size of the company, this function may be kept entirely separate from the existing marketing team or it may draw on members of that team to provide expertise as and when required. New products are, of course, the future of the industry and this area is one to which many aspire. There can be frustrations because projects are often 'handed on' before a product is ready to market and thus those who have nursed the drug through development may never be directly involved in its early success. Some scientists, however, enjoy the ever-changing aspects of developing new concepts and prefer not to partake in the day-to-day tactical planning of a launch and sales campaign.

The ability to review data critically and make judgements about the viability of products is important. A respected marketing manager will often be involved in the decision to move a new product into the next stage of development based upon his or her market knowledge. The multidisciplinary development teams which many companies now run help to bring good products to the market more quickly by using the commercial representatives to make enlightened judgements about market potential. Many organisations have resolved that the involvement of marketing early in the development process can be highly beneficial to the final outcome of the product. Companies can save development resources by only progressing viable—i.e. profitable—products, and marketeers have a significant role to play in these decisions.

## INTER-DEPARTMENTAL LIAISON

As already mentioned, there are many approaches that the skilful sales/marketing person can use to develop his or her brand. Most of these will require the support of others both inside and outside the company.

An understanding of the many different job functions and their inter-relationship will help to facilitate good communication and speed the progress of projects. 'Wars' and inter-departmental strife are to be avoided at all costs. Medical and marketing departments which liaise well produce better campaigns and probably more successful products in the long run.

A medical adviser who is involved with the concept of an advertisement and then sees it through to production is more likely to approve it. Medical departments which are willing to discuss and understand the demands of marketing find that they are more often presented with designs that they can approve. Graduate scientists working in the commercial arm of the company can, and should, digest detail about their products, know the background papers and be able to argue their corners from a position of credible strength.

## ABPI CODE OF PRACTICE

Above all, in the UK it is important not to see the ABPI Code of Practice as something to be simply adhered to but rather to work with it. The combined creative, scientific and analytical skills of the company personnel and their agencies can work happily and successfully within its bounds to produce blockbuster drugs with accompanying blockbuster campaigns.

## THE FUTURE

The challenge of successful sales and marketing careers and the long-term prospects for those who embark upon them represents the story of today's pharmaceutical industry. Drugs do not sell themselves. The market is highly sophisticated, with customers becoming more commercially aware and governments looking to save money and restrict health spending. Health economics, prescribing formularies, the increasing importance of over-the-counter medication, single market marketing and global harmonisation will all have their impact on the 'bottom line' of the world's pharmaceutical companies. Increasing computerisation, improved electronic communications and a reduction in user resistance will see a change in the way information is exchanged both nationally and internationally. It is possible that medical conferences in exotic locations will decline, with interactive satellite links between opinion leaders becoming the norm. Paper use will decline with journals on disc. The representative may become a thing of the past but drugs and products of biotechnology will still need to be marketed to ensure continued R&D investment and return. Those able to take on the challenge of the new and see a clear way forward will prosper. The industry will need good scientists in sales and marketing in the future.

# 33
# Consultant in Pharmaceutical Medicine

## Brian Gennery

Gennery Associates, Bracknell, UK

The idea of being a totally independent person who both earns their living and obtains job satisfaction by using their own intellectual and personal resources is an attractive one for many people. Some such people leave the environs of a pharmaceutical company or contract research organisation and set themselves up as a consultant in pharmaceutical medicine. It is difficult to quantify how many individuals have taken this step but the number is growing on both sides of the Atlantic. The reasons for this growth are partly because of the numbers of separations or lay-offs of even quite senior medical staff from corporations who are struggling to cut back costs in view of the squeeze in health care budgets in all developed countries. In this chapter an attempt will be made to analyse the reasons for people going into consultancy, the planning required and the steps that need to be taken, the characteristics and qualities needed to succeed, the types of work which are available and finally the problems and risks of making this particular choice of career.

This chapter will not cover consultancy work carried out by contract research organisations or by full-time academic and hospital physicians who offer part-time consultancy services to various companies.

*Discovering New Medicines: Careers in Pharmaceutical Research and Development.*
Edited by P.D. Stonier
© 1994 John Wiley & Sons Ltd

## REASONS FOR GOING INTO CONSULTANCY

Anyone entering consultancy or contemplating a career in this direction should always look upon it as part of a career plan. It is a step which should only be taken after a careful analysis of the various career opportunities open to an individual and a thought-out decision that this is absolutely the right step for that person. It is no use going into consultancy just to have a 'try at it'. Unless one is committed to this career option it is not likely that anyone would be successful at it.

Having said this it is not at all uncommon, and this is a quite different scenario, for people who have reached retirement age and are in receipt of a full company pension to do some occasional or part-time consultancy as a way of maintaining an intellectual challenge. This is, of course, open to anyone who so desires to take up such a challenge, and the risks from it are obviously considerably less than if consultancy is considered to be a deliberate career move from which one wishes to earn sufficient money to replace a salary or a pension.

Assuming that one is moving into consultancy as part of a planned career move, it is important as part of the analysis to look at the risks and benefits of the opportunity and to ensure that at least in the medium to long term the benefits are likely to outweigh the risks.

### Risks

The biggest risk of moving into consultancy from a company position is the immediate cessation of all the benefits package associated with working for a large company. One no longer has the comfort of a regular and predictable monthly income which would normally be expected to take care of all the necessities of life and perhaps having a little bit over. Equally there will be no further bonuses which in the past may have been an important source of income and form the basis of such important events as family holidays and Christmas presents. The car will almost certainly have gone, as will the pension, contributory or non-contributory, free life assurance, chronic sickness benefit packages and private health care insurance. Suddenly you are on your own and you have to provide for all of this list of things. Clearly some priorities will be decided as to which are the most important and this will vary as to an individual's personal circumstances.

### Benefits

The potential benefits of being a consultant is the idea of being able to plan one's own life pattern; associated with this is being one's own boss! In practice of course one no longer has a single boss but hopefully a multitude of bosses who are all pulling for their project to be done at the fastest possible pace and for the least possible cost. A consultant would hope to do only those jobs which are really of interest and have a variety of different projects moving forward at the same time which provide intellectual challenge and a large amount of interest in work. There is also the hope and possibility of working with a variety of different companies and benefiting from seeing their various corporate cultures in operation. Finally, if one is successful, there is the hope of considerable personal reward both financial and in terms of job satisfaction.

## CONSULTANCY BY DEFAULT

It is becoming increasingly common to come across individuals who are setting themselves up in a consultancy operation not out of choice or desire but because they have been the victim of a major corporate reorganisation or merger and are unable to find employment in any other company. This is not the way to move into consultancy because it means that the individual is probably not committed to that type of career, has not planned for such a move and thought through the type of services that they are able or prepared to offer, and has not got the necessary resources behind them to enable them to establish their position within the scope of consultancy opportunities before they become successful.

## PLANNING FOR CONSULTANCY

As with any business a consultancy package offered by an individual should be viewed as *product* and as such should be marketed, preferably with some unique features about it which makes it attractive to potential clients, who will usually be pharmaceutical companies. As with any product launch the product needs to be thoroughly researched and worked out, and the time of the launch planned so as to maximise the opportunity available. This usually means reviewing the attributes of the individual providing the consultancy service and seeing what they can offer potential clients.

### 'Product' Characteristics

The following is a list of experiences and skills that a pharmaceutical physician might have had and that might be appropriate for him or her to use as part of their consultancy product package which they are going to offer to clients.

The first of these is the amount of time spent in the industry. As in so many aspects of life, time means experience gained and types of events experienced, both of which may be unique to an individual and if in demand will put that individual into a good position to offer a consultancy service. All too often people who have spent three to five years in the industry set themselves up in a consultancy position, only to find they have almost nothing to offer beyond the experience of a few clinical trials, putting together one or two CTXs (Clinical Trial Certificate Exemption) and attending a few symposia. Whilst there can be no hard and fast rules on timing, it is difficult to imagine that anyone who has done less than 15–20 years experience in the industry has had sufficient variety and depth of experience to make what they have of value to potential clients.

The types of experience that should have been acquired during a career in pharmaceutical medicine will inevitably include those in clinical research and associated activities such as product registration. It would have been important to list the number of products for which one has had responsibility in phases I, II, III and IV, whether there is any experience with post-marketing surveillance studies, activities with the Code of Practice Committee, putting together CTX applications and product license applications, and finally what experience an individual has with the various European procedures.

It will also be important to list the breadth of an individual's experience in the clinical research and registration arena, taking into account not only Europe but also the USA and Japan.

Other attributes that need to be examined and brought together are an analysis of training programmes that have been undertaken and the length and depth of an individual's management experience in a variety of different positions.

Other important aspects that will be helpful in demonstrating one's stature within the environment of pharmaceutical medicine is to have demonstrated wide experience in a number of organisations, such as serving on committees and helping with activities of various organisations such as the British Association of Pharmaceutical Physicians, the Society of Pharmaceutical Medicine, the Faculty of Pharmaceutical Medicine and finally the Association of the British Pharmaceutical Industry.

Also of importance will be a list of publications demonstrating an individual's knowledge and experience and whether or not a person serves on the editorial board of a journal.

These then are the elements that go to make the 'product'. It now needs to be put in the context of the market in which it is to operate and merchandised and presented to potential clients so that they take advantage of the opportunity presented.

## Resources

It is important to view a pharmaceutical consultancy as a business and the content of the type of consultancy being offered as a product. The elements which go to make up the product have already been discussed, but it needs to be presented in the same way as any other product.

The first thing to do is to write out a business plan in exactly the same way as one would for a large multinational corporation. This should include a mission statement, a set of objectives against which you can measure your own performance, and a financial plan including a cash flow analysis for at least the first three years.

The next thing to look at is to determine what finance is going to be needed to be invested into the business before it becomes a viable self-sustaining operation. This is where long-term planning for consultancy comes into play, as few people are likely to be able to sustain themselves by generating enough income over the first few months or a year and therefore need some personal financial resources to fall back on to carry them through this period. The only alternative of course is to solicit a bank loan, which may be perfectly possible but inevitably involves interest charges and arrangement fees. These come more expensive for a business than for a personal loan and this option should be avoided if at all possible.

The business plan should be shared widely with a variety of professional people such as legal advisers, financial advisers, accountants and any financial backer or bank manager. The reason for doing this is two-fold: one is to solicit their views as they will often have considerable experience in helping people start up small businesses, and secondly to show that you have a grasp of what you are trying to do and that you are setting about it in a structured, organised way.

The next decision is to decide whether one is going to work from home or to find a small office. This will often be determined by availability of space at home, the price of office accommodation to be found in the locality and finally personal preference. Some people just cannot work at home and feel that they have to go to an office in order to be able to change their mind-set into a work mode. Others can happily get up and work at home just as though they were going out into an office environment. Wherever one is going to work from, it is important to get the necessary facilities to be able to operate effectively; as a minimum, these include a high-quality computer with a considerable range of software, a fax machine and in the absence of full-time secretarial help an answer-phone. It may also be necessary to get a mobile phone in order to be able to stay in contact at all times.

The next thing is to register with the Customs and Excise for Value Added Tax. This is not a critical requirement in the first instance, but as soon as one is approaching the thresholds for VAT it is important to register so as not to fall foul of the law.

The next exercise is to market the product, and this should be approached in exactly the same way as with any other marketing operation. There should be efforts at direct selling by personal contact with colleagues either individually in their offices or at meetings; this network can be widened by writing personal letters to colleagues explaining the types of consultancy on offer and if appropriate asking for a personal meeting. It may be appropriate to produce a brochure describing the range of facilities being offered, and this can be mailed widely across the industry either to personal contacts and friends or just in a somewhat more blind fashion. Finally it may be appropriate to take out advertisements in journals to make sure that everybody knows exactly what programmes and facilities are being offered.

## CHARACTERISTICS AND QUALITIES REQUIRED FOR SUCCESS

As with any marketing operation, it will only be as successful as the quality of the product on offer and the way it is presented to potential clients. There are a number of characteristics about the consultancy business which make it somewhat distinctive from many other areas of endeavour and there are qualities required of somebody going into consultancy which are probably a prerequisite to success.

### What Is On Offer

In order to be successful in consultancy it is necessary to have a long history of achievements in the pharmaceutical industry. It is better if these are in more than one company, cover a wide range of functions within pharmaceutical medicine, include some experience in management at a senior level, and cover a wide geographical area and are not just confined to the UK. It is also helpful to have served on a wide variety of committees and organisations as this establishes a substantial network. This network is necessary not just for potential clients but also as a resource to be called upon for help when uncertainty about a particular issue or problem arises and it is important to get reassurance from a senior colleague or friend. This network should include other consultants in pharmaceutical medicine. Obviously to some extent one is in competition with such individuals but to exclude them from one's network of contacts is not in one's own interest and there is no harm in offering sound advice to a colleague who hopefully one day will return the favour.

### Defining Areas of Expertise

It is crucial only to offer services in areas in which one has experience and know-how and something to offer. In the common jargon this means bringing 'added value'. Developing and maintaining credibility is critical and there is nothing better designed to destroy such credibility than to offer services ranging from discovery research, through clinical R&D, registration, post-marketing surveillance, sales, marketing, public relations, crisis management and treasury operations when one has worked in only one or two of these areas and has no knowledge of any of the others. This means going back to the simple basics of knowing one's own strengths and weaknesses and having the courage to turn away work that is simply outside one's experience. This is clearly difficult to do early on when the number of projects on offer may be somewhat limited, but it never does any good to take on a project that clearly cannot be tackled effectively and with the appropriate degree of skill and knowledge. One's credibility as a consultant can rapidly be destroyed by totally letting a client down with regard to a particular project.

### Being Resourceful

The first thing that one learns on leaving a corporate organisation is that suddenly you have none of the facilities available in the way of secretarial resources, computer back-up resources, library facilities etc. Therefore one has to do everything from arranging hotels and travel plans through to carrying out literature searches and writing up reports. Many of the resources that one would want are not immediately to hand. Examples are a lack of the wide range of journals normally found in most companies and access to critical documents such as those coming from the European Community Commission and from the Medicines Control Agency. Somehow one has to go out and find these, as it is very important to keep up to date with the rapidly evolving discipline of pharmaceutical medicine.

### Work Ethic

Most consultants will say that their time in consultancy is the busiest of their life. With luck they are working harder than ever before but this in its own way brings a number of problems. There is sometimes great difficulty in managing one's time effectively. Work comes in peaks and troughs, at least early on in consultancy, and the tendency is to take anything and everything that comes along, thereby creating continuous peaks and fewer and fewer troughs. The ideal of being one's own boss, planning one's own lifestyle, and controlling one's own work-load rapidly evaporates as one quickly realises that one no longer has a single boss but a hundred people pulling in different directions, all wanting their project done by the day before yesterday. This is an important point and needs to be continuously borne in mind, particularly as the temptation early on in the consultancy career is to take any project that becomes available.

## TYPES OF WORK

Companies will only employ consultants when they have to fill some type of gap in their resources. These gaps occur in a variety of interesting and unusual areas and different consultants will feel that they are better able to fill one gap than another.

### Gaps in Head Count

With the increasing uncertainty in the health care area and the various pressures being put on pharmaceutical companies, most managements these days are trying to man for the troughs and manage the peaks. However, the work that comes with the peaks has to be done and this is where consultants can usefully be employed. It is possible that a consultant will simply be asked to act as a 'locum' to fill the role of a medical adviser or senior medical adviser for a particular project over a defined period of time. This may be whilst the company is recruiting a new full-time member of staff or it may be on a longer contract, with the consultant spending one or two days a week in the company. Other projects which require this type of gap to be filled include protocol writing, report writing, monitoring studies and sites, and ghost-writing either expert opinions or articles for journal publication.

### Gaps and Experience

Whilst most of the very large companies find that within their staff they have people with experience in most areas of therapeutics, many medium to small companies do not have this luxury. Therefore they will seek outside help in order to find out about a new therapeutic area, and a pharmaceutical medicine consultant with wide experience can often fill this gap. These projects tend to be somewhat short term and involve explaining the area, offering some kind of training for people within the company and leaving them able to cope with the new challenges ahead of them. Another gap in experience is in the limitation of territory in which a company has operated, and a consultant with wide international experience may be able to help a company start new programmes in new territories. The third gap in experience is with registration problems, often of a trans-national nature, and a consultant with a great depth of experience will be able to help a company through some of these issues. Finally a consultant with wide experience in different types of organisations may be able to help a company which is trying to reorganise its medical function to cope with the developing concept of globalisation.

## Gaps in Expertise

Whilst most large companies will have within their organisation the necessary resources to tackle all aspects of pharmaceutical medicines, there are still a number of areas which are rapidly developing and changing where a consultant may be of use to both large companies and smaller ones. The first of these is training, and whilst many organisations run a variety of training programmes sometimes a consultant has a particular area of expertise and knowledge which is valuable to a company and is able to offer training in that particular area. Indeed sometimes companies may ask consultants to run significant training programmes for them covering many layers of staff and embracing many aspects of pharmaceutical medicine. The second area is in quality assurance and the need to be able to satisfy registration authorities that clinical studies have been done to Good Clinical Practice standards and a certificate of quality assurance inspection can be proffered. Even some quite big companies do not yet have quality assurance units in place who are capable of carrying out this function, and even those companies that do have such units in place may find themselves short of resources on occasions. Therefore consultants with the appropriate know-how and expertise in this area will be invited in to fulfil this growingly important function. Thirdly, some companies still do not have full sets of standard operating procedures (SOPs) in place and even those who have sometimes feel unhappy with what they have available to them. They might therefore invite in a consultant to review their SOPs and to advise how these may be changed and developed so as to be more user friendly and therefore used more frequently. Finally, in this age of medicolegal problems and a litiginous society, companies are frequently finding themselves faced with not only the threat but also the reality of litigation and all the crisis management issues that surround that problem, and often will bring in a consultant who has had some experience in this area to help them through a variety of aspects of this difficulty.

## Bridging a Gap

An interesting and somewhat surprising function of a consultant is sometimes to act as a reconciling person within a company. There are situations where there are strong divisions of opinion as to how a particular project should be developed within a company, and a consultant is sometimes brought in to act as the 'referee'. The consultant has no face to lose either way and can quite often bring new light to bear on the problem, reconciling the different opinions within the company and hopefully helping the company to develop its product in a more effective way.

## PITFALLS AND MINEFIELDS

As with any business there are a number of pitfalls and minefields which need to be avoided if the business is to thrive and be successful.

## Size of Operation

If a consultant is successful there will be the temptation to expand the organisation and operation so as to cope with bigger and bigger projects, perhaps branching out into contract clinical research, and offering a variety of other services. This will be perhaps the most important decision the consultant ever has to make about the way he or she is going to manage the business and how they are going to let it develop and grow. Most companies when they call in a consultant expect the undivided and personal attention of that individual and not for the programme to be delegated down to junior member staff of or associate of some sort. Whilst other members of staff may be useful in terms of carrying out background research, in the end a consultant and his or her organisation only thrives on reputation and that can be destroyed very quickly. Therefore the decision to stay small as a one-person organisation or to expand into a small group is a critical one from a business point of view and it is also a risky one from a financial point of view. If one has been operating without an outside office previously this now becomes necessary and one also becomes responsible for other people's mortgages, pension plans, life assurance, etc., as well as one's own. This means that the revenue generated by the business has to expand very dramatically and whilst what has been coming in up to date has been perfectly adequate to support the consultant and his or her immediate family, whether it can take the quantum leap to support other members of staff is something that needs to be looked at very critically. An alternative may be to go and seek financial backing to help the business to expand but again this requires critical review and analysis before making such a decision.

## Buffers

Inevitably with consultancy, work tends to come in peaks and troughs and it is essential when there are a number of good peaks to put some of that income into a high-interest deposit account so as to cope with the troughs. As has been stated previously, one of the great difficulties is not having that regular salaried income coming in every month from a company and therefore one has to plan financially on a somewhat longer term than when working for a corporate organisation. Another part of having a buffer is to ensure that there is enough 'work' available to cover the troughs. This may mean storing up articles and other literature that needs to be read, having some pet project which one can never quite get round to but could cope with if there was no other work to be done for a few days or weeks, going to meetings and training courses if the opportunities avail themselves and doing something very lateral such as learning a new language.

## Speaking

If one has expertise in one or more areas it is not uncommon to be invited to speak at a variety of seminars and meetings. This is a very good method of meeting potential clients and demonstrating one's skills and expertise in a particular area. However, invitations to speak should be reviewed critically and carefully as for every hour of presentation one needs something like one working day of preparation. As the fees for speaking at many such seminars tend to be somewhat mediocre, to say the least, one has to weigh up very carefully if the potential value of accepting an invitation to speak is justified in view of the potential lost income that it involves.

## Conflict of Interest

Clients of consultants assume that the work that they ask their consultants to do will be treated as confidential and some companies will ask for a confidentiality agreement to be signed. Indeed it may be as well for the consultant to have their own confidentiality agreement prepared and offered to clients so as to demonstrate their commitment to confidentiality. However, there is another type of conflict of interest which must be borne in mind and that is not to accept assignments on products from two or more companies which clearly are in conflict with each other. This would be highly unethical and would rapidly destroy one's credibility. Equally important is for the consultant to protect their own long-term interest and ensure that the reports that they produce for clients are exclusive to the client only inasmuch as they are particular to that product under investigation and evaluation and not the consultant's generic skills.

## CONCLUSION

If one goes into consultancy for the right reasons and it has been properly planned for it is very likely that the individual will succeed. They will probably have the right qualities and resourcefulness to find appropriate projects and they will eventually find enough to provide an interesting, wide variety of work which is both enjoyable and rewarding.

# Useful Information

## GENERAL AND PROFESSIONAL

*Association of the British Pharmaceutical Industry (ABPI)*
12 Whitehall, London SW1A 2DY, UK
Tel: 071 930 3477
Fax: 071 930 3290

*European Federation of Pharmaceutical Industry Associations (EFPIA)*
Avenue Louise 250, Boite 91, 1050 Brussels, Belgium
Tel: (32)2 6406815
Fax: (32)2 6476049

*Association of Independent Clinical Research Contractors (AICRC)*
15–16 King Charles House, Cavalier Court, Bumpers Farm,
Chippenham, Wilts SN14 6LH, UK
Tel: 0249 444212
Fax: 0249 444189

*International Federation of Associations of Pharmaceutical Physicians*
*(IFAPP)*
President: Prof. Anders Rosén, Bristol-Myers Squibb Scandinavia,
PO Box 15200, 16115 Bromma, Sweden
Tel: (46)8 7047100
Fax: (46)8 7048931

*Discovering New Medicines: Careers in Pharmaceutical Research and Development.*
Edited by P.D. Stonier
© 1994 John Wiley & Sons Ltd

*Regulatory Affairs Professional Society (RAPS)*
83 Avenue E. Mounier, B-1200 Brussels, Belgium
Tel: (32)2 7729247
Fax: (32)2 7727237

*British Association of Pharmaceutical Physicians (BrAPP)*
1 Wimpole Street, London W1M 8AE, UK
Tel: 071 491 8610
Fax: 071 499 2405

*Association for Clinical Research in the Pharmaceutical Industry (ACRPI)*
c/o Institute of Biology, 20 Queensberry Place, London SW7 2DZ, UK
Tel: 071 581 8333

*Statisticians in the Pharmaceutical Industry (PSI)*
Executive Secretary, PO Box 37, Ely, Cambridgeshire CB6 3XW, UK
Tel/Fax: 0353 648740

*Association of Clinical Data Managers (ACDM)*
PO Box 1208, Maidenhead, Berkshire SL6 2YH, UK
Tel: 0628 789450
Fax: 0628 21230

*Association of Information Officers in the Pharmaceutical Industry (AIOPI)*
Secretary, Merck Sharp & Dohme Ltd, Neuroscience Research
Centre, Terlings Park, Eastwick Road, Harlow, Essex CM20 1QR, UK

*The British Institute of Regulatory Affairs (BIRA)*
34 Dover Street, London WX1 3RA
Tel: 071 499 2797
Fax: 071 499 1628

*American Academy of Pharmaceutical Physicians*
c/o Schnader, Harrison, Segal & Lewis, Suite 1400, 330 Madison
Avenue, New York, NY 10017, USA
Tel: (1)212 973 8054
Fax: (1)212 972 8798

*Association des Médecines de l'Industrie Pharmaceutique (AMIP)*
Secrétariat permanent de l'AMIP, 83 av. André Morizet, 92100
Boulogne, France
Tel: (33)1 46 030345
Fax: (33)1 46 032002

*Association Belge des Médecines de l'Industry Pharmaceutique
(ABEMIP/BEVAFI)*
Belgische Vereniging der Artsen van de Farmaceutische Industrie,
11 avenue des Hannetons, 1170 Brussels, Belgium

*Asociación de Medicos de la Industrial Farmacéutica Española (AMIFE)*
Villanueva, 11, 3°, 28001 Madrid, Spain

*Società di Scienze Farmacologiche Applicate (SSFA)*
PO Box 10741, 20110 Milano, Italy
Fax: (39)2 29 520179

*Landelijke Vereniging van Farmaceutische Industrie-Artsen (FIA)*
Secretariaat FIA, Kamgras 10, 36–48 HM Wilnis, The Netherlands
Tel: (31)2979 81121
Fax: (31)2979 41401

*Fachgesellschaft der Ärzte in der Pharmazeutischen Industrie (FÄPI)*
Dr Volker Gladigau, Medical Department, Boehringer Ingelheim,
Postfach 200, D-55216 Ingelheim am Rhein, Germany
Tel: (49)6132 772041
Fax: (49)6132 773818

*Läkemedelsindustrins Läkarförening (LL)*
(Swedish Association of Physicians in the Pharmaceutical Industry),
Prof. Anders Rosén, Bristol-Myers Squibb Scandinavia, PO Box
15200, 16115 Bromma, Sweden
Tel: (46)8 7047100
Fax: (46)8 7048931

*Society of Pharmaceutical Medicine (SPM)*
Institute of Biology, 20–22 Queensberry Place, London SW7 2DZ,
UK
Tel: 071 493 7825

*Faculty of Pharmaceutical Medicine of the Royal Colleges of Physicians of
the United Kingdom (FMP)*
1 St Andrew's Place, Regent's Park, London NW1 4LB, UK
Tel: 071 224 0343
Fax: 071 224 5381

*Drug Information Association (DIA)*
PO Box 3113, Ambler, PA 19002, USA
Tel: (1)215 628 2288
Fax: (1)215 641 1229

*American Medical Writers Association*
9650 Rockville Pike, Bethesda, MD 21814, USA

*Society of Freelance Editors and Proofreaders*
Membership Secretary: Kathleen Lyle, 43 Brighton Terrace Road,
Sheffield S10 1NT, UK

*Australian Medical Writers Association*
PO Box 423, Broadway, New South Wales 2007, Australia

*European Medical Writers Association*
(a chapter of the American Medical Writers Association)
Secretary: Dr Remy Brossel, Director, Biologie et Industrie, 150 Ave
de Paris, 94300 Vincennes, France

*Centre for Medicines Research (CMR)*
Woodmansterne Road, Carshalton, Surrey SM5 4DS, UK
Tel: 081 643 4411
Fax: 081 770 7958

*Office of Health Economics (OHE)*
12 Whitehall, London SW1A 2DY, UK
Tel: 071 930 9203

*Royal Society of Medicine Library (RSM)*
1 Wimpole Street, London W1M 8AE, UK
Tel: 071 408 2119
Fax: 071 408 0062

## COURSES AND QUALIFICATIONS

*Faculty of Pharmaceutical Medicine of the Royal Colleges of Physicians of
the United Kingdom (FPM)*
The Administrator, 1 St Andrew's Place, Regent's Park, London
NW1 4LB, UK
Tel: 071 224 0343
Fax: 071 224 5381

*Postgraduate Course in Pharmaceutical Medicine*
Director: Professor David Luscombe, Division of Clinical Pharmacy,
Welsh School of Pharmacy, University of Wales, Redwood Building,
King Edward VII Avenue, Cardiff CF1 3XF, UK
Tel: 0222 874783
Fax: 0222 874149

*Diploma in Clinical Science*
Director: Dr Bailey, Division of Clinical Pharmacy, Welsh School of
Pharmacy, University of Wales, Redwood Building, King Edward VII
Avenue, Cardiff CF1 3XF, UK
Tel: 0222 874783
Fax: 0222 874149

*Diploma in Regulatory Affairs*
Director: Dr I. Harrison, Division of Clinical Pharmacy, Welsh School
of Pharmacy, University of Wales, Redwood Building, King Edward
VII Avenue, Cardiff CF1 3XF, UK
Tel: 0222 874783
Fax: 0222 874149

*European Course in Pharmaceutical Medicine (ECPM)*
Under auspices of EUCOR (European Confederation of the Upper
Rhine Universities)
Information: ECPM Secretariat, Department of Research, University
Hospitals, CH-4031 Basel, Switzerland
Tel: (41)61 265 23 63
Fax: (41)61 261 15 00

*Pharmed*
Post-graduate Programme in Pharmacology and Pharmaceutical
Medicine, Universite Libre de Bruxelles
Information: Pharmed, Campus Grasme, Building C, CP602, Route
de Lennik 808, B-1070 Brussels, Belgium
Tel: (32)2 555 42 20
Fax: (32)2 555 46 55

*The British Toxicology Society*
20–22 Queensberry Place, London SW7 2D2, UK
Tel: 071 581 8333

*MSc in Pharmaceutical Medicine*
MSc Course Administrator, HPRU, University of Surrey, Milford
Hospital, Godalming, Surrey GU7 1UF, UK
Tel: 0483 418208
Fax: 0483 418453

## Recruitment/Employment

*AXESS*
AXESS House, Forest Road, Kew, Richmond, Surrey TW9 3BY, UK
Tel: 081 332 9944
Fax: 081 332 0697

*Clinpharm Ltd*
St Ives House, St Ives Road, Maidenhead, Berkshire SL6 1QS, UK
Tel: 0628 778994
Fax: 0628 778430

*Eames Jones Judge Hawkings*
29 High Street, Welwyn, Hertfordshire AL6 0EE, UK
Tel: 0438 840984
Fax: 0438 840429

*'Improving Health, Preventing Disease' (Booklet)*
Careers for graduates in the Pharmaceutical Industry
Information: Health Industry Information Officer, ABPI, 12
Whitehall, London SW1A 2DY, UK
Tel: 071 930 3477

*Innovex Limited*
Innovex House, Reading Road, Henley-on-Thames, Oxon RG9 1EL,
UK
Tel: 0491 578171
Fax: 0491 575057

*Roger Stephens & Associates*
Chequers House, 3 Park Street, Old Hatfield, Hertfordshire AL9
5AT, UK
Tel: 07072 75361

*Talentmark Limited*
King House, 5–11 Westbourne Grove, London W2 4UA, UK
Tel: 071 229 2266
Fax: 071 229 3549

# Bibliography

## REFERENCES

Adam, H.M. and Passmore, R. (1980) Introduction, in *A Companion to Medical Studies: Vol. 2. Pharmacology, Microbiology, General Pathology and Related Subjects* (eds R. Passmore and J.S. Robson), Blackwell Scientific Publications, London.

Anderson, S. (1993) *Pharm. J.*, **251**, 210.

Armitage, P. and Berry, G. (1987) The scope of statistics, Ch. 1 in *Statistical Methods in Medical Research*, Blackwell Scientific Publications, London.

ASA Committee on Training of Statisticians for Industry (1980) Preparing statisticians for careers in industry: report of the ASA Section on Statistical Education Committee on Training of Statisticians for Industry. *Am. Statist.*, **34** (2), 65–75.

Baber, N.S. (1991) The scope of clinical pharmacology in the pharmaceutical industry. *Br. J. Clin. Pharmacol.*, **31**, 495–496.

Bailey, D.G., Spence, J.D., Munro, C. and Arnold, J.M.O. (1991) Interactions of citrus juices with felodipine and nifedipine. *Lancet*, **337**, 268–269.

Barrett, C., Tugwell, C. and Jones, C. (1992) Preparing realistic 'budgets' for medicines: a need for change. *Hosp. Update Plus*, Oct., 148–151.

Bax, R.P., McCulley, D. and Wheeley, M.St.G. (1982) The diploma in pharmaceutical medicine. *J. R. Coll. Physician Lond.*, **16**, 105–106.

Blackburn, S.C.F., Ellis, R., George, C.F. and Kirwan, J.R. The impact and treatment of arthritis in general practice. Accepted for publication by *Pharmacoepidemiology and Drug Safety*.

Bradford Hill, Sir A. (1937) *Principles of Medical Statistics*, Edward Arnold, London.

Buckley, C., Curtin, D., Walsh, T. and O'Malley, K. (1986). Ageing and platelet $\alpha_2$ adrenoceptors. *Br. J. Clin. Pharmacol.*, **21**, 721–722.

Burley, D. (1987) Pharmaceutical medicine: foundations and future. *Lancet*, **ii**, 1222.

Burley, D.M., Clarke, J.M. and Lasagna, L. (1993) Preface, in *Pharmaceutical Medicine (second edition)* (eds D.M. Burley, J.M. Clarke and L. Lasagna), Edward Arnold, London.

Capewell, S., Freestone, S., Critchley, J.A.J.H., Pottage, A. and Prescott, L.F. (1988) Reduced felodipine bioavailability in patients taking anticonvulsants. *Lancet*, **ii**, 480–482.

Cartwright, A. and Smith, C. (1988) *Elderly People, their Medicines and their Doctors*. Routledge, London.

Castleden, C.M., George, C.F., Marcer, D. and Hallett, C. (1977) Increased sensitivity to nitrazepam in old age. *Br. Med. J.*, **i**, 10–12.

Challenor, V.F., Waller, D.G., Renwick, A.G. and George, C.F. (1989) Slow release nifedipine plus atenolol in chronic stable angina pectoris. *Br. J. Clin. Pharmacol.*, **28**, 509–516.

Cholerton, S., Daly, A.K. and Idle, J.R. (1992) The role of individual human cytochromes P-450 in drug metabolism and clinical response. *Trends Pharmacol. Sci.*, **13**, 434–439.

Clay, T. (1990) *The Politics of Nursing*. Scutari Press, London.

CPMP Working Party on Efficacy of Medicinal Products (1990) EEC Note for Guidance: Good Clinical Practice for Trials on Medicinal Products in the European Community. *Pharmacol. Toxicol.*, **67**, 361–372.

Cranston, W.I., Juel-Jensen, B.E., Semmence, A.M., Handfield Jones, R.P.C., Forbes, J.A. and Mutch, L.M.M. (1963). Effects of oral diuretics on raised arterial pressure. *Lancet*, **ii**, 966–970.

Criteria for Accreditation of Degrees in Pharmacy (1992) Royal Pharmaceutical Society of Great Britain, London.

Cromie, B. (1993) The evolution of pharmaceutical medicine since the 1950s. *Pharmacol. Med.*, **7**, 127–137.

Crow, J. (1980) *Effects of Preparation on Problem Solving*. RCN Research Monograph, London.

Darbourne, A. (1993) Room at the top for clinicians. *Scrip Magazine*, **15**, 21–22.

Douglas, F. (1993) Dilemmas in clinical research. *Scrip Magazine*, **15**, 10–12.

Drayer, J.I. and Newman, T.J. (1993). People are depending on us (letter to the editor). *Appl. Clin. Trials*, **2**(8), 16.

Drummond, M., Teeling Smith, G. and Wells, N. (1988) *Economic Evaluation in the Development of Medicines*, OHE, London.

European Council Directive 92/28/EEC (31 March 1992) *Advertising of Medicinal Products for Human use.*

Feely, M., Cooke, J., Price, D., Singleton, S., Mehta, A., Bradford, L. and Calvert, R. (1987) Low-dose phenobarbitone as an indicator of compliance with drug therapy. *Br. J. Clin. Pharmacol.*, **24**, 77–83.

Gabbay, F.J. and Goldberg, A. (1991) The faculty of pharmaceutical medicine. *Br. J. Clin. Pharmacol.*, **32**, 265–266.

Gascon, M.-P. and Dayer, P. (1991) In vitro forecasting of drugs which may interfere with the biotransformation of midazolam. *Eur. J. Clin. Pharmacol.*, **41**, 573–578.

George, C.F. (1980) Amiloride handling in renal failure. *Br. J. Clin. Pharmacol.*, **9**, 94–95.

George, C.F. and Waller, D.G. (1993) Drug treatment, in *Clinical Heart Disease in Old Age* (eds. A. Martin and J. Camm), Wiley, Chichester.

George, C.F., Renwick, A.G., Darragh, A.S., Hosie, J., Black, D., van Marle W. and Frank, G.J. (1986) A comparison of isoxicam pharmacokinetics in young and elderly subjects. *Br. J. Clin. Pharmacol.*, **22**, 129S–134S.

George, C.F., George, R.H. and Howden, C.W. (1992) The liver and response to drugs, in *Wright's Liver and Biliary Disease, 3rd edn* (eds G.H. Millward-Sadler, R. Wright and M. Arthur), Saunders, London.

Goldberg, A. and Smith, R.N. (1985) Pharmaceutical medicine. *Lancet*, i, 447–448.

Greenblatt, D.J., Harmatz, J.S., Shapiro, L., Engelhardt, N., Gouthro, T.A. and Shader, R.I. (1991) Sensitivity to triazolam in the elderly. *N. Engl. J. Med.*, **324**, 1691–1698.

Grevel, J., Thomas, P. and Whiting, B. (1989) Population pharmacokinetic analysis of bisoprolol. *Clin. Pharmacokinet.*, **17**, 53–63.

Hamdy, R.C., Murnane, B., Perera, N., Woodcock, K. and Koch, I.M. (1982) The pharmacokinetics of benoxaprofen in elderly subjects. *Eur. J. Rheumatol. Inflamm.*, **5**, 69–75.

Hampton, S.R. and Julian, D.G. (1987) Role of the pharmaceutical industry in major clinical trials. *Lancet*, Nov. 28, 1258–1259.

Hayward J. (1992) *Of Graduates and Kings*. Winifred Memorial Lecture. RCN Research Monograph, London.

Health Trends (1972) Medical and dental staffing prospects in the NHS in England and Wales. *Health Trends*, **4**, 47–49.

Health Trends (1993) Medical and dental staffing prospects in the NHS in England and Wales, 1991. *Health Trends*, **25**, 4–12.

Honing, P.K., Woosley, R.L., Zamoni, K., Conner, D.P. and Cantilena, L.R. (1992) Changes in the pharmacokinetics and electrocardiographic pharmacodynamics of terfenadine with concomitant administration of erythromycin. *Clin. Pharmacol. Ther.*, **52**, 231–238.

House of Lords Select Committee on Science and Technology (1988) *Priorities in Medical Research*. HMSO London.

Ilett, K.F., Blythe, T.H., Hackett, L.P., Ong, R.T.T. and Clarke, T.M.F. (1993) Plasma concentrations of dothiepin and its metabolites are not correlated with clinical efficacy in major depressive illness. *Ther. Drug Monit.*, **5**, 351–357.

Jackson, G., Pierscianowski, T.A., Mahon, W. and Condon, J. (1976). Inappropriate hypertensive therapy in the elderly. *Lancet*, **ii**, 1317–18.

Jackson, P.R., Tucker, G.T. and Woods, H.F. (1989) Testing for bimodality in frequency distributions of data suggesting polymorphisms of drug metabolism: histograms and probit plots. *Br. J. Clin. Pharmacol*, **28**, 647–653.

King, L. (1993) *A Study of Critical Care: Nurses' Assessment Strategies*. Ongoing PhD study, King's College London.

Kronbach. T., Mathys, D., Umeno, M., Gonzales, F.J. and Meyer, U.A. (1989) Oxidation of midazolam and triazolam by human liver cytochrome P450IIIA4. *Mol. Pharmacol.*, **36**, 89–96.

Lant, A.F. (1987) Evolution of diuretics and ACE inhibitors, their renal and antihypertensive actions: parallels and contrasts. *Br. J. Clin. Pharmacol.*, **23**, 27S–41S.

Lawrence D.R. (1966a) Drug control, drug names, in *Clinical Pharmacology*, Churchill, London.

Lawrence D.R. (1966b) Drug therapy: the thalidomide disaster, in *Clinical Pharmacology*, Churchill, London.

Lightfoot, G. (1992) The evolving role of the CROs in drug development. Presented at International Business Communications Workshop. *Clinical Trials: Cost Control Design Operational Strategies*, July 7–9, Philadelphia.

Lis, Y. and Walker, S.R. (1989) Novel medicines marketed in the UK (1960–1980) *Br. J. Clin. Pharmacol.*, **28**, 333–343.

Lovatt, B. (1993) Organizational needs and new internal relationships, in *Economic Evaluation of Medicines*. IBC, London.

LoVerde, M., Prochazka, A. and Byyny, R.L. (1993) Investigators and CROs: partners or adversaries? *Appl. Clin. Trials*, **2** (1), 24–27.

Macleod, H.M. and Goldberg, A. (1981) Diploma in pharmaceutical medicine. *Br. J. Clin. Pharmacol.*, **12**, 3–4.

Macleod Clark, J., Wilson-Barnett, J., Latter S. and Maben, J. (1993) *Health Education and Health Promotion in Nursing: A Study of Practice in Acute Areas*. DoH Report.

Mahgoub, A., Idle, J.R., Dring, L.G., Lancaster, R. and Smith, R.L. (1977) Polymorphic hydroxylation of debrisoquine in man. *Lancet*, **ii**, 584–586.

Maloney, A.M. (1990) Training The Clinical Research Scientist, in *Proceedings of 7th International Conference on Pharmaceutical Medicine* (eds J. Ruiz Ferrán, J. Lahuerta Dal Rè and R. Lardinois), Prous Science Publishers.

Mann, R.D., Lis, Y., Chukwujindu, J. and Spitzer W.O. (1992) *Triazolam and Psychiatric Events: An Interim Report*. 8th Int. Congr. Pharmacoepidemiology, Minnesota, USA. 30 Aug. to 2 Sept. 1992.

Mann, R.D., Lis, Y , Chukwujindu, J. and Chanter, D. (1993) *A Study of the Association between Hormone Replacement Therapy, Smoking, and the Occurrence of Myocardial Infarction in Women.* 9th Int. Congr. Pharmacoepidemiology, Washington DC, USA, 29 Aug. to 1 Sept. 1993.

Montamat, S.C. and Davies, A.O. (1989). Physiological response to isoproterenol and coupling of beta-adrenergic receptors in young and elderly human subjects. *J. Gerontol.*, **44**, M100–105.

Mullinger, B.M. (1990) Training in the pharmaceutical industry for CRAs. *Pharm. Med.*, **4**, 235–247.

Murphy, M.B., Lewis, P.J., Kohner, E., Schumer, B. and Dollery, C.T. (1982) Glucose intolerance in hypertensive patients treated with diuretics: a fourteen year follow-up. *Lancet*, **ii**, 1293–1295.

Ontario (1991) *Draft Guidelines*, Toronto.

Parke Davis (1939) *Analecta Therapeutica*. Parke Davis & Co., London.

Paterson, J.W., Conolly, M.E., Dollery, C.T. and Hayes, A. (1970) The pharmacodynamics and metabolism of propranolol in man. *Pharmacol. Clin.*, **2**, 127–133.

Pembrey, S. (1980) *The Ward Sister: Key to Nursing.* RCN Research Monograph, London.

*Pharm. Ind.* (1990) Good Clinical Practice: CPMP Working Party on Efficacy of Medicinal Products. *Pharm. Ind.*, **52**(12).

Porter, S. (1992) The poverty of professionalism: a critical analysis of strategies for the occupational advancement of nursing. *J. Adv. Nurs.*, **17**, 6, 720–726.

Pritchard, B.N.C. and Gillam, P.M.S. (1971) Assessment of propranolol in angina pectoris: clinical dose–response curve and effect on electrocardiogram at rest and on exercise. *Br. Heart J.*, **33**, 473–480.

PSI (1989) Careers for Statisticians in the Pharmaceutical Industry. PSI, PO Box 37, Ely, Cambs CB6 3XW, UK.

Reid, J.L., Calne, D.B., George, C.F., Pallis, C. and Vakil, S.D. (1971) Cardiovascular reflexes in Parkinsonism. *Clin. Sci.*, **41**, 63–67.

*Research Assessment Exercise* (1992) The outcome (University Funding Council Circular 26/92, December 1992), Department for Education, London.

Ridout, S., Waters, W.E. and George, C.F. (1986) Knowledge of and attitudes to medicines in the Southampton community. *Br. J. Clin. Pharmacol.*, **21**, 701–712.

Robertson, D.R.C. and George, C.F. (1990) Drug therapy for Parkinson's disease. *Br. Med. Bull.*, **46**, 124–146.

Robertson, D.R.C., Waller, D.G., Renwick, A.G. and George, C.F. (1988) Age related changes in the pharmacokinetics and pharmacodynamics of nifedipine. *Br. J. Clin. Pharmacol.*, **25**, 297–305.

Robertson, D.R.C., Wood, N.D., Everest, H., Monks, K., Waller, D.G., Renwick, A.G. and George, C.F. (1989) The effect of age on the pharmacokinetics of levodopa administered alone and in the presence of carbidopa. *Br. J. Clin. Pharmacol.*, **28**, 61–69.

Romankiewicj, J.A., Brogden, R.N., Heel, R.C., Speight, J.M. and Avery, G.S. (1983) Captopril: an update review of its pharmacological properties and therapeutic efficacy in congestive heart failure. *Drugs*, **25**, 6–40.

Rondel, R. K. (1993) Quality Assurance and Clinical Data Management, in, *Clinical Data Management* (eds. R.K. Rondel, S.A. Varley and C.F. Webb) John Wiley & Sons, Chichester.

Salter, A.J. and Gabbay, F.J (1990) The Society of Pharmaceutical Medicine: development of the discipline. *J. Pharm. Med.*, **1**, 53–60.

Sampson, M. (1984) Career opportunities in industrial clinical research, in *The Clinical Research Process in the Pharmaceutical Industry* (ed. G. Matoren), Marcel Dekker, New York.

Scarpace, P.J (1986) Decreased β-adrenoceptor responsiveness during senescence. *Fed. Proc.*, **45**, 51–54.

Schering-Plough Corporation (1992) *Annual Report*. Maddison, New Jersey.

Shand, D.G., Nuckolls, E.M. and Oates, J.A. (1970) Plasma propranolol levels in adults, with observations in four children. *Clin. Pharmacol. Ther.*, **11**, 112–120.

Shelley, J.H. (1991) Changes to the regulations for the diploma in pharmaceutical medicine. *Pharm. Med.*, **5**, 81–86.

Smith, R.S., Warren, D.J., Renwick, A.G. and George, C.F. (1983) Acebutolol pharmacokinetics in renal failure. *Br. J. Clin. Pharmacol.*, **16**, 253–258.

Snell, E.S. (1970) The value and range of jobs in companies. *Med. News Tribune*, Oct. 30, 14.

Snell, E.S. (1985) Education, information and promotion, in *Pharmaceutical Medicine* (eds D.M. Burley and T.B. Binns), Edward Arnold, London.

Spencer, P.S.J. (1992) Development of academic audit in the United Kingdom: a pharmacy example. *Am. J. Pharm. Ed.*, **57**, 76–80.

Spilker, B. (1991) *Guide to Clinical Trials*. Raven Press, New York.

Spilker, B. (1994) *Multinational Pharmaceutical Companies: Principles and Practices (Second Edition)*. Raven Press, New York.

Stonier, P.D. and Gabbay, F.J. (1992) Training requirements in relation to the scope of pharmaceutical medicine: a survey of practitioners. *J. Pharm. Med.*, **2**, 263–276.

Strom, B.L. (ed.) (1989) *Pharmacoepidemiology*. Churchill Livingstone, Edinburgh.

*Teaching Standards and Excellence in Higher Education* (Occasional Green Paper, No 1, October, 1991), Committee for Vice Chancellors and Principals, London.

Teeling Smith, G. (1992) The British pharmaceutical industry: 1961–1991, in *Innovative Competition in Medicine* (ed. G. Teeling Smith), Office Health Economics, London.

*The Measurement of Value Added in Higher Education* (Report of joint working party of Polytechnic and Colleges Funding Council, and the Council for National Academic Awards, October 1989), Department for Education, London.

Trigg, A. and Bosanquet, N. (1992) Tax harmonization and the reduction of European smoking rates. *J. Health Econ.*, **11**, 329–346.

Tucker, G.T., Silas, J.H., Iyun, A.O., Lennard, M.S. and Smith, A.J. (1977) Polymorphic hydroxylation of debrisoquine. *Lancet*, **ii**, 718.

Turner, P. (1993) Clinical pharmacology: its efficacy and prospect. The Lilly Lecture, 1992. *Br. J. Clin. Pharmacol.*, **36**, 13–17.

Veterans Administration Cooperative Study Group on Antihypertensive Agents (1967) Effects of treatment on morbidity in hypertension. *JAMA*, **202**, 1028–1034.

Vogel, J.R. (1993) Achieving results with contract research organizations: pharmaceutical industry view. *Appl. Clin. Trials*, **1**, 44–49.

Watson, D. (1989) *Managing the Modular Course*. Oxford University Press.

Webb, C. (1993) Feminist research: definitions, methodology, methods and evaluation. *J. Adv. Nursing*, **18** (3), 416–423.

Wells, F. (1993a) Fraud and misconduct in clinical research, in *The Textbook of Pharmaceutical Medicine* (eds J.P. Griffin, J. O'Grady and F.O. Wells), Queen's University, Belfast.

Wells, N. (1993b) Pharmaceuticals: is economic evaluation relevant?, in *Economic Evaluation of Medicines*. IBC, London.

Wellstein, A., Essig, J. and Belz, G.G. (1987). A method for estimating the potency of angiotensin converting enzyme inhibitors in man. *Br. J. Clin. Pharmacol.*, **24**, 397–399.

Williamson, J. and Chopin, J.M. (1980) Adverse reactions to prescribed drugs in the elderly: a multicentre investigation. *Age Ageing*, **9**, 73–80.

Woosley, R.L., Kornhauser, D., Smith, R., Reele, S., Higgins, S.B., Nies, A.S., Shand, D.G. and Oates, J.A. (1979) Suppression of chronic ventricular arrhythmias with propranolol. *Circulation*, **60**, 819–827.

## FURTHER READING

### Chapter 4   Contributions of Schools of Pharmacy to the Pharmaceutical Industry

*Criteria for Accreditation of Degrees in Pharmacy* (1992). Royal Pharmaceutical Society of Great Britain, London.

*Research Assessment Exercise (1992): The Outcome*. (University Funding Council Circular 26/92, December 1992). Department for Education, London.

Spencer, P.S.J. (1992) Development of Academic Audit in the United Kingdom: A Pharmacy Example. *Am. J. of Pharm. Educ.* 57: 76–80.

*Teaching Standards and Excellence in Higher Education* (Occasional Green Paper, No. 1, October, 1991), Committee for Vice Chancellors and Principals, London.

*The Measurement of Value Added in Higher Education* (Report of joint working party of Polytechnic & Colleges Funding Council, and the Council for National Academic Awards, October 1989), Department for Education, London.

Watson, D., for the Society for Research into Higher Education (1989) *Managing the Modular Course*. Oxford University Press.

## Chapter 13   The Phamaceutical Physician in Clinical Research

Burley, D. (1985) The pharmaceutical physician and the company medical department, in *Pharmaceutical Medicine* (eds D. Burley and T. Binns), Edward Arnold, London, pp. 260–282.

Burley, D. and Lasagna, L. (1993) Clinical trials, in *Pharmaceutical Medicine 2nd Edition* (eds D. Burley, J. Clarke and L. Lasagna), Edward Arnold, London, pp. 65–106.

Drury, M. (1993) Clinical trials of drugs in general practice. *Prescribers J.*, **33** (1), 8–15.

*European GCP Guidelines* (1993) Brookwood Medical Publications, Brookwood, Surrey.

Padfield, J. (1993) Making drugs into medicines, in *Pharmaceutical Medicine 2nd Edition* (eds D. Burley, J. Clarke and L. Lasagna), Edward Arnold, London, pp. 33–64.

Symposium: Drug development and clinical trials (1991) *Prescribers J.*, **31** (6), 219–257.

Warlow, C. (1990) Organise a multicentre trial. *Br. Med. J.*, **300**, 180–183.

## Chapter 21   Careers in Medical Information

*United Kingdom*

Huntingford, A.L. (1990) INF/0145, A survey of industry medical information departments' activity. *Pharm. J.*, **245**, 238–239.

*USA*

Colvin, C.L. (1990) INF/0146, Drug information services provided by the pharmaceutical industry. *Am. J. Hosp. Pharm.*, **47** (9), 1989–2001.

## Chapter 30: Career Development in Pharmaceutical Medicine

*Defining Yourself as a Product: Aims and Objectives*

Francis, D. (1985) *Managing your own Career*. Fontana–ATM, London.

Golzen, G. and Garner, A. (1992) *Smart Moves*. Penguin, London.

Maslow, A. (1970) *Motivation and Personality*. Harper & Row, New York.

Nelson Bolles, R. (1985) *What Colour is Your Parachute?*. Umbrella Publishing, London.

Nicholson, N. and West, M. (1988) *Managerial Job Change: Men and Women in Transition*. Cambridge University Press.

Sheehey, G. (1977) *Passages: Predictable Crises of Adult Life*. Bantam, New York.

Yeager, N. (1991) *The Career Doctor*. John Wiley, New York.


*The Market for Your Product*

de Bono, E. (1980) *Opportunities*. Pelican, Harmondsworth.

McCormack, M.H. (1984) *What They Don't Teach You at Harvard Business School*. Collins, London.

Mintzberg, H. (1993) *The Nature Of Managerial Work*. Prentice-Hall, Englewood Cliffs, N.J.

*Pharma Facts & Figures* (1992) ABPI, London

*Scrip League Tables* (1992) PJB Publishing, Richmond.

Townsend, R. (1971) *Up The Organisation*. Coronet, London.

Whyte, W. H. (1980) *The Organisation Man*. Penguin, Harmondsworth.

## Chapter 32   Scientists in Sales and Marketing

Bangs, D.H. (1989) *Practical Marketing*. Kogan Page, London.

Bell, G. (1987) *The Secrets of Successful Speaking and Business Presentations*. Heinemann, London.

Holden, P. (1992) *Marketing Communications in the Pharmaceutical Industry*. Radcliffe Professional Press, Oxford.

Hunt, J.W. (1987) *Managing People at Work*. McGraw Hill, Maidenhead.

Pedlar, M., Burgoyne J. and Boydell, T (1986) *A Manager's Guide to Self-Development*. McGraw Hill, Maidenhead.

Sweeney, N.R. (1982) *Managing a Sales Team*. Kogan Page, London.

# Index

nb – page numbers in *italics* refer to figures and tables

*Index compiled by Jill Halliday*